# Manual of Head and Neck Reconstruction

Fiyin Sokoya • Aurora G. Vincent
Editors

# Manual of Head and Neck Reconstruction

## A Step-by-Step Guide

Springer

*Editors*
Fiyin Sokoya
Wellstar Health Systems
Atlanta, GA, USA

Aurora G. Vincent
Eisenhower Army Medical Center
Fort Gordon, GA, USA

ISBN 978-3-031-65998-0 ISBN 978-3-031-65999-7 (eBook)
https://doi.org/10.1007/978-3-031-65999-7



This Springer imprint is published by the registered company Springer Nature Switzerland AG
The registered company address is: Gewerbestrasse 11, 6330 Cham, Switzerland

# Foreword

Thank you for having an open mind as you read this excellent book. I commend Dr. Fiyin Sokoya and Dr. Aurora Vincent for their outstanding effort in putting together a collection of techniques that should help improve outcomes for surgeons looking to improve efficiency and results with their surgical techniques. These are techniques that we have developed over the past 25 years in a high-volume tertiary referral practice. They are focused on allowing surgeons in both private practice and university settings to have equally high quality outcomes. The authors in this text have varied practice models but are able to provide cost-efficient excellent care for even the most complex and challenging patients. I am proud of all of the authors contributions not only in the chapters they have chronicled herein, but also in how they each continue to contribute to their communities and the field of Facial Plastic and Reconstructive Surgery. At the end of the day, our time as individual surgeons is limited. We have all stood on the shoulders of giants in surgery. But we should never be content in our expectations of results and surgical speed. Constant improvement should be the goal and continual dissemination of knowledge is the only way we, as a specialty, will continue to thrive. I pray that you enjoy this volume as much as the authors did putting it together.

Otolaryngology and Facial Plastic Surgery Associates
Fort Worth, TX, USA

Yadranko Ducic

# Contents

# Contributors

**Yusuf M. Agamawi** Department of Otolaryngology—Head and Neck Surgery, Saint Louis University School of Medicine, Saint Louis, MO, USA

Otolaryngology and Facial Plastic Surgery Associates, Fort Worth, TX, USA

**Spenceer R. Anderson** Department of Orthopedic and Plastic Surgery, Boonshoft School of Medicine at Wright State University, Dayton, OH, USA

Division of Plastic and Reconstructive Surgery, Wright State University Boonshoft School of Medicine, Dayton, OH, USA

**Luka Bahra** College of Osteopathic Medicine, Rocky Vista University, Englewood, CO, USA

**Ryan F. Brown** Department of Head and Neck Surgery/Facial Plastic and Reconstructive Surgery, Denver, CO, USA

Department of Head and Neck Surgery/Facial Plastic Surgery, The Permanente Medical Group, Santa Rosa, CA, USA

**Ricardo L. Carrau** Department of Otolaryngology—Head and Neck Surgery, The Ohio State University Wexner Medical Center, Columbus, OH, USA

**David Chan** Department of Surgery, Section of Otolaryngology—Head and Neck Surgery, The University of Chicago Medicine, Chicago, IL, USA

Century Ear, Nose, and Throat—Head and Neck Surgery, Orland Park, IL, USA

Section of Otolaryngology—Head and Neck Surgery, University of Chicago, Chicago, IL, USA

**Jason Cohn, DO, FACS** Cohn Plastic Surgery, PC, Smithtown, NY, USA

Sunrise ENT and Facial Plastics, Lindenhurst, NY, USA

**Yadranko Ducic** Otolaryngology and Facial Plastic Surgery Associates, Fort Worth, TX, USA

**Eli Gordin** Department of Otolaryngology—Head and Neck Surgery, UT Southwestern Medical Center, Dallas, TX, USA

**Marc H. Hohman** Baghdad Diplomatic Support Center, Baghdad, Iraq

Department of Surgery, Uniformed Services University of the Health Sciences, Bethesda, MD, USA

**Sameep P. Kadakia** Department of Orthopedic and Plastic Surgery, Boonshoft School of Medicine at Wright State University, Dayton, OH, USA

Premier Comprehensive Head and Neck Oncology and Reconstructive Surgery Program, Miami Valley Hospital, Dayton, OH, USA

Department of Plastic and Reconstructive Surgery, Wright State University Boonshoft College of Medicine, Dayton, OH, USA

**Scott Kohlert** CHRISTUS Health, Tyler, TX, USA

**Seung Lee** Department of Otolaryngology, Virginia Commonwealth University Medical Center, Richmond, VA, USA

Department of Otolaryngology, Virginia Commonwealth University Hospital, Richmond, VA, USA

**Thomas S. Lee** Department of Otolaryngology, Virginia Commonwealth University Medical Center, Richmond, VA, USA

Department of Otolaryngology, Virginia Commonwealth University Hospital, Richmond, VA, USA

**Wesley Mcilwain** Otolaryngology and Facial Plastic Surgery Associates, Fort Worth, TX, USA

**Fatemeh Mirzamohammadi** Department of Orthopedic and Plastic Surgery, Boonshoft School of Medicine at Wright State University, Dayton, OH, USA

**Arya Namin** Otolaryngology and Facial Plastic Surgery Associates, Fort Worth, TX, USA

**Adrian A. Ong** Otolaryngology and Facial Plastic Surgery Associates, Fort Worth, TX, USA

**Sammy Othman, MD** Division of Plastic and Reconstructive Surgery, Department of Surgery, Northwell Health, New York, NY, USA

**Kaitlynne Pak** Boonshoft School of Medicine at Wright State University, Dayton, OH, USA

**Laura Petrauskas** Section of Otolaryngology—Head and Neck Surgery, University of Chicago, Chicago, IL, USA

**Kevin Quinn** Department of Otolaryngology, Ohio State University Medical Center, Columbus, OH, USA

Department of Otolaryngology, Virginia Commonwealth University Hospital, Richmond, VA, USA

**David A. Rengifo** Department of Otolaryngology, Head and Neck Surgery, University of Florida, Gainesville, FL, USA

**Masoud Saman** DallasFaceDoc, PLLC, Dallas, TX, USA

**Raja Sawhney** Department of Otolaryngology, Head and Neck Surgery, University of Florida, Gainesville, FL, USA

**Britney Scott** Department of Otolaryngology—Head and Neck Surgery, Kettering Health, Kettering, OH, USA

**Derek Sheen** Department of Otolaryngology Head and Neck Surgery, University of Texas Southwestern Medical Center, Dallas, TX, USA

**Alexander P. Simko** University of Florida School of Medicine, Gainesville, FL, USA

**Collin Smith** Department of Otolaryngology—Head and Neck Surgery, Kettering Health, Kettering, OH, USA

**Fiyin Sokoya** Wellstar Health Systems, Atlanta, GA, USA

**Ugochukwu Umeh** Medical University of Lublin, Lublin, Poland

**Nima Vahidi** Department of Otolaryngology, Virginia Commonwealth University Medical Center, Richmond, VA, USA

Department of Otolaryngology, Virginia Commonwealth University Hospital, Richmond, VA, USA

**Aurora G. Vincent** Eisenhower Army Medical Center, Fort Gordon, GA, USA

**Weitao Wang** Department of Otolaryngology Head and Neck Surgery, University of Rochester, Rochester, NY, USA

**Kathryn Bradburn Wie** Department of Otolaryngology Head and Neck Surgery, University of Rochester, Rochester, NY, USA

**Sunishka M. Wimalawansa** Department of Orthopedic and Plastic Surgery, Boonshoft School of Medicine at Wright State University, Dayton, OH, USA

**Cheryl Yu** Department of Otolaryngology, Virginia Commonwealth University Medical Center, Richmond, VA, USA

Department of Otolaryngology, Virginia Commonwealth University Hospital, Richmond, VA, USA

# Part I

# Facial Reconstruction

# Local Flaps

# 1

Adrian A. Ong, Ugochukwu Umeh, and Arya Namin

## Introduction

Local flap reconstruction is utilized when simple primary closure cannot be achieved, when there is excessive tension on the wound, or when primary closure would result in significant functional deficits. These are especially important to consider in the reconstruction of the head and neck, which are the most visible structures of the body. A local flap is described as a skin and subcutaneous tissue that is transferred from its original position to an area adjacent to the flap. Due to the robust blood supply of the face, many local flap options are available and proper execution of the flap is dependent on the specific defect location, available adjacent tissue, patient-specific factors, and surgeon comfort. Local flaps can be classified by their vascular supply, composition, or method of transfer and design. Successful local flap reconstruction relies on an organized and methodical approach to defect analysis to determine the optimal method of reconstruction.

## Anatomy

To successfully reconstruct facial defects with local flaps, a firm understanding of cutaneous anatomy is imperative (Fig. 1.1). The most superficial layer of the skin is the epidermis. Immediately underneath this is the dermis, which consists of the superficial papillary and deeper reticular layers. The vascular supply is composed of a superficial dermal plexus between the reticular and papillary dermis and a deep

A. A. Ong (✉) · A. Namin
Otolaryngology and Facial Plastic Surgery Associates, Fort Worth, TX, USA

U. Umeh
Medical University of Lublin, Lublin, Poland



F. Sokoya, A. G. Vincent (eds.), *Manual of Head and Neck Reconstruction*,
https://doi.org/10.1007/978-3-031-65999-7_1

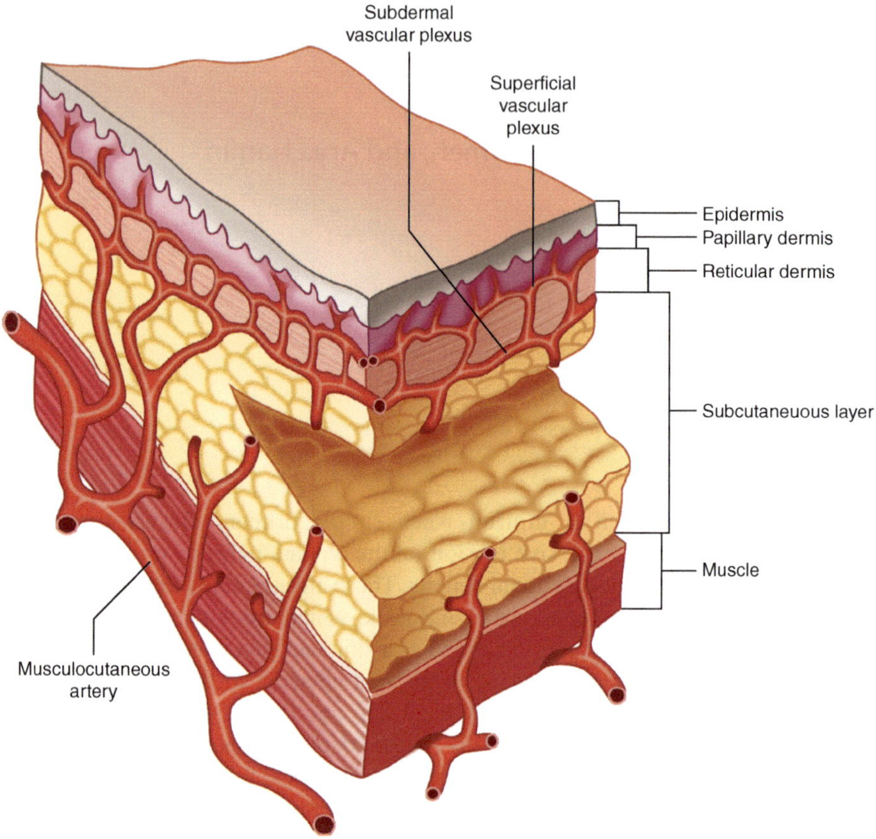


**Fig. 1.1** Schematic of the skin/soft tissue layers. A random flap is depicted being elevated in the subcutaneous layer, and shows the vascular supply of the flap through the subdermal plexus

"subdermal" plexus between the reticular dermis and the subcutaneous tissue, the latter allows for random pattern donor flaps.

As mentioned earlier, flaps can be classified in many ways, including by their vascular supply. The majority of local flaps are based on a random vascular supply and rely on the subdermal plexus and not a named skin perforator [1]. These flaps depend on the vascular perfusion pressure. To ensure flap survival, the perfusion pressure through the flap must exceed the critical closing pressure of the capillary vessels and prevent distal flap ischemia [2]. Historically, it was thought that a wider-based flap would allow for increased length; however, a wider flap that only increases the number of included vessels without changing the perfusion pressure will not affect the length of the viable flap. Alternatively, flaps can also be classified by their vascular supply; for example, axial flaps are named for a specific direct cutaneous artery. Specific axial flaps include the paramedian forehead flap and the pectoralis major myocutaneous flap, which are further discussed in Chaps. 2 and 7, respectively.

Flaps are also classified by the method of transfer and design, which is a more commonly used classification when discussing local flaps [3]. An advancement flap depends on the advancement of adjacent tissue along a linear axis to close the defect. This type of flap often creates standing cutaneous deformities or "dog-ear" deformities, which must be addressed. Rotational flaps pivot around a fixed point along an arc to close the defect. Oftentimes, local flaps in the head and neck have elements of both rotation and advancement flaps. Transposition flaps refer to a flap that is elevated and mobilized from adjacent donor tissue and transposed over an incomplete bridge of skin to close the primary defect. During transposition of the donor tissue, the secondary defect created the donor site is closed primarily. Examples of transposition flaps include the rhombic flap, bilobed flap, and Z-plasty. Finally, interpolated flaps are similar to transposition flaps; however, the donor tissue is transposed over a complete bridge tissue, creating a cutaneous pedicle and requiring pedicle division at a second stage. An example of this type of flap is the paramedian forehead flap, which is further discussed in Chaps. 2 and 3.

An understanding of the facial anatomy is also important when considering local flap reconstruction. The relaxed skin tension lines (RSTL) reflect the intrinsic orientation of tension and relaxation of the skin at rest and represent areas along which scars should be placed [4]. The lines of maximum extensibility, which run perpendicular to the RSTLs, are also considered when designing local flaps and signify the direction in which closure should be performed with the least tension. In addition to RSTLs, scars can also be hidden within the borders of aesthetic subunits. These borders represent imaginary lines along which scars can hide inconspicuously, based on how the eye processes faces as block images that are spatially organized [5]. The major aesthetic subunits of the face include the forehead, eyes, nose, lips, chin, ears, and neck. These units can be further subdivided based on less discrete borders. For example, the nose is further subdivided into the dorsum, sidewall, tip, ala, columella, and soft tissue facet or soft tissue triangle [6].

## Indications/Contraindications

The major indication for local flap reconstruction in the head and neck is reconstruction after Mohs micrographic surgery for cutaneous malignancies for which primary closure is either inadequate or would result in functional deficits. Local flaps may also be used to reconstruct other types of cancer defects as well as traumatic wounds.

An absolute contraindication to local flap reconstruction includes positive margins at the site of the defect. In addition, proper patient selection is important as local flaps taken from areas of scar or that have undergone radiation may have compromised vascular supply, and other reconstructive options should be considered. Relative contraindications to local flap reconstruction include the risk of hemorrhage and current smoking status. Patients on anticoagulant therapy are at increased risk of perioperative and postoperative bleeding, which can impair the perfusion pressure and thus the viability of the local flap [7]. In general, smokers are at increased risk of complications and should be advised [8]. Those who continue to smoke are at increased risk of flap necrosis.

## Preoperative Planning

The preoperative assessment is essential for optimal reconstruction with a local flap [9, 10]. The defect should be analyzed carefully and characterized. This includes the determination of skin color and thickness, defect composition and thickness, and involvement of subunits. If the defect involves greater than 50% of an aesthetic subunit, consideration can be given to resection of the entire subunit to improve the aesthetic outcome. Landmarks that must not be distorted or placed under significant amounts of tension, such as the hairline, eyelid, nasal ala, or nasolabial fold, should be identified. Areas of recruitment are assessed for adjacent tissue that is easily accessible and has sufficient laxity to reconstruct the defect. Donor site considerations include prior operations or trauma as well as prior radiation. Flaps are then designed such that the resultant scar will rest along RSTLs or along aesthetic subunit borders. Before any incisions are created, it is important to review outcomes after the planned adjacent tissue transfer: Will there be any limiting anatomic and physiologic restraints and are there consequences of tissue movement? If the planned local flap results in untoward outcomes, other flap options can be considered. Following these steps will result in an organized approach to defect analysis and optimal flap choice, leading to excellent function and aesthetic outcomes.

## Instrument/Equipment Set

In general, a soft tissue instrument set is used for dissection. Depending on the location of the defect, additional equipment may be required, such as a basic oculoplastic or septorhinoplasty surgical set. Monopolar and bipolar cautery, skin hooks, and fine dissecting scissors are utilized to assist in flap elevation. Closure of the donor and recipient sites is achieved with a combination of deep dermal dissolvable sutures and non-absorbable skin sutures.

## Flap Design/Surgical Technique/Ducic Pearls

### Advancement Flap

Advancement flaps rely on the recruitment of adjacent tissue that is moved along a linear axis to close a defect. Examples of advancement flaps include primary fusiform closure, unilateral unipedicle and bilateral unipedicle (H-plasty) advancement flaps, A-T or O-T flap, V-Y or Y-V flap, and subcutaneous tissue pedicle island flap. Examples can be seen in Fig. 1.2.

In both unilateral and bilateral unipedicle advancement flaps, the flap pedicle width is determined by the operative defect size; however, the flap width should be slightly wider than the defect size as the flap width decreases slightly with advancement in the defect size. The flap length is dictated by the pliability of nearby tissue. As a test, if the defect cannot be closed with forceful pushing, another flap option

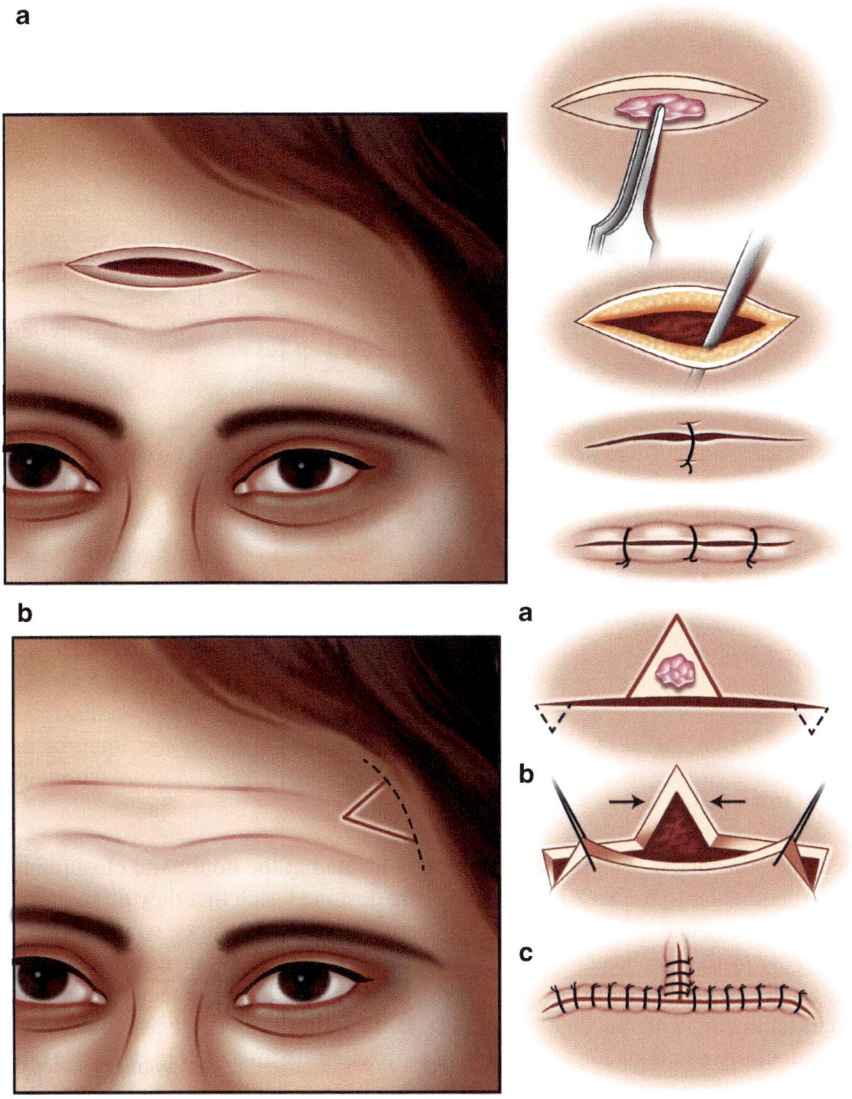


**Fig. 1.2** Examples of local advancement flaps. (**a**) Closure of an ellipse, which represents the simplest advancement flap. (**b**) A-T advancement flap. (**c**) V-Y advancement flap. (**d**) Unilateral advancement flap. (**e**) Bilateral advancement flap

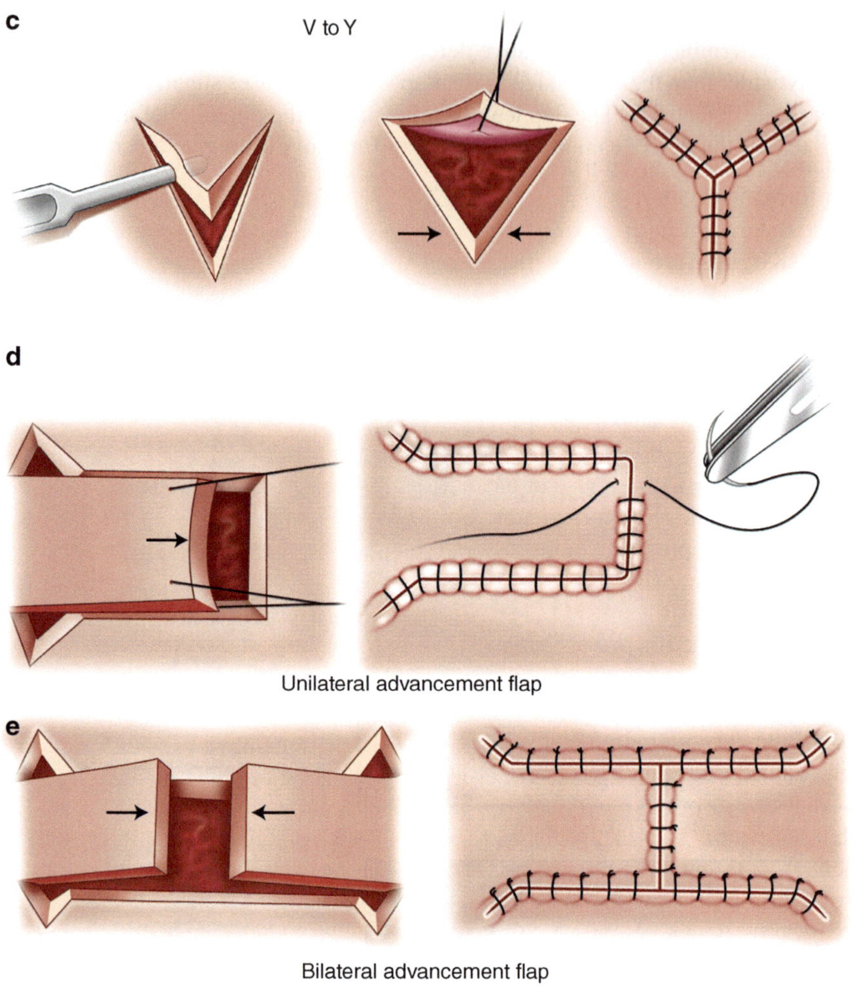


**Fig. 1.2** (continued)

should be considered. The primary tension is located at the donor site closure and lies perpendicular to the incision. Incisions are designed such that they lie within or parallel to horizontal creases or along borders of natural landmarks, which is useful for defects in the forehead. Typically, a unipedicle advancement flap is designed with a ratio of defect width to flap length of 1:3, with larger defects requiring a bilateral unipedicle advancement flap [11]. Bilateral unipedicle advancement flaps are particularly advantageous in the closure of "central" lip and chin defects as the two flaps "pull" equally, reducing the potential for tissue distortion and midline structure deviation. In both instances, a standing cutaneous deformity is created at the base of the flap and often requires the removal of the Burow triangles.

The A-T and O-T advancement flaps (T-plasty) are named for their transformation of triangular A-shaped) or round (O-shaped) defects into a T-shaped scar after closure. Both require two flaps on either side of the defect, which are advanced toward each other, representing a modification of the bilateral unipedicle advancement flaps. The advantages of the T-plasty include dividing the defect in half by using two flaps for closure and using a single incision for each flap, thereby decreasing scar formation, which is typically hidden at the border of a natural landmark.

In the V-Y advancement flap, a triangular incision is made and the broad base of the triangle is advanced into the defect. The resultant scar results in a Y-shape. Conversely, in a Y-V advancement flap, the tip of the triangle is advanced toward the defect, resulting in a V-shaped scar.

## Rotational Flap

When advancement flaps are unable to close a defect in one direction, consideration can be given to rotational flaps which redistribute the tension vectors from the primary defect site closure to the secondary donor site along the arc of rotation. Rotation flaps are ideal for the closure of triangular-shaped defects. The classic definition of a rotation flap includes an arc of 30 degrees or less, with a radius of two to three times the diameter of the defect, and an arc length approximately four to five times the diameter of the defect [11]. Examples of rotational flaps include the O-Z flap for scalp repairs, the dorsal nasal flap, and the cervicofacial flap (Fig. 1.3). Rotational flaps are often the preferred method of repair for most scalp defects, which accommodate curvilinear incisions well and do not require planning around RSTLs or aesthetic subunits. Disadvantages of the rotational flap method include the necessity for a flap much larger than the original defect, extensive undermining of the flap, and incisions that often cross RSTLs or aesthetic subunits.

## Transposition Flap

Transposition flaps recruit tissue from an area of laxity, which is then transferred into the defect over an incomplete bridge of tissue, and allows for tension redirection and redistribution. Common examples of transposition flaps include the rhombic flap (including the Duformental and Webster modifications), the bilobe flap, and Z-plasty. The Z-plasty is most commonly used in scar revision to change the scar direction, interrupt the scar linearity, or release scar contracture; this will be further discussed in Chap. 30.

In the classic rhombic flap described by Limberg (Fig. 1.4), an equilateral parallelogram is designed to close a defect with the same shape and size, and classically is designed with two 60-degree angles and two 120-degree angles [12]. The first line is drawn extending from one of the 120-degree angles, with a length approximating the size of the defect. A second line is then drawn from the end of the first line at a 60-degree angle and parallel to the adjacent side of the defect. The choice of the flap design is based on the location of the donor site closure, which should approximate the RSTLs, and be perpendicular to the lines of maximal extensibility. Once the defect and proposed flap design are finalized, the flap incisions are made and the flap is undermined. The first deep dermal suture for closure should be at the donor

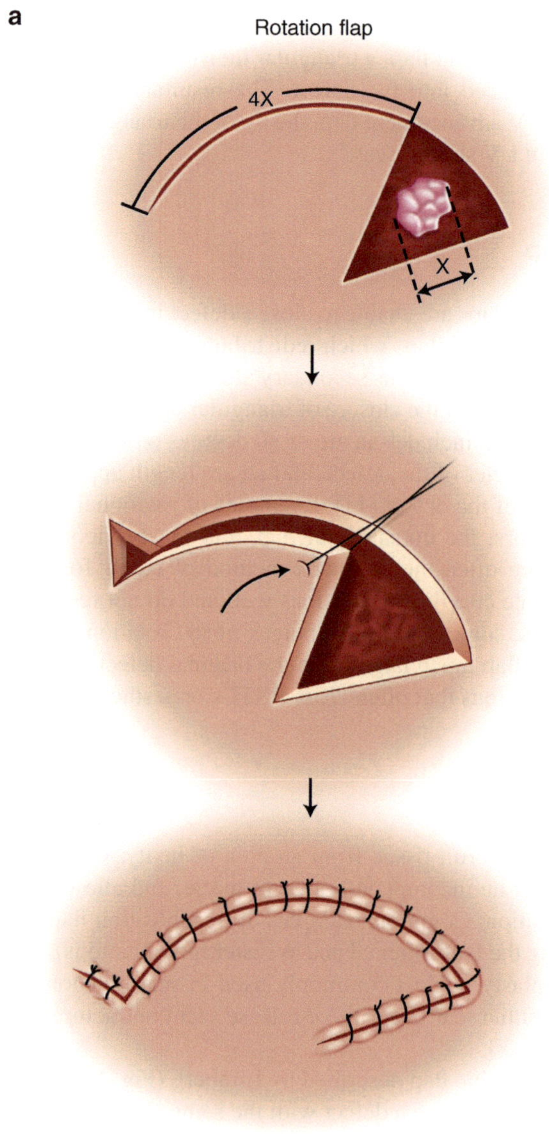


**Fig. 1.3** Examples of local rotation flaps. (**a**) Basic rotation flap. Note the length of the arc which is approximately 4 times the diameter of the defect. (**b**) O-Z flap. This involves two opposing rotation flaps that are closed at a central point in the defect

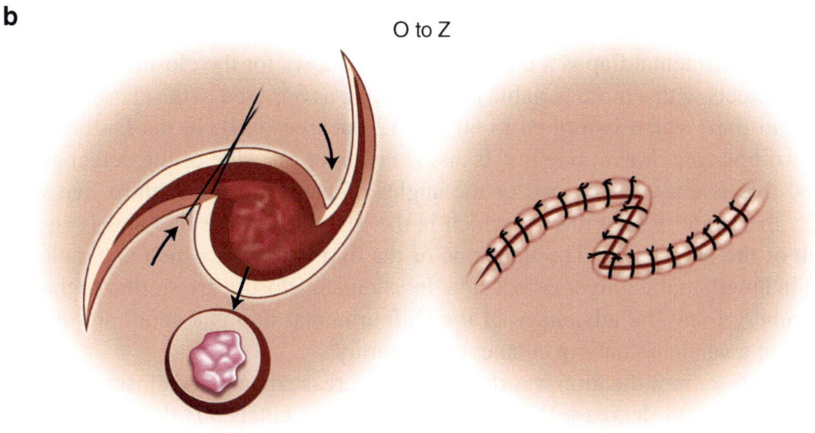


**Fig. 1.3** (continued)

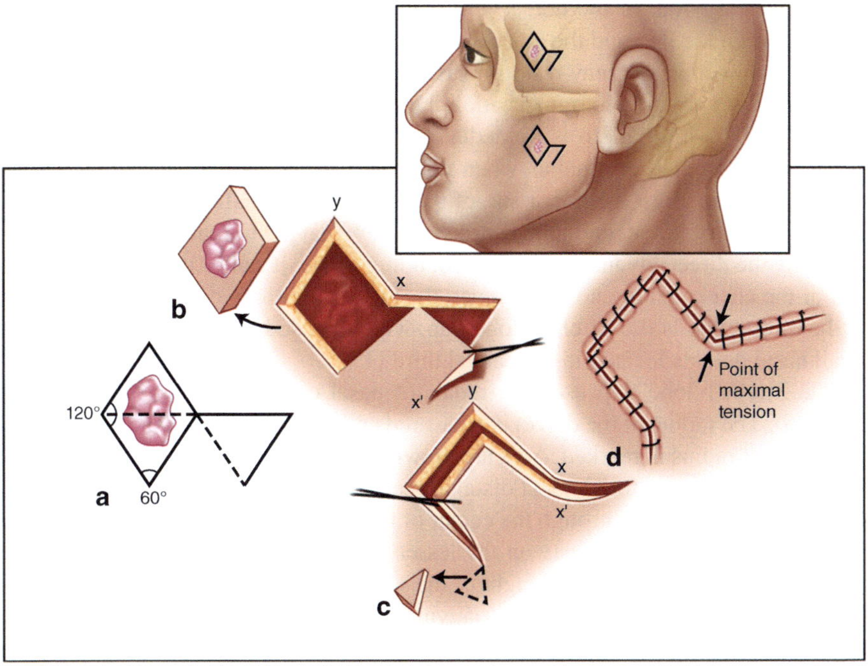


**Fig. 1.4** Limberg rhombic flap

site closure, which is the point of maximal tension. Disadvantages of the classic rhomboid flap include the creation of a secondary defect with the same size and shape as the primary defect and the creation of standing cutaneous deformities due to the angle of closure.

The Dufourmental flap is a modification that allows for the closure of rhombus-shaped defects with a more variable internal angle as opposed to the classic Limberg rhomboid flap, which is limited to 60 and 120 degrees [13]. In the Dufourmental flap, two lines are drawn: one line is an extension of one side of the defect and the second line is drawn from one of the angles of the rhombus. A third line which bisects the angle is then drawn, which is the first side of the flap and is equal in length of the defect size. The final side of the flap is drawn, which is parallel and equal in length to the longer defect side. Incision and closure are similar to the classic Limberg flap. The advantage of the Dufourmental flap is a small arc of pivot, leading to a smaller standing cutaneous deformity.

The Webster modification was designed to decrease the wound closure tension at the donor site and decrease the size of the standing cutaneous deformity [14]. A W-plasty is designed where the standing cutaneous deformity would be excised. In addition, the apex of the proposed flap is designed at an angle of approximately 30 degrees, leading to a narrow-angled donor site. The length of the flaps still equals the length of a side of the defect; however, the base of the flap is approximately half of the greatest width of the defect. Prior to incision, the surgeon must ensure the angle between the flap and the adjacent side of the defect approximates at least 110 degrees as lesser angles may result in vascular compromise of the flap.

Bilobe flaps are double transposition flaps with a common base. In general, the first lobe of the bilobe flap is immediately adjacent to the defect and is approximately equal in size or smaller when compared to the defect. The second lobe, which is used to close the donor site of the first lobe, is smaller than the first lobe. The donor site of the second lobe is designed such that the remaining defects can be closed by the direct advancement of surrounding tissue. It can be used in reconstruction of the cheek and the nose; however, the most commonly described application of the bilobe flap is the Zitelli bilobe flap, which is used for the reconstruction of small nasal defects located in the caudal third [15].

The Zitelli bilobe flap used for repair of nasal defects is geometrically exact (Fig. 1.5). The radius of the defect is measured and a point lateral to the defect equal to the defect radius is marked. Arcs are drawn using the marked point as the center: the first arc is tangent to the most distal aspect of the defect from the marked point, and a second arc passes through the center of the defect. These arcs are important as the base of the two lobes rests on the lesser arc while the height of the first lobe extends to the greater arc. The height of the second lobe is approximately 1.5 to 2.0 times greater than the first lobe and triangular in shape. The width of the first lobe is equal to the width of the defect, while the width of the second lobe is similar to slightly less than the first lobe. Due to the positioning of the bilobe flap, the axis between the defect and first lobe and axis between the first lobe and second are approximately 45 degrees apart. After designing the flap, a standing cutaneous deformity is expected near the pivot of the first lobe and drawn; the base is typically

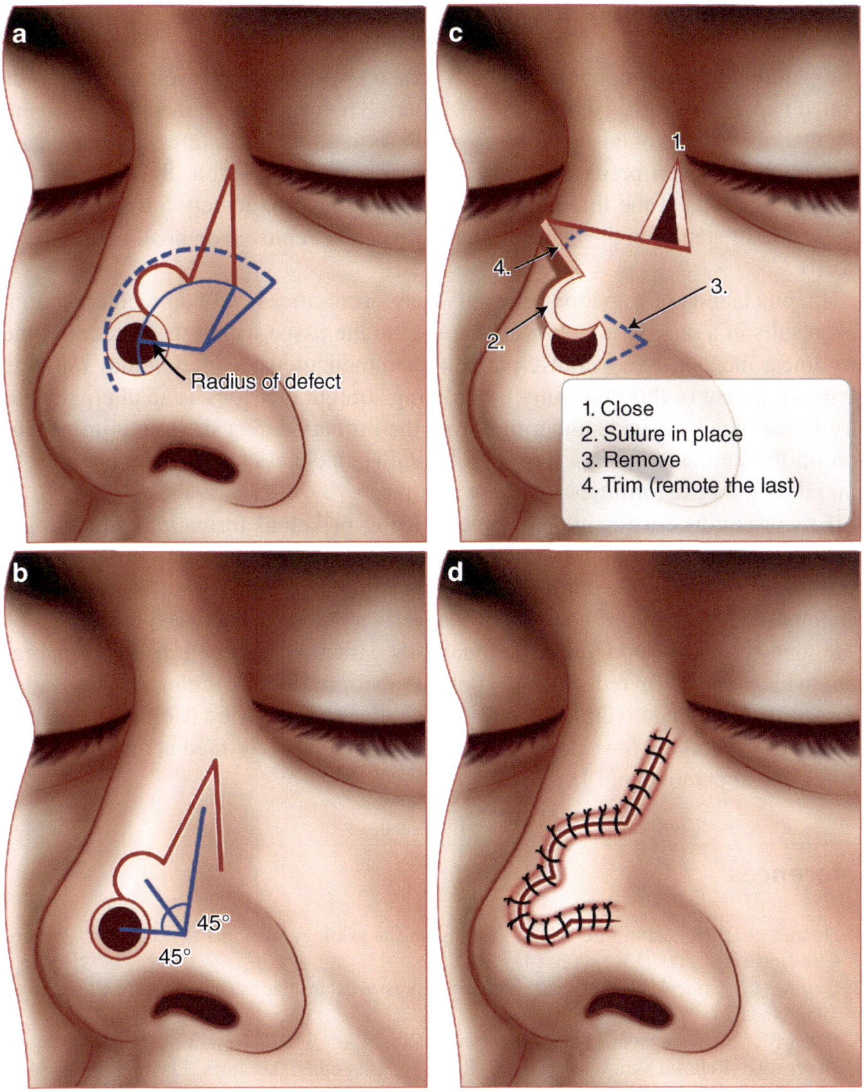


**Fig. 1.5** Zitelli bilobe flap

the diameter of the defect and one side of the expected standing cutaneous deformity is planned to rest along the alar groove. After incision and wide undermining of the flap, the defect from the second lobe is closed first, followed by insetting the first lobe into the defect. The expected standing cutaneous deformity at the base of the first lobe is then excised, followed by the excision of the excess tissue at the tip of the second lobe.

## Postoperative Management

Postoperatively, the wound is typically coated with antibiotic ointment and is applied two to three times daily for 48 h. After 48 h, the patient can apply petroleum jelly to moisten the wound and minimize scab formation. Suture lines can be cleaned with dilute hydrogen peroxide to also minimize scab formation. Skin sutures are typically removed at the first postoperative visit in approximately 5 to 7 days, and any sutures or staples in the hair-bearing scalp can be removed on postoperative day 7 to 10.

The pincushion or trapdoor deformity may occur after local flap reconstruction. This results in a raised, domelike appearance to the tissue within the borders of the curvilinear incision. Preoperative planning and meticulous dissection may mitigate the development of this deformity by utilizing straight incisions as an alternative to curvilinear incisions, wide undermining of the primary defect site to minimize tension on the flap, and using a flap with a similar thickness to the recipient site. In general, trapdoor deformities resolve with time.

If there is concern for hypertrophic scarring or keloid formation, silicone gel sheeting can be applied to the wound [16, 17]. Patients are advised to use the sheeting for as long as possible during the day and at night for 2 to 3 months. In addition, triamcinolone can be injected into the scar at 4- to 6- week intervals [16, 18].

In many cases of flap reconstruction, many patients will benefit from dermabrasion, which can help reduce any contour abnormalities or color discrepancies between the donor and recipient site. For local flaps, the incision itself can be dermabraded at the earliest 6 weeks after surgery but can be performed at any time after 6 weeks postoperatively [19].

## References

1. Honrado CP, Murakami CS. Wound healing and physiology of skin flaps. Facial Plast Surg Clin North Am. 2005;13(2):203–14, v.
2. Cutting C. Critical closing and perfusion pressures in flap survival. Ann Plast Surg. 1982;9(6):524.
3. Baker SR. Local cutaneous flaps. Otolaryngol Clin N Am. 1994;27(1):139–59.
4. Borges AF. Relaxed skin tension lines (RSTL) versus other skin lines. Plast Reconstr Surg. 1984;73(1):144–50.
5. Burget GC. Modification of the subunit principle. Arch Facial Plast Surg. 1999;1(1):16–8.
6. Burget GC, Menick FJ. The subunit principle in nasal reconstruction. Plast Reconstr Surg. 1985;76(2):239–47.
7. Lewis KG, Dufresne RG Jr. A meta-analysis of complications attributed to anticoagulation among patients following cutaneous surgery. Dermatol Surg. 2008;34(2):160–4; discussion 4–5.
8. Kinsella JB, Rassekh CH, Wassmuth ZD, Hokanson JA, Calhoun KH. Smoking increases facial skin flap complications. Ann Otol Rhinol Laryngol. 1999;108(2):139–42.
9. Clevens RA, Baker SR. Conceptual considerations in head & neck reconstruction. Defect analysis and options for reconstruction. Otolaryngol Clin N Am. 1997;30(4):495–517.
10. Larrabee WF Jr. Design of local skin flaps. Otolaryngol Clin N Am. 1990;23(5):899–923.

11. Larrabee WF Jr, Sutton D. The biomechanics of advancement and rotation flaps. Laryngoscope. 1981;91(5):726–34.
12. Limberg AA. Design of local flaps. Mod Trends Plast Surg. 1966;2:38–61.
13. Dufourmentel C. [The L-shaped flap for lozenge-shaped defects. Interview with Claude Dufourmentel by E. Achard]. Ann Chir Plast 1979;24(4):397–9.
14. Webster RC, Davidson TM, Smith RC. The thirty degree transposition flap. Laryngoscope. 1978;88(1 Pt 1):85–94.
15. Zitelli JA. The bilobed flap for nasal reconstruction. Arch Dermatol. 1989;125(7):957–9.
16. Mustoe TA, Cooter RD, Gold MH, Hobbs FD, Ramelet AA, Shakespeare PG, et al. International clinical recommendations on scar management. Plast Reconstr Surg. 2002;110(2):560–71.
17. Ohmori S. Effectiveness of silastic sheet coverage in the treatment of scar keloid (hypertrophic scar). Aesthet Plast Surg. 1988;12(2):95–9.
18. Darougheh A, Asilian A, Shariati F. Intralesional triamcinolone alone or in combination with 5-fluorouracil for the treatment of keloid and hypertrophic scars. Clin Exp Dermatol. 2009;34(2):219–23.
19. Katz BE, Oca AG. A controlled study of the effectiveness of spot dermabrasion ('scarabrasion') on the appearance of surgical scars. J Am Acad Dermatol. 1991;24(3):462–6.

# 2 Facial Regional Flaps

Arya Namin, Adrian A. Ong, and David Chan

## Introduction

The regional flaps of the face are axial flaps based off the branches of the external and internal carotid artery systems. The facial artery, supratrochlear artery, deep temporal artery, and superficial temporal artery allow for the transfer of axial patterned flaps that typically match the skin thickness and quality of the surrounding defect. These regional flaps include the paramedian forehead flap, melolabial flap, temporoparietal fascia flap, and temporalis muscle flap. The melolabial flap is most commonly utilized as an interpolated flap or transposition flap in nasal, lip, and cheek reconstruction. The paramedian forehead flap is the workhorse of nasal reconstruction. The temporalis and temporoparietal fascia flaps are utilized in orbital, auricular, lip, and skull base reconstruction [1–6].

The forehead flap has an illustrious history dating back three millennia and continues to be a modern-day workhorse in nasal reconstruction [7–9]. The technique has evolved with time and saw particular advances and more widespread utilization after World War I [9]. The forehead flap is a robust flap with an axial blood supply from the supratrochlear artery, and forehead flap necrosis is exceptionally rare [10]. The median forehead flap was championed during the first part of the twentieth century; however, as time went on, the pedicle location and width were modified in order to improve the mobility of the flap [8, 11, 12]. A subcutaneous tissue pedicle was described in order to decrease the width of the pedicle allowing for increased mobility as well as obviating the need for a second stage given that the pedicle was tunneled under the glabellar skin into the nasal defect [13]. Towards the end of the

A. Namin (✉) · A. A. Ong
Otolaryngology and Facial Plastic Surgery Associates, Fort Worth, TX, USA

D. Chan
Department of Surgery, Section of Otolaryngology—Head and Neck Surgery, The University of Chicago Medicine, Chicago, IL, USA





F. Sokoya, A. G. Vincent (eds.), *Manual of Head and Neck Reconstruction*,
https://doi.org/10.1007/978-3-031-65999-7_2

twentieth century, the paramedian forehead flap became the workhorse of nasal reconstructions, and the importance of reconstructing the nasal lining and structural framework also became apparent [14–17].

The melolabial flap has been extensively described in the literature for nasal reconstruction dating back to the late nineteenth and early twentieth centuries [18–23]. The melolabial flap can be utilized as an advancement, rotation, transposition, and interpolated flap for the reconstruction of cutaneous defects [24, 25]. The melolabial flap can be tunneled into the oral cavity or nasal cavity [21]. The melolabial flap is an important flap to consider in lip reconstruction, particularly reconstruction of the lateral lip [18, 26, 27]. The superiorly based melolabial interpolated flap was described by Baker et al. in 1995 with the primary objective of preserving the alar-facial sulcus [28]. While transposition, rotation, and advancement melolabial flaps are best suited for lip and cheek reconstruction, the interpolated melolabial flap is best suited for reconstruction of the lower third of the nose.

The temporal fossa offers two vascular pedicles, the superficial temporal artery and vein and the deep temporal artery and vein. The temporoparietal fascia flap, based off the superficial temporal artery and vein, can be transferred as either a pedicled flap or free flap based off the superficial temporal artery and vein. It can be transferred as a fascial flap, fasciocutaneous flap, or osseofasciocutaneous flap. The temporal muscle flap, based off the deep temporal artery and vein, is transferred as a pedicled flap and has been described in reconstruction of facial paralysis, orbital defects, lateral and anterior skull base defects, and facial defects [29–32].

## Anatomy

Understanding the anatomy of facial regional flaps hinges on an understanding of the relationships of surface landmarks to terminal branches of the external and internal carotid artery branches and knowing the course of these vessels as they transition from the sub-superficial musculoaponeurotic system plane to the subcutaneous plane. In this section, the anatomy of the supratrochlear, facial, superficial temporal, and deep temporal arteries will be discussed.

The supratrochlear artery is a terminal branch of the ophthalmic artery and typically exits the orbit in line with the medial canthus and medial brow. This can be found 1.7–2.2 cm from midline [33]. The supratrochlear artery typically courses superficial to the corrugator muscle and deep to the orbicularis muscle as it exits the orbit. As it courses vertically in the paramedian position, it pierces the frontalis muscle and can be found within the subcutaneous tissue plane at the level of the brow [33].

The facial artery is a branch of the external carotid artery that courses anteriorly. The facial artery then passes deep to the digastric and stylohyoid muscles before contacting the posterior aspect of the submandibular gland and typically sending multiple branches to this gland [34–36]. The facial artery is typically palpable at the anterior aspect of the masseter as it courses over the mandible in the sub-superficial musculoaponeurotic system plane. As the facial artery courses superiorly, it gives off the inferior and superior labial arteries and becomes more superficial distally. The facial artery is typically found in close proximity to the nasolabial fold and transitions from the sub-superficial musculoaponeurotic system plane below the oral commissure to very superficial in the subcutaneous plane at the level of the nasal base [37]. At its most distal aspect, the facial artery becomes more superficial, and the branches lateral to the melolabial fold allow for the versatility of the melolabial flap. The venous drainage is via the facial angular vein.

The soft tissue layers of the temporal fossa are the skin, subcutaneous tissue, temporoparietal fascia, loose areolar plane, temporalis muscle fascia, temporalis muscle, and pericranium. The skin, subcutaneous tissue, temporoparietal fascia, and temporalis muscle fascia are all vascularized by the superficial temporal artery [5, 38]. The temporoparietal fascia is continuous as the galea superiorly and the superficial musculoaponeurotic system in the face. These fascial layers do have dense attachments along the temporal line of fusion and the zygomatic arch. At its point of origin, the superficial temporal artery lies within or deep to the parotid gland behind the ramus of the mandible [38]. The superficial temporal artery then enters the temporoparietal fascial layer approximately 4–5 mm anterior to the tragus [38]. During the proximal 2–3 cm of the superficial temporal artery within the temporoparietal fascia, the middle temporal artery branches and supplies the temporalis muscle fascia. The superficial temporal artery then divides into the frontal and parietal branches about 2–3 cm above the root of the helix [38]. The temporalis muscle arises from the superior temporal line, inserts into the coronoid process, and is innervated by the branches of the trigeminal nerve. The temporalis muscle is thickest in its anterior third and thinner in the middle and posterior thirds. The middle third of the muscle is the longest portion. The deep temporal arteries, branches of the internal maxillary artery, supply the temporalis muscle.

## Indications/Contraindications

The most common indication for a paramedian forehead flap is nasal defects that are not amenable or would have poor cosmetic outcomes with secondary intention healing, primary closure, skin grafting, or local skin flaps. The paramedian forehead flap is able to resurface the entire middle and lower thirds of the nose. The vascularity of the paramedian forehead flap can support extensive cartilaginous grafting. For small internal lining defects in the lower third of the nose, the forehead flap can be folded [39, 40]. However, multiple alternatives to the folded forehead flap exist for nasal lining defects, including septal flaps, turbinate flaps, bipedicled vestibular flaps, and free tissue transfer (see Chap. 3). An additional option for nasal lining defects includes bilateral simultaneous paramedian flaps [41]. The pedicle can be either tunneled under the glabellar skin, passed over the intervening skin bridge, or via a lateral rhinotomy approach resulting in a temporary nasal fistula. In these cases where dual paramedian flaps are utilized, an extensive reconstructed osseocartilaginous framework typically exists which requires neovascularization as well as minimal contact with defect edges along the periphery. It is therefore necessary to delay pedicle division much longer than the typical 2 to 3 weeks. In these cases, it has been suggested to divide the lining pedicle at 2 months and then divide the external flap pedicle and complete inset an additional 2 months following this [41]. Regardless of the technique utilized to address full thickness nasal defects, the number of procedures is typically more numerous, and the time until completed result is typically longer. However, the chimeric paramedian-pericranial forehead flap allows for reconstruction of the nasal lining and external skin using a single flap [42]. The pericranium is utilized to reconstruct the nasal lining defect, and the forehead skin is utilized to reconstruct the cutaneous defect, which allows for significant structural grafting during the first stage of reconstruction [42]. Pedicle division and inset of this chimeric flap were completed at 1 month given the patient's history of nicotine use. There are multiple other techniques that have been described allowing for reconstruction of full thickness nasal defects with prelaminated forehead flaps [43–45]. During a preliminary stage of reconstruction, the subcutaneous tissue plane can be dissected and a silicone sheet can be placed in this plane, therefore separating the galea from the cutaneous layer, and a split thickness skin graft can be applied to the deep surface of the galea which will serve as the nasal lining reconstruction [43].

The melolabial flap is an excellent option for nasal alar defects given the similarity in skin thickness and quality; however, it is less well suited for defects in the middle third of the nose given that the skin thickness tends to decrease in this area [24, 28]. The melolabial flap is also well suited for a variety of cheek and upper lip defects [18, 26, 27, 46, 47]. When utilized for nasal reconstruction, the melolabial flap is most commonly interpolated; however, in cases of upper lip and cheek reconstruction, the flap can be rotated, advanced, transposed, or interpolated depending on size and location of the defect. Although there is a rare application of this flap, the melolabial flap can be tunneled into the oral cavity or nasal cavity [21].

The temporoparietal and temporalis flaps have been applied to a variety of defects. The temporoparietal fascia flap is a thin, pliable, and well-vascularized flap that has a variety of uses in the head and neck [5]. It can be transferred as a fascial, fasciocutaneous, and osseofasciocutaneous flap. The temporoparietal flap can be transferred as a fasciocutaneous flap in order to reconstruct the upper lip in men with hair-bearing tissue [1]. When transferred as a fascial flap, it has been used in reconstructing lateral skull base, anterior skull base, auricular, orbitomaxillary, facial, and oral cavity defects among others [1, 2, 5, 38, 48]. Although uncommonly utilized in the twenty-first century, both the temporal muscle flap and the temporoparietal fascial flap have been transferred with attached split calvaria bone grafts [49, 50]. Both the paramedian forehead flap and the temporoparietal flap are useful in complex eyelid reconstructions [48, 51–53]. The temporoparietal fascial flap has been extensively described for auricular reconstruction [3, 4]. The temporalis muscle can be utilized in orbitomaxillary defects, anterior and lateral skull base defects, facial defects, and oral cavity defects [29, 30, 54–56]. The temporalis muscle has some bulk to it allowing for partial obliteration of orbital and temporal cavities with vascularized tissue and can act as a well-vascularized tissue bed to be skin grafted.

The primary disadvantage of the temporalis muscle flap is the temporal hollowing that is seen postoperatively.

## Preoperative Planning

When assessing a defect and considering a facial regional flap for reconstruction, multiple considerations must be made. The size of the defect, depth of the defect, and need for structural reconstruction in addition to cutaneous and/or mucosal reconstruction should be noted. The presence of hair-bearing skin in the area as well as skin thickness and quality should be taken into account. If it a nasal defect, the nasal subunits should be considered, and any concurrent adjacent lip and cheek defect should be reconstructed first prior to undertaking the nasal reconstruction. If it is a facial defect, involvement of the various facial subunits should be noted. The interpolated paramedian forehead flap, melolabial flap, and temporoparietal flap all have a period of at least 2 to 3 weeks when there is obvious facial deformity. For interpolated flaps, distance from the defect to the hinge point of the flap pedicle is measured to ensure that the pedicled flap can reach the defect and also ensure proper positioning of the skin paddle. Preoperative discussion with the patient will determine if this type of reconstruction is deemed acceptable to both surgeon and patient. Facial regional flaps are typically robust, and identification of the axial vessel can be confirmed with Doppler.

## Instrument/Equipment Set

- Bipolar electrocautery
- Monopolar electrocautery
- Skin hooks
- Fine tip dissecting scissors
- Dissolvable and permanent sutures
- Doppler probe

## Flap Design/Surgical Technique

### Paramedian Forehead Flap

A template of the defect is created typically using aluminum suture packaging. If the forehead flap will be folded in order to replace a lining defect, a separate template is made for the lining defect [15]. This allows for the necessary redundancy when folding the flap on itself. Once the defect template is created, the flap is most commonly designed based off the ipsilateral supratrochlear artery with a planned medial rotation of the pedicle (Fig. 2.1). A sterile gauze is used to measure the distance from the pivot point of the flap, the medial eyebrow, to the defect so that the

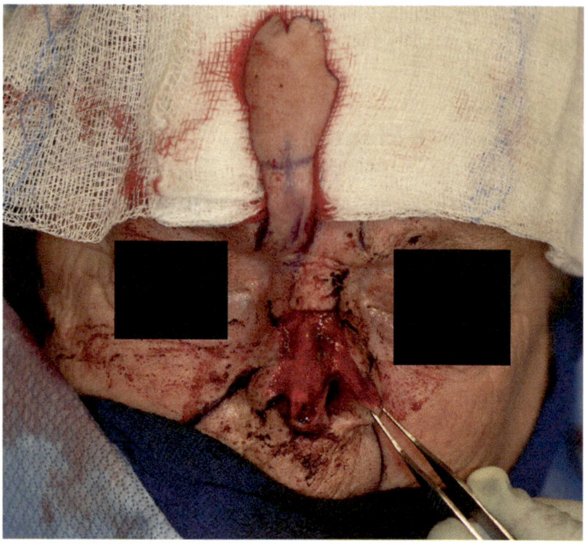

**Fig. 2.1** Defect involving nasal dorsum, nasal tip, bilateral soft tissue triangles, and left more than right ala. The paramedian forehead flap is demonstrated with planned medial rotation. (Courtesy of David Chan MD)

flap can be designed in the appropriate cranial caudal position on the forehead. The flap is then designed on the forehead using the created template. If a folded forehead flap is being performed, an additional 2–3 mm of length is added between the planned external defect and internal lining components [15]. If the flap is designed to incorporate hair-bearing scalp, then the individual follicles should be cauterized in the subcutaneous plane after elevation of the flap in order to minimize the transfer of hair-bearing skin to the nose [40, 41]. The base of the pedicle is centered over the supratrochlear which corresponds to a vertical axis 1.7–2.2 cm from midline and is typically 1.5 cm in width [40, 41].

The edges of the flap are then incised, and the flap is elevated in a distal to proximal fashion. Distally, in the area of the skin to be interpolated into the defect, the flap elevation can take place in the subcutaneous or subgaleal plane. Dissection in the subgaleal plane is a tissue plane that is more easily dissected, and the distal skin paddle can be appropriately thinned after flap elevation but prior to insetting into the defect. As dissection proceeds more proximally, the subgaleal plane is entered as the supratrochlear artery becomes subcutaneous approximately 15–25 mm above the supraorbital rim [57]. Most proximally, a subperiosteal dissection plane is performed as the orbital rim is approached [9]. Closure of the donor site is accomplished with extensive undermining of the forehead in the subgaleal plane from superficial temporal line of fusion to contralateral superficial temporal line of fusion. A pulley stitch can be applied to facilitate closure of the donor site. In addition, vertical galeotomies can be made at the level of the frontalis muscle taking care to avoid the supraorbital neurovascular bundle in the vertical plane of the medial limbus [33, 57]. A standing cutaneous deformity typically develops at the superior aspect of the donor site defect, and this is excised during closure of the donor site defect. Donor site defects which are unable to be closed primarily are allowed to heal by secondary intention given the poor cosmetic outcome of skin grafts for this particular defect [40]. The flap is then inset into the defect (Fig. 2.2).

If a two-stage forehead flap is planned, the pedicle is typically divided in 2 to 3 weeks. In a recent study, the forehead flap pedicle was divided in 1 week in ten patients who were not nicotine users and whose defects required less than 50% structural grafting within the defect [58]. Prior to division of the pedicle, the pedicle was atraumatically clamped, and using laser-assisted indocyanine green angiography to ensure adequate neovascularization [58]. The process of neovascularization has been found to take longer in the presence of cartilaginous grafting, and therefore, a 2- to 3-week delay prior to pedicle division may be more prudent in these cases [58, 59]. The pedicle is divided slightly cephalad to the cephalic margin of the nasal defect, and the cephalic 25% of the flap inset is incised in order to appropriately thin out the thickness of the flap, trim the flap to precisely fit the defect size, and then complete the inset. A triangular portion of the most proximal pedicle is then returned to the medial eyebrow in order to prevent height mismatch of the eyebrows (Fig. 2.3) [41]. The proximal portion of the donor site is incised and widely elevated in order to reposition the eyebrow. A triangular portion of the proximal portion of the pedicle, consisting of the medial brow, is fashion and advanced superiorly to position the brow approximately 2 mm superior to the contralateral brow in order to counteract the depression of the brow that is seen postoperatively [41].

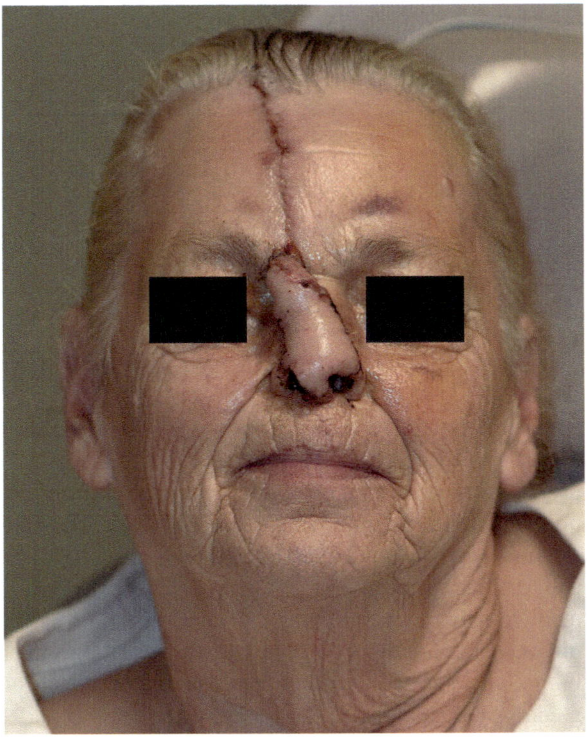

**Fig. 2.2** Paramedian forehead flap inset into defect after first stage with primary closure of the forehead. (Courtesy of David Chan MD)

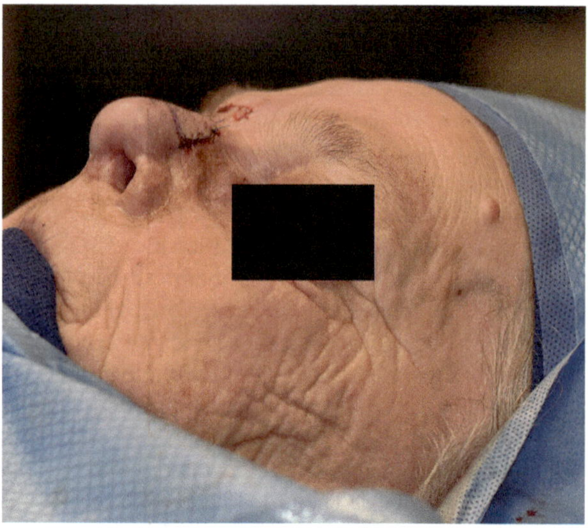

**Fig. 2.3** Pedicle division and completion of flap inset during third stage. A triangular portion of the most proximal pedicle is returned to the medial eyebrow in order to prevent height mismatch of the eyebrows. (Courtesy of David Chan MD)

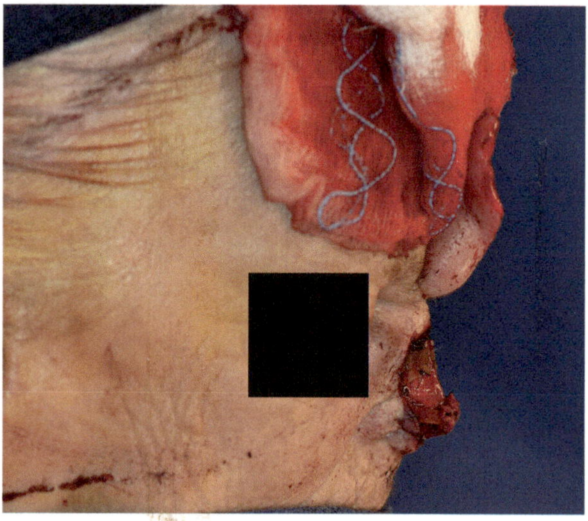

**Fig. 2.4** Intermediate stage. Paramedian forehead flap is elevated off the defect, and cartilage grafting is placed. (Courtesy of David Chan MD)

An intermediate stage can be added to forehead flap reconstruction of nasal defects in order to more aggressively thin and contour the flap [15, 40]. In nicotine users and in cases with extensive structural grafting, this intermediate stage may be prudent in order to train the flap and provide additional time for neovascularization. The intermediate stage can also allow for more flap thinning as well as soft tissue and cartilaginous sculpting (Fig. 2.4). The obvious disadvantage of adding an intermediate stage is prolonging the social isolation and the related consequences of obvious external deformity. In cases where the forehead flap is folded for internal lining, an intermediate stage becomes necessary in order to incise the flap at the planned alar rim, excise the excess skin that was added to account for the folding, debulk the internal and external components of the flap, and add structural grafts [15, 40].

## Melolabial Flap

The melolabial flap can be utilized as a tunneled, advancement, transposition, and interpolated flap [41]. When utilized as a transposition flap, it can reconstruct a variety of cheek defects and can be based either superiorly or inferiorly. The flap can be tunneled for reconstruction of oral cavity and nasal cavity defects; however, this is less commonly utilized [21]. The melolabial advancement flap is well suited for lateral upper lip defects and medial cheek defects adjacent to the nasal base [26, 27].

The melolabial flap can be interpolated either on a subcutaneous or cutaneous tissue pedicle. The interpolated melolabial flap offers an excellent option in the reconstruction of nasal alar defects because it preserves the alar facial sulcus [24, 28, 41]. A template of the defect is created, and the flap is then designed. The center of the flap is centered in the cranial caudal dimension 1 cm above the horizontal plane of the oral commissure [24, 28, 41]. The pedicled melolabial flap is superiorly based, and the superior aspect of this flap remains 5 mm inferior to the alar facial sulcus [24, 28, 41]. The medial aspect of the melolabial flap is positioned in or parallel to the melolabial crease. The flap is designed with a planned rotation medially. Standing cutaneous deformities are also marked out both superiorly and inferiorly. The edges of the flap are then incised, and in cases where a subcutaneous pedicle is planned, dissection is carried down to the zygomaticus major and levator labii superioris muscles [41]. The benefit of the subcutaneous tissue pedicle is improved mobility of the flap; however, it does require a deeper plane of dissection and entails some risk of damage to the terminal branches of the facial nerve as they innervate the zygomaticus major and levator labii superioris muscles [41]. If the flap is planned as a cutaneous pedicle flap, it is based superiorly with the width of the pedicle matching the width of planned flap. The flap is incised while leaving the base of the cutaneous pedicle intact, and the flap is elevated in the subcutaneous tissue plane leaving a few millimeters of subcutaneous fat on the pedicle. The melolabial flap pedicle is typically divided in 2 to 3 weeks; however, in a study of ten patients, using laser-assisted indocyanine green angiography demonstrated no association of improved neovascularization with time from first to second stage, which ranged from 19 to 30 days in this study [60]. This suggests that in select patients, earlier pedicle division may be safe [59, 60]. However, structural grafting is commonly needed in alar reconstructions in order to prevent alar retraction and external valve dysfunction, which would preclude earlier pedicle division.

## Temporoparietal Fascia Flap and Temporalis Muscle Flap

When designing the temporoparietal flap, the superficial temporal artery is identified with the use of a Doppler, and then the frontal and parietal branches can be typically identified with the Doppler approximately 3 cm above the root of the helix [1, 5, 38]. The anterior extent of the temporoparietal fascia flap harvest is limited by the course of the frontal branch of the facial nerve as it courses within the temporoparietal fascial along a line 0.5 cm below the tragus to 1.5 cm above the lateral brow [61]. A vertical incision is then marked out extending from the root of the helix. The incision can be continued inferiorly along the preauricular sulcus. If a fasciocutaneous flap is planned, the skin paddle is marked out based on a template of the defect. It is designed at a cranial-caudal level that would allow for transfer of the skin paddle into the defect with the pedicle based at the root of the helix. The planned incision is then made, and subcutaneous flaps are elevated. The temporoparietal fascia is immediately deep to the subcutaneous fat, and therefore, meticulous subcutaneous flap elevation must be performed in order to prevent damage to the vascular pedicle, fascial flap, and hair follicles [1, 5, 38]. The vascular pedicle is identified 4–5 mm anterior to the tragus, and the base of the flap is typically kept about 2 cm in width [1, 5, 38]. The frontal branch of the superficial temporal artery is ligated rather proximally in order to avoid injury to the frontal branch of the facial nerve. The temporoparietal fascia is then incised along the periphery of the flap margins and the superior temporal line. The flap is then elevated in the loose areolar tissue plane superficial to the temporalis muscle fascia. However, the temporalis muscle fascia can be incorporated with the temporoparietal flap given that the middle temporal artery supplies this fascial layer [38]. The flap is then transferred into the defect, and the donor site is closed primarily in layers. A suction drain is typically placed.

## Postoperative Management

Standard postoperative care is undertaken. Depending on the ablative portion of the procedure, most patients undergoing reconstructive surgery with facial regional flaps can be discharged to home on the same day. Wound care instructions regarding the incision lines and the exposed surfaces of interpolated flaps are given to the patients. Patients are typically seen at 1 week postoperatively for suture removal, and assessment of healing. Signs of flap loss, infection, and dehiscence are identified. In cases of staged procedures, the patient is prepared for the next stage of the reconstruction.

## References

1. Kim JC, Hadlock T, Varvares MA, Cheney ML. Hair-bearing temporoparietal fascial flap reconstruction of upper lip and scalp defects. Arch Facial Plast Surg. 2001;3(3):170–7.
2. Kim JYS, Buck DW, Johnson SA, Butler CE. The temporoparietal fascial flap is an alternative to free flaps for orbitomaxillary reconstruction. Plast Reconstr Surg. 2010;126(3):880–8.
3. Brent B, Byrd HS. Secondary ear reconstruction with cartilage grafts covered by axial, random, and free flaps of temporoparietal fascia. Plast Reconstr Surg. 1983;72(2):141–52.

4. Brent B. Auricular repair with autogenous rib cartilage grafts: two decades of experience with 600 cases. Plast Reconstr Surg. 1992;90(3):355–74; discussion 375–6.
5. Cheney ML, Varvares MA, Nadol JB. The temporoparietal fascial flap in head and neck reconstruction. Arch Otolaryngol Head Neck Surg. 1993;119(6):618–23.
6. Cheney ML, Megerian CA, Brown MT, McKenna MJ, Nadol JB. The use of the temporoparietal fascial flap in temporal bone reconstruction. Am J Otol. 1996;17(1):137–42.
7. Mcdowell F, Valone JA, Brown JB. Bibliography and historical note on plastic surgery of the nose. Plast Reconstr Surg 1946. 1952;10(3):149–85.
8. Kazanjian VH. The repair of nasal defects with the median forehead flap; primary closure of forehead wound. Surg Gynecol Obstet. 1946;83:37–49.
9. Shokri T, Kadakia S, Saman M, Habal MB, Kohlert S, Sokoya M, et al. The paramedian forehead flap for nasal reconstruction: from antiquity to present. J Craniofac Surg. 2019;30(2):330–3.
10. Boyd CM, Baker SR, Fader DJ, Wang TS, Johnson TM. The forehead flap for nasal reconstruction. Arch Dermatol. 2000;136(11):1365–70.
11. Blair VP, Byars LT. Hits, strikes and outs in the use of pedicle flaps for nasal restoration or correction. Surg Gynecol Obstet. 1946;82:367–85.
12. Conley JJ, Price JC. The midline vertical forehead flap. Otolaryngol Head Neck Surg. 1981;89(1):38–44.
13. Converse JM, Wood-Smith D. Experiences with the forehead Island flap with a subcutaneous pedicle. Plast Reconstr Surg. 1963;31:521–7.
14. Burget GC, Menick FJ. Nasal support and lining: the marriage of beauty and blood supply. Plast Reconstr Surg. 1989;84(2):189–202.
15. Menick FJ. A 10-year experience in nasal reconstruction with the three-stage forehead flap. Plast Reconstr Surg. 2002;109(6):1839–55; discussion 1856–61.
16. Burget GC, Menick FJ. Nasal reconstruction: seeking a fourth dimension. Plast Reconstr Surg. 1986;78(2):145–57.
17. Menick FJ. The use of skin grafts for nasal lining. Clin Plast Surg. 2001;28(2):311–21. viii
18. Cameron RR, Latham WD, Dowling JA. Reconstructions of the nose and upper lip with nasolabial flaps. Plast Reconstr Surg. 1973;52(2):145–50.
19. Climo MS. Nasolabial flap for alar defect. Case report. Plast Reconstr Surg. 1969;44(3):303–4.
20. Da Silva G. A new method of reconstructing the columella with a NASO-labial flap. Plast Reconstr Surg. 1964;34:63–5.
21. Georgiade NG, Mladick RA, Thorne FL. The nasolabial tunnel flap. Plast Reconstr Surg. 1969;43(5):463–6.
22. Macfee WF. The surgical treatment of cancer of the nose, with emphasis on methods of repair. Ann Surg. 1954;140(4):475–96.
23. Wesser DR, Burt GB. Nasolabial flap for losses of the nasal ala and columella. Case report. Plast Reconstr Surg. 1969;44(3):300–2.
24. Fader DJ, Baker SR, Johnson TM. The staged cheek-to-nose interpolation flap for reconstruction of the nasal alar rim/lobule. J Am Acad Dermatol. 1997;37(4):614–9.
25. Hagerty RF, Smith W. The nasolabial cheek flap. Am Surg. 1958;24(7):506–10.
26. Burget GC, Hsiao Y-C. Nasolabial rotation flaps based on the upper lateral lip subunit for superficial and large defects of the upper lateral lip. Plast Reconstr Surg. 2012;130(3):556–60.
27. Burget GC, Menick FJ. Aesthetic restoration of one-half the upper lip. Plast Reconstr Surg. 1986;78(5):583–93.
28. Baker SR, Johnson TM, Nelson BR. The importance of maintaining the alar-facial sulcus in nasal reconstruction. Arch Otolaryngol Head Neck Surg. 1995;121(6):617–22.
29. Renner G, Davis WE, Templer J. Temporalis pericranial muscle flap for reconstruction of the lateral face and head. Laryngoscope. 1984;94(11 Pt 1):1418–22.
30. Naquin HA. Orbital reconstruction utilizing temporalis muscle. Am J Ophthalmol. 1956;41(3):519–21.
31. Hallock GG. Reconstruction of a lower eyelid defect using the temporalis muscle. Ann Plast Surg. 1984;13(2):157–62.

32. Cheney ML, McKenna MJ, Megerian CA, Ojemann RG. Early temporalis muscle transposition for the management of facial paralysis. Laryngoscope. 1995;105(9 Pt 1):993–1000.
33. Shumrick KA, Smith TL. The anatomic basis for the design of forehead flaps in nasal reconstruction. Arch Otolaryngol Head Neck Surg. 1992;118(4):373–9.
34. Lee H-J, Won S-Y, Jehoon O, Hu K-S, Mun S-Y, Yang H-M, et al. The facial artery: a comprehensive anatomical review. Clin Anat. 2018;31(1):99–108.
35. Yang H-M, Lee J-G, Hu K-S, Gil Y-C, Choi Y-J, Lee H-K, et al. New anatomical insights on the course and branching patterns of the facial artery: clinical implications of injectable treatments to the nasolabial fold and nasojugal groove. Plast Reconstr Surg. 2014;133(5):1077–82.
36. Garcia-Serrano G, Moñux A, Maranillo E, Simon C, Sanudo JR, Vázquez MT, et al. Vascular clinical anatomy of the submandibular gland. J Cranio-Maxillofac Surg. 2020;48(6):582–9.
37. Lee J-G, Yang H-M, Choi Y-J, Favero V, Kim Y-S, Hu K-S, et al. Facial arterial depth and relationship with the facial musculature layer. Plast Reconstr Surg. 2015;135(2):437–44.
38. David SK, Cheney ML. An anatomic study of the temporoparietal fascial flap. Arch Otolaryngol Head Neck Surg. 1995;121(10):1153–6.
39. Mazzola RF, Marcus S. History of total nasal reconstruction with particular emphasis on the folded forehead flap technique. Plast Reconstr Surg. 1983;72(3):408–14.
40. Menick FJ. Nasal reconstruction art and practice. 1st ed. Amsterdam: Elsevier; 2008.
41. Baker SR. Local flaps in facial reconstruction. 4th ed. Amsterdam: Elsevier; 2021.
42. Harrison L, Sieffert M, Kadakia S, Kadakia S, Johnson RM, Ducic Y. Reconstruction of a subtotal septorhinectomy defect with a chimeric paramedian-pericranial forehead flap. Am J Otolaryngol. 2019;40(3):445–7.
43. Alagöz MS, Işken T, Sen C, Onyedi M, Izmirli H, Yücel E. Three-dimensional nasal reconstruction using a prefabricated forehead flap: case report. Aesthet Plast Surg. 2008;32(1):166–71.
44. Potter JK, Ducic Y, Ellis E. Extended bilaminar forehead flap with cantilevered bone grafts for reconstruction of full-thickness nasal defects. J Oral Maxillofac Surg. 2005;63(4):566–70.
45. Brackley PTH, Jones NS. The use of a periosteal/forehead flap with sandwiched conchal cartilage graft: a novel approach for nasal reconstruction in the absence of a nasal septum. Plast Reconstr Surg. 2002;110(3):831–5.
46. Bi H, Xing X, Li J. Nasolabial-alar crease: a natural line to facilitate transposition of the nasolabial flap for lower nasal reconstruction. Ann Plast Surg. 2014;73(5):520–4.
47. Durgun M, Özakpinar HR, Sari E, Selçuk CT, Seven E, Tellioğlu AT. The versatile facial artery perforator-based nasolabial flap in midface reconstruction. J Craniofac Surg. 2015;26(4):1283–6.
48. Hocaoğlu E, Özden BÇ, Aydın H. Lower eyelid reconstruction in a paediatric face: a one-stage aesthetic approach using the versatile temporoparietal fascia flap. J Plast Reconstr Aesthetic Surg. 2012;65(9):e246–9.
49. Bite U, Jackson IT, Wahner HW, Marsh RW. Vascularized skull bone grafts in craniofacial surgery. Ann Plast Surg. 1987;19(1):3–15.
50. Casanova R, Cavalcante D, Grotting JC, Vasconez LO, Psillakis JM. Anatomic basis for vascularized outer-table calvarial bone flaps. Plast Reconstr Surg. 1986;78(3):300–8.
51. Patel V, Osborne S, Morley AMS, Malhotra R. The use of pericranial flaps for reconstruction and elevation of the lower eyelid. Orbit Amst Neth. 2010;29(1):1–6.
52. Bababeygy SR, Kao AR, Kokot NC, Chang EL. Reconstruction of total lower eyelid defects with the temporoparietal fascial flap. Case Rep Ophthalmol Med. 2012;2012:927260.
53. Weerdt GD, Luyten P, Dubrulle F, Loonen M. Reconstruction of an extensive periocular and bilamellar defect of the lower and upper eyelid using local, regional and free chondral graft techniques: a case report. World J Plast Surg. 2021;10(1):125–31.
54. Byrne PJ, Kim M, Boahene K, Millar J, Moe K. Temporalis tendon transfer as part of a comprehensive approach to facial reanimation. Arch Facial Plast Surg. 2007;9(4):234–41.
55. Bradley P, Brockbank J. The temporalis muscle flap in oral reconstruction. A cadaveric, animal and clinical study. J Maxillofac Surg. 1981;9(3):139–45.
56. Bakamjian VY, Souther SG. Use of temporal muscle flap for reconstruction after orbitomaxillary resections for cancer. Plast Reconstr Surg. 1975;56(2):171–7.

57. Kleintjes WG. Forehead anatomy: arterial variations and venous link of the midline forehead flap. J Plast Reconstr Aesthetic Surg. 2007;60(6):593–606.
58. Rudy SF, Abdelwahab M, Kandathil CK, Most SP. Paramedian forehead flap pedicle division after 7 days using laser-assisted indocyanine green angiography. J Plast Reconstr Aesthetic Surg. 2021;74(1):116–22.
59. Abdelwahab M, Kandathil CK, Most SP, Spataro EA. Utility of indocyanine green angiography to identify clinical factors associated with perfusion of paramedian forehead flaps during nasal reconstruction surgery. JAMA Facial Plast Surg. 2019;21(3):206–12.
60. Abdelwahab M, Spataro EA, Kandathil CK, Most SP. Neovascularization perfusion of melolabial flaps using intraoperative indocyanine green angiography. JAMA Facial Plast Surg. 2019;21(3):230–6.
61. Pitanguy I, Ramos AS. The frontal branch of the facial nerve: the importance of its variations in face lifting. Plast Reconstr Surg. 1966;38(4):352–6.

# Nasal Reconstruction

# 3

Arya Namin and David Chan

## Introduction

Nasal reconstruction has been a major focus point of plastic surgery during the past three millennia [1]. Many reconstructive surgeons throughout history and around the globe have embraced the challenge of nasal reconstruction and shared their experiences, making the foundation of knowledge we have today [2]. Various flaps for nasal defects have been described, including a pedicled arm flap from Sicilian surgeons in the fifteenth and sixteenth centuries [2]. However, the forehead flap and melolabial flap have played an integral part in the evolution of nasal reconstruction (Chap. 2) [1–4]. The injuries of World War I and II resulted in more widespread dissemination of these techniques [5]. Millard describes modern nasal reconstruction as having three stages: the first two main stages are restoring the covering and lining of the nose, and the third stage is restoring nasal support [5]. It was during the late nineteenth and early twentieth centuries that the importance of nasal lining to prevent contraction was reported on in the literature [5]. Throughout the nineteenth and twentieth centuries, various methods to restore the nasal framework were attempted, including metallic implants, pedicled frontal bone flaps, pedicled clavicular flaps, bone grafts, and cartilage grafts [5]. Despite these old, even ancient techniques, our improved modern understanding of the form and function of the nose, vascular anatomy of the head and neck, and microvascular surgery allows for continued refinement of these techniques and improved outcomes [1, 6–10].

Nasal reconstruction is challenging because the nose is critical to the form and function of the craniofacial skeleton, and its complex three-dimensional anatomy consists of a very thin vascular internal lining that is tightly adherent to a thin flexible

A. Namin
Otolaryngology and Facial Plastic Surgery Associates, Fort Worth, TX, USA

D. Chan (✉)
Century Ear, Nose, and Throat—Head and Neck Surgery, Orland Park, IL, USA



F. Sokoya, A. G. Vincent (eds.), *Manual of Head and Neck Reconstruction*,
https://doi.org/10.1007/978-3-031-65999-7_3

cartilaginous structure. Additionally, it has an overlying soft tissue envelope consisting of the superficial musculoaponeurotic system, dermis, and epidermis [11]. There are several examples that illustrate the many challenges of nasal reconstruction. The structural relationships that the osseocartilaginous framework has with both the internal and external lining is one. When placing a lateral crural strut graft in an underlay fashion between the vestibular lining and the alar cartilage during rhinoplasty, the surgeon is required to dissect the vestibular lining off the alar cartilage [12]. Simply the disruption of the vestibular lining from the lower lateral cartilage changes the competence of the external nasal valve necessitating structure grafting to reconstruct the external valve, implying that the native relationship between the vestibular lining and lower lateral cartilages contribute to the form and function of the nose. Likewise, the importance of the ligamentous system (vertical and longitudinal scroll ligaments, Pitanguy's ligament, and interdomal ligaments) in the relationship between the underlying osseocartilaginous framework and the overlying soft tissue envelope has been described and is a component of preservation rhinoplasty [11, 13]. These examples demonstrate that the form and function of the nose is not dependent solely on the presence of the vestibular lining, osseocartilaginous framework, superficial musculoaponeurotic system, and skin, but also on an inherent relationship among these layers that the reconstructive surgeon cannot replicate.

Despite these challenges, it is remarkable how far nasal reconstruction has developed during the past century, particularly in regard to full thickness and total nasal defects [5, 8–10, 14, 15]. Millard utilized a combination of nasal turn-in flaps, dual forehead flaps, and melolabial flaps for lining defects, and cantilevered autologous bony rib grafts for structural support with excellent results [5]. Millard's critique of prior full thickness and total nasal reconstructions was the bulky appearance of the columella and alar areas [5]. Burget and Menick noted these challenges, explaining that nasal reconstruction is much more than recreating the three-dimensional structure [16]. The importance and challenge of reconstructing the nasal lining with thin and well-vascularized tissue were noted, and vestibular flaps and septal mucoperichondrial flaps were described [16]. Various methods have subsequently been described for repairing internal lining defects, including skin grafts, folded forehead flaps, dual forehead flaps, chimeric paramedian-pericranial forehead flap, turbinate flaps, and free flaps [6, 8–10, 14, 15, 17]. A multitude of nasal reconstructive options exist; however, successful execution of these requires an understanding of the form and function of the nose, visualization of planned result, and meticulous preoperative planning and patient preparation.

## Anatomy

The nose consists of four basic layers: the skin, superficial musculoaponeurotic layer, osseocartilaginous framework, and lining. When assessing surface landmarks for nasal reconstruction, the nose is typically broken down into subunits: paired nasal sidewalls, soft tissue triangles, and alars as well as midline dorsum, tip, and columellar subunits (Fig. 3.1) [18]. The soft tissue envelope consists of the skin and

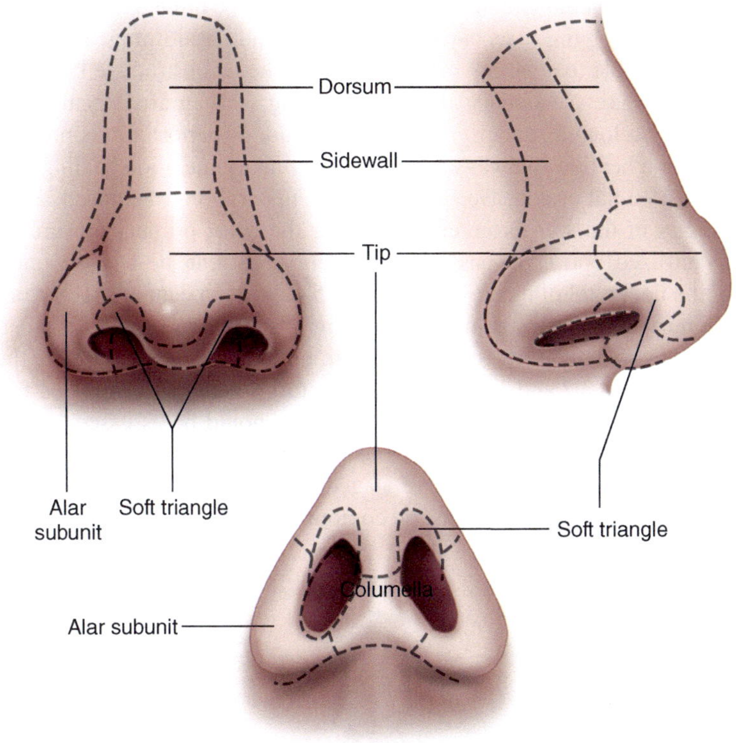


**Fig. 3.1** Nasal subunits. Paired nasal sidewalls, soft tissue triangles, and alars. Midline dorsum, tip, and columellar subunits

the superficial musculoaponeurotic layers, and the thickness of these layers varies significantly in different areas of the nose and between patients. The thickness of the soft tissue envelope and the defect are important variables when choosing a reconstructive option. The soft tissue envelope is typically thickest in the upper third, thinnest in the middle third over the rhinion, and then quite variable in the lower third [19]. While the alar subunit does not have any cartilaginous structure, it does contain the tela subcutanea cutis, which provides structure to the alar lobule [20]. The osseocartilaginous vault consists of the nasal bones, frontal process of maxilla, septum, upper lateral cartilages, and lower lateral cartilages. At the keystone area, the upper lateral cartilages pass under the nasal bones to meet the dorsal septum where it transitions to the perpendicular plate of the ethmoid. At the scroll area, the lower lateral and upper lateral cartilages connect via the horizontal scroll ligament in a variable fashion [21]. The internal lining of the nose consists largely of mucoperichondrium and mucoperiosteum, with skin lining the nasal vestibule.

## Indications

Most nasal defects encountered in clinical practice will be limited to external defects with an intact underlying osseocartilaginous vault and nasal lining. These external defects are amenable to a variety of options along the reconstructive ladder including primary closure, secondary intention healing, skin grafts, local flaps, and regional flaps. So long as underlying perichondrium or periosteum is present, secondary intention healing is always an option. Secondary intention healing serves as a better option on flat or concave surfaces of the upper 2/3 of the nose [22]. Due to the inelasticity of the soft tissue envelope over the nose, primary closure is not a frequently utilized option in nasal reconstruction but can be a good option for defects of the upper 2/3 of the nose measuring 5–10 mm in diameter. If the underlying perichondrium or periosteum is intact, skin grafts are an option for most nasal defects. Even large defects involving the upper, middle, and lower thirds of the nose can be grafted (Figs. 3.2 and 3.3). When a skin graft is being contemplated for nasal reconstruction, the patient's remaining nasal skin should be assessed, and patient desires should be understood. The obvious advantages of skin grafts are minimal donor site morbidity and avoidance of staged procedures, with the disadvantages being higher risk for color mismatch and contour irregularities. With that being said,

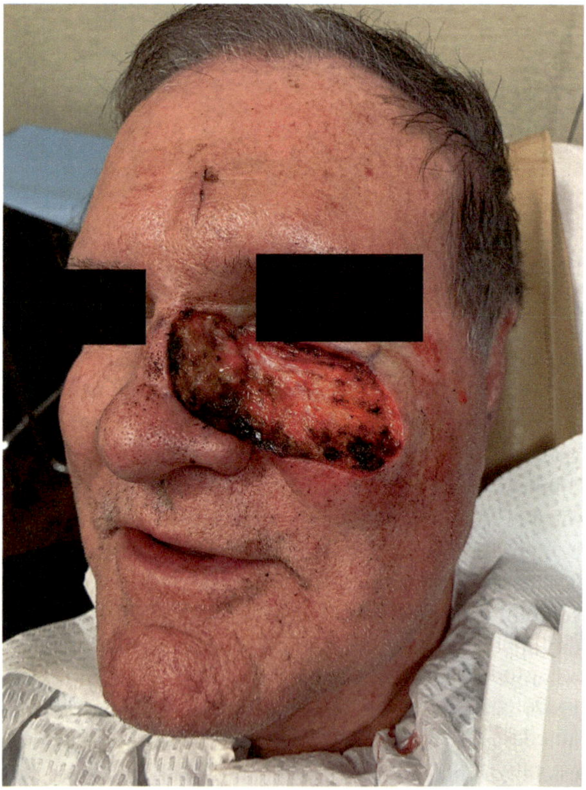

**Fig. 3.2** Nasal defect involving nasal sidewall, a small portion of the alar, cheek, and lower eyelid

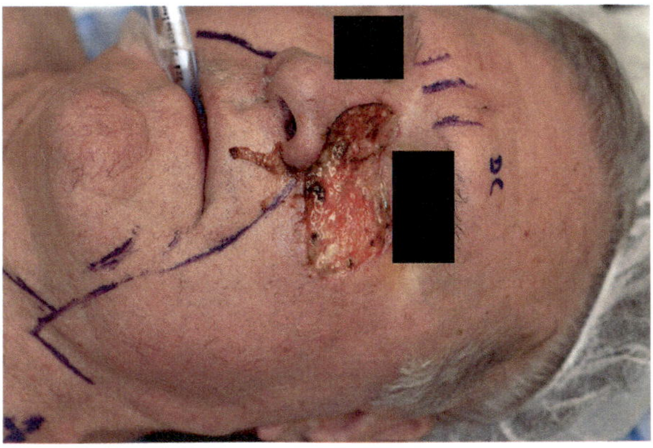

**Fig. 3.3** Planned reconstruction with cervicofacial advancement flap for the cheek and lower eyelid defect and split thickness skin graft for the nasal sidewall defect

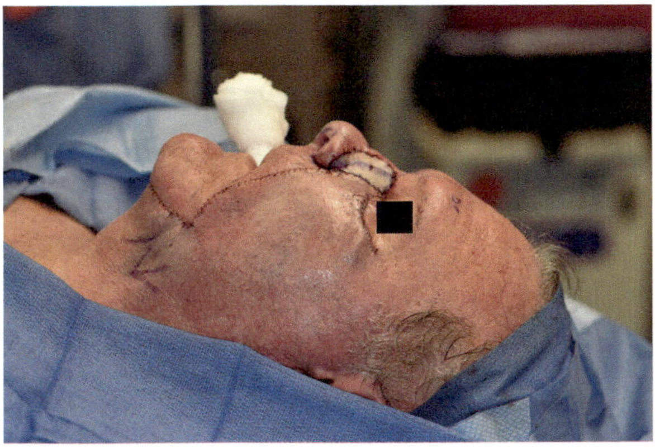

**Fig. 3.4** Immediate postoperative result demonstrating cervicofacial advancement flap inset and split thickness skin graft

excellent cosmetic results can be obtained when skin grafts are utilized in appropriately selected candidates (Figs. 3.4 and 3.5). Common skin graft donor sites for nasal reconstruction are the forehead, preauricular region, and supraclavicular region [22, 23]. Small defects (<1 cm) along the columella, soft tissue triangle, and alar margin pose unique challenges. While they are small defects, they are often times full thickness and particularly prone to contraction and distortion. Therefore, structural grafting and staged regional flaps are often utilized to obtain the best result. However, an alternative for small defects (<1 cm) along the columella, soft tissue triangle, and alar margin is a composite graft taken from the root of the helix or conchal bowl [23]. Composite grafts have high metabolic demands and are therefore more prone to failure than skin grafts [23]. Ideal defects for compositive grafts would be less than 1 cm in size in a healthy patient less than 65 years of age [23]. Postoperatively, a steroid taper should be prescribed, and icing should be applied in order to help decrease the metabolic demands of the graft [23].

Defects of the middle and upper thirds of the nose measuring 1.0–1.5 cm are well suited for transposition flaps. Once these defects are larger than 1 cm, primary closure typically is less than ideal as it requires significant tension and possible structural

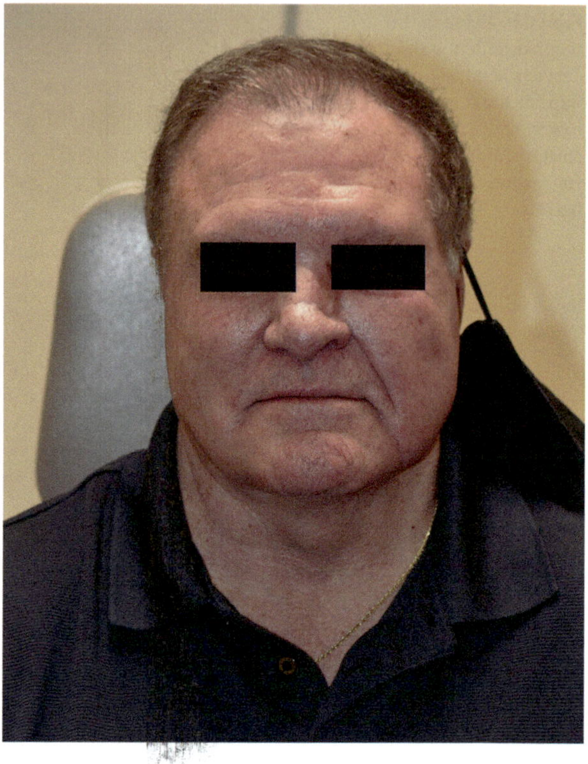

**Fig. 3.5** Four-month postoperative result

deformation to be achieved. Skin grafting and healing by secondary intention are acceptable considerations for defects measuring 1.0–1.5 cm of the upper and middle thirds. The nasal skin of the lower third is the least mobile, so extensive undermining is required if defects in this area are to be reconstructed with local tissue rearrangement. The bilobe flap is classically described as an option for nasal defects measuring up to 1.5 cm in the lower third of the nose but not extending into the ala or within 0.5 cm of the nostril margin [23]. The V-Y advancement flap is an option for defects <1.5 cm in the supra alar groove [24]. The dorsal nasal flap is a good single-stage reconstruction for defects of the middle third measuring up to 2.5 cm in diameter [25]. The advantage of this flap is that it is only one stage and can reconstruct fairly large defects. The primary disadvantage of the dorsal nasal flap is that the incision lines typically cross nasal subunits making scars more noticeable postoperatively. It also carries the possibility of increased tip rotation, which may be welcomed by older patients. The paramedian forehead flap will often result in the best cosmetic outcome for larger defects of the lower 2/3 of the nose with the disadvantage being a multiple stage reconstruction. Most nasal defects will have multiple reconstructive options, and the surgeon should discuss the advantages and disadvantages of each with the patient to come to a shared reconstructive path forward that meets patient's goals.

The complexity of nasal reconstruction increases exponentially once a lining defect exists. Options available to repair lining defects include nasal turn-in flaps, bipedicled vestibular flaps, septal mucoperichondrial flaps, composite septal chondromucosal flaps, inferior turbinate flaps, skin grafts, dual forehead flaps, melolabial flaps, folded forehead flaps, chimeric paramedian-pericranial forehead flaps, and a variety of free flaps [8–10, 14, 15, 17, 23]. Nasal turn-in flaps are not commonly utilized given the poor vascularity of these flaps; however, they can be considered for small internal lining defects limited to the upper and middle thirds of the nose. For full thickness defects of the alar margin up to 1.0–1.5 cm in vertical height, both the bipedicled vestibular skin advancement flap and folded forehead flap can be considered [9, 23, 26]. The advantages of the bipedicled vestibular skin advancement flap include its thinness and vascularity, which support cartilaginous grafting without distorting the reconstructed alar margin [26]. Utilizing a folded forehead flap in a two-stage approach would undoubtedly leave the patient with a poorly defined alar margin. However, utilizing a folded forehead flap in a three-stage approach can obtain a well-defined alar margin in full thickness defects of the alar margin up to 1.5 cm in vertical height [9]. In this approach, an intermediate stage is added to incise the flap at the designed alar margin, excise the planned excess cutaneous portion of the flap, place cartilaginous grafting, and sculpt the external portion of the flap [9]. The pedicle is then divided, and inset is completed during an additional third stage 3 weeks later.

When present, nasal lining flaps are an ideal option for larger lining defects. Nasal lining flaps are thin, pliable, and vascular. They can support cartilaginous grafting without creating a bulky or stiff reconstruction. The disadvantages include significant postoperative crusting while the donor site heals by secondary intention, the increased risk of epistaxis, and the possibility for temporary nasal obstruction depending on the lining flap utilized. For lining defects larger than 1.5 cm of the lower third, the septal mucoperichondrial hinge flap provides an excellent option, albeit at the expense of temporary complete nasal obstruction until the hinge pedicle is divided. For lining defects of the middle third, the dorsal septal mucoperichondrial hinge flap can be used and is transposed from the contralateral septum necessitating a septal fistula [23]. The ipsilateral caudal septal mucoperichondrial hinge flap and contralateral dorsal septal mucoperichondrial hinge flap can be used concurrently to repair large unilateral lining defects involving the middle and lower thirds [23]. An alternative nasal lining flap is the inferior turbinate mucosal flap [17].

Skin grafts have been utilized in a variety of ways for reconstructing the nasal lining [14, 27]. The challenge of using skin grafts for lining reconstruction is that it can limit the extent and precision of structural grafting and is more prone to failure and cicatricial forces. When combined with paramedian forehead flap reconstruction of the nasal skin, one technique to mitigate limited structural grafting is to place a skin graft in a preliminary operation on the deep surface of the frontalis muscle. In this initial operation, a plane between the subcutaneous tissue layer and frontalis, is dissected and a silicone sheet or graft is placed. This area is allowed to heal, essentially creating two vascularized soft tissue paddles that will have some degree of independent mobility and allowing for structural grafting to be placed between the subcutaneous and frontalis tissue planes during a later procedure [27]. Menick describes a similar method for larger unilateral lining defects involving the alar margin using full thickness skin grafts and a concomitant three-stage forehead flap technique [14]. A full thickness skin graft is designed for the lining defect and sutured in place [14]. A forehead flap is utilized and transferred into the defect providing the vascular supply to the skin graft [14]. During the second, intermediate stage, the plane between the frontalis and subcutaneous tissue is dissected in the area of the middle and upper thirds, and structural grafting is placed [14]. Inset completion, soft tissue sculpting, and pedicle division are then completed during the third stage 3 weeks later.

In cases of extensive unilateral lining defects where the nasal mucosal flap options are depleted, or in cases of bilateral nasal defects, options to restore the nasal lining include skin grafting, dual forehead flaps, or free tissue transfer. In these larger defects requiring extensive structural grafting, skin grafts have many disadvantages and typically are not an option. Both the anterolateral thigh fascial flap and the radial forearm free flap have been described with good outcomes in reconstructing lining defects in total nasal reconstruction while concomitantly using paramedian forehead flaps for the external defect [8, 10, 15].

## Preoperative Planning

When assessing a nasal defect, there are multiple variables to consider prior to designing and finalizing a reconstruction plan. An interview with the patient should explore prior satisfaction with nasal appearance, prior photos of the patient before the current deformity, and patient expectations. A discussion of the various options and advantages/disadvantages must be had. The surgeon should begin to visualize the planned outcome and the steps necessary to obtain that outcome [22]. The patient should then be prepared for the reconstructive process, particularly staged procedures that often times require weeks of deformity that the patient may find unacceptable for public appearance. One of the first variables that should be assessed is to determine if the defect extends into the adjacent lip, cheek, or periorbital subunits. If the defect does extend into adjacent facial subunits, these should be reconstructed first in order to restore the nasal platform prior to embarking on the nasal reconstruction [22]. The nasal subunits should be carefully evaluated [18, 22]. If the defect involves more than 50% of a convex subunit, particularly the tip or alar subunits, excision of the remaining portion of that subunit should be considered, paired with a reconstruction that resurfaces the entire subunit [18, 22]. This prevents scarring and trap door defects within subunits, a deformity that is more noticeable when looking at an individual's face. When examining a defect, it can be helpful to outline the nasal subunits.

The depth of the defect should be assessed. The extent of missing epidermis/dermis, superficial musculoaponeurotic system, osseocartilaginous framework, and nasal lining is assessed. The extent and depth of missing soft tissue envelope should be carefully assessed. The thickness of the dermis and superficial musculoaponeurotic system varies significantly based on location within the nose and skin thickness of the patient. Defects in patients with thick skin or those involving the superficial musculoaponeurotic system are less favorable for secondary intention healing or skin graft reconstruction. The location of the various defects should be noted, and the relationship both in terms of size and location between the nasal lining defect and cutaneous defect should be assessed in order to devise a reconstructive plan for both the external and lining defects.

Finally, the need for structural grafting should be assessed. Although the alar subunits do not typically contain cartilage, structural grafting to these defects is prudent in order to prevent alar retraction during the healing process. The alar lobule does contain the tela subcutaneous cutis, which provides structural support to the alar lobule and is disrupted after trauma or oncologic procedures to the alar lobule [20]. Missing portions of the osseocartilaginous framework are then assessed, and a reconstructive plan to replace or repair the osseocartilaginous framework should be devised. The osseocartilaginous framework can be reconstructed with split calvarial bone grafts, rib grafts, septal grafts, conchal cartilage grafts, and free tissue transfer. When reconstructing the osseocartilaginous framework, the contralateral side can serve as a mirrored template. An additional consideration when reconstructing the osseocartilaginous framework, particularly the tip, is the polygon concept, which correlates underlying structural anatomy with surface aesthetics [28]. The ideal tip shape can be broken down into underlying structural polygons: paired dome triangles, paired lateral crurual polygons, interdomal triangle, paired facet polygons, infralobular polygon, columellar polygon, and footplate polygon [28]. This concept may be particularly helpful in cases where the defect is bilateral.

The presence, size, and location of lining defects are then assessed. The extent of the septal defect, if present, should be analyzed, and any remaining septal cartilage and/or mucoperichondrium is assessed. Involvement of the nasal floor mucosa and turbinate should be assessed as well.

## Instrument/Equipment Set

- Bipolar electrocautery
- Monopolar electrocautery
- Skin hooks
- Fine-tip dissecting scissors
- Dissolvable and permanent sutures
- Doppler probe
- Flap Design/Surgical Technique

The reconstructive surgeon will encounter a wide variety of nasal defects, ranging from small cutaneous defects that are amenable to secondary intention healing to septorhinectomy defects that often times require free tissue transfer, structural grafting, and regional tissue transfer to resurface the defect. Both local (Chap. 1) and regional flaps (Chap. 2) are excellent tools in a variety of nasal defects, and the techniques for these reconstructions are discussed elsewhere in this text. In this section, the surgical technique of various lining flaps will be discussed.

The *bipedicled vestibular skin advancement flap* is based off a pedicle to the septum at the anterior septal angle and a pedicle at the lateral floor of the vestibule [26]. The dimensions of the lining defect are measured, and the remaining vestibular skin up to the planned intercartilaginous incision is then assessed to ensure adequate flap dimension. The vestibular skin is then infiltrated with local anesthesia prior to incision and elevation. An intercartilaginous incision is then made extending from the anterior septal angle to the lateral floor of the nasal vestibule [23, 26]. The pedicled flap is then elevated off the underlying lower lateral cartilage, which is a difficult dissection if hydrodissection with local anesthesia was not performed first. Structural grafting is then placed along the planned alar margin and secured to the pedicled vestibular skin advancement flap. Depending on the extent of the cutaneous deformity and operative plans, a paramedian forehead flap or melolabial flap is then utilized to reconstruct the cutaneous defect and secured to the pedicled vestibular flap along the alar margin.

The *septal mucoperichondrial hinge flap* is based along the caudal septum supplied by the septal branch of the labial artery [23, 26]. The plane between the septal cartilage and mucoperichondrium is infiltrated with local anesthesia ipsilateral to the side of the defect. The dorsal incision parallels the nasal dorsum and is begun about 1 cm posterior to the anterior septal angle and 1 cm inferior to the roof of the middle vault [23]. The caudal incision begins 1 cm posterior to the anterior nasal spine and continues posteriorly parallel to the nasal crest [23]. The posterior incision connects the dorsal and caudal incisions and is typically designed in a fashion so that flap length is at least 4 cm [23]. The flap is then elevated from the septal cartilage in standard fashion and hinged inferiorly to reconstruct the lining defect. The *dorsal septal mucoperichondrial hinge flap* is based off the contralateral septum and hinged dorsally [23]. This reconstruction necessitates a septal fistula. The *inferior turbinate mucosal flap* is based anteriorly and is an additional nasal lining flap. The turbinate is liberally injected with local anesthesia and is then separated from the nasal sidewall from posterior to anterior [17]. Once the bony turbinate is separated from the nasal sidewall, the mucosa is dissected off the turbinate bone keeping its pedicle attached anteriorly [17]. The bony turbinate is then removed and can be used for grafting if deemed useful [17].

## Postoperative Management

Standard postoperative care is undertaken. Depending on the ablative portion of the procedure, most patients undergoing reconstructive surgery with facial regional flaps can be discharged home on the same day. Wound care instructions regarding the incision lines and the exposed surfaces of interpolated flaps are given to the patients. Patients are typically seen at 1 week postoperatively for suture removal and an initial assessment of healing. Signs of flap loss, infection, and dehiscence are examined for. In cases of staged procedures, the patient is prepared for the next stage of the reconstruction.

## References


1. Shokri T, Kadakia S, Saman M, Habal MB, Kohlert S, Sokoya M, et al. The paramedian forehead flap for nasal reconstruction: from antiquity to present. J Craniofac Surg. 2019;30(2):330–3.
2. Mcdowell F, Valone JA, Brown JB. Bibliography and historical note on plastic surgery of the nose. Plast Reconstr Surg 1946. 1952;10(3):149–85.
3. Kazanjian VH. The repair of nasal defects with the median forehead flap; primary closure of forehead wound. Surg Gynecol Obstet. 1946;83:37–49.
4. Baker SR, Johnson TM, Nelson BR. The importance of maintaining the alar-facial sulcus in nasal reconstruction. Arch Otolaryngol Head Neck Surg. 1995;121(6):617–22.
5. Millard DR. Total reconstructive rhinoplasty and a missing link. Plast Reconstr Surg. 1966;37(3):167–83.
6. Harrison L, Sieffert M, Kadakia S, Kadakia S, Johnson RM, Ducic Y. Reconstruction of a subtotal septorhinectomy defect with a chimeric paramedian-pericranial forehead flap. Am J Otolaryngol. 2019;40(3):445–7.
7. Abdelwahab M, Kandathil CK, Most SP, Spataro EA. Utility of indocyanine green angiography to identify clinical factors associated with perfusion of paramedian forehead flaps during nasal reconstruction surgery. JAMA Facial Plast Surg. 2019;21(3):206–12.
8. Seth R, Revenaugh PC, Scharpf J, Shipchandler TZ, Fritz MA. Free anterolateral thigh fascia lata flap for complex nasal lining defects. JAMA Facial Plast Surg. 2013;15(1):21–8.
9. Menick FJ. A 10-year experience in nasal reconstruction with the three-stage forehead flap. Plast Reconstr Surg. 2002;109(6):1839–55; discussion 1856–61.
10. Salibian AH, Menick FJ, Talley J. Microvascular reconstruction of the nose with the radial forearm flap: a 17-year experience in 47 patients. Plast Reconstr Surg. 2019;144(1):199–210.
11. Saban Y, Andretto Amodeo C, Hammou JC, Polselli R. An anatomical study of the nasal superficial musculoaponeurotic system: surgical applications in rhinoplasty. Arch Facial Plast Surg. 2008;10(2):109–15.
12. Samra S, Steitz JT, Hajnas N, Toriumi DM. Surgical management of nasal valve collapse. Otolaryngol Clin N Am. 2018;51(5):929–44.
13. Kosins AM, Daniel RK. Decision making in preservation rhinoplasty: a 100 case series with one-year follow-up. Aesthet Surg J. 2020;40(1):34–48.
14. Menick FJ. The use of skin grafts for nasal lining. Clin Plast Surg. 2001;28(2):311–21. viii
15. Winslow CP, Cook TA, Burke A, Wax MK. Total nasal reconstruction: utility of the free radial forearm fascial flap. Arch Facial Plast Surg. 2003;5(2):159–63.
16. Burget GC, Menick FJ. Nasal reconstruction: seeking a fourth dimension. Plast Reconstr Surg. 1986;78(2):145–57.
17. Murakami CS, Kriet JD, Ierokomos AP. Nasal reconstruction using the inferior turbinate mucosal flap. Arch Facial Plast Surg. 1999;1(2):97–100.
18. Burget GC, Menick FJ. The subunit principle in nasal reconstruction. Plast Reconstr Surg. 1985;76(2):239–47.
19. Daniel RK, Palhazi P. Rhinoplasty: an anatomical and clinical atlas. 2018. Springer Publishers.
20. Daniel RK, Glasz T, Molnar G, Palhazi P, Saban Y, Journel B. The lower nasal base: an anatomical study. Aesthet Surg J. 2013;33(2):222–32.
21. Saban Y, Daniel RK, Polselli R, Trapasso M, Palhazi P. Dorsal preservation: the push down technique reassessed. Aesthet Surg J. 2018;38(2):117–31.
22. Menick FJ. Nasal reconstruction: art and practice. 2009. Elsevier Health Sciences.
23. Baker SR. Local flaps in facial reconstruction. 2021. Elsevier Publishing.
24. Viciana EJ, Lessard A-S. V-Y flap for nasal reconstruction. Plast Reconstr Surg Glob Open. 2020;8(8):e3040.
25. Johnson TM, Swanson NA, Baker SR, Brown MD, Nelson BR. The rieger flap for nasal reconstruction. Arch Otolaryngol Head Neck Surg. 1995;121(6):634–7.
26. Burget GC, Menick FJ. Nasal support and lining: the marriage of beauty and blood supply. Plast Reconstr Surg. 1989;84(2):189–202.

27. Alagöz MS, Işken T, Sen C, Onyedi M, Izmirli H, Yücel E. Three-dimensional nasal reconstruction using a prefabricated forehead flap: case report. Aesthet Plast Surg. 2008;32(1):166–71.
28. Çakır B, Öreroğlu AR, Daniel RK. Surface aesthetics in tip rhinoplasty: a step-by-step guide. Aesthet Surg J. 2014;34(6):941–55.

# Patient-Specific Implants and Prosthetics

4

David A. Rengifo, Alexander P. Simko, and Raja Sawhney

## Introduction and History

Major facial defects are typically repaired with autologous reconstructive techniques. There are situations, however, where prosthetic rehabilitation is preferable as a primary or complementary reconstruction method for facial defects. The advancement of technologies in imaging and biocompatible materials has allowed patient-specific implants and prostheses to become an integral part of facial reconstructive surgery. By providing a synthetic replacement of traumatic, ablative, or congenital defects, the transformative role of these prosthetics can provide a robust combination of function and aesthetics.

Initially, the historical breakthroughs in prosthetics were limited to biomaterials. The earliest prosthetics were largely composed of shells and animal xenografts; however, extensive use and experience with these materials showed poor integration and high infection rates. Rapid improvement and utilization of implants and prosthetics began during the world wars of the twentieth century. Advancements in antibiotics and anesthesia meant patients surviving what were once mortal injuries. These patients presented with morbid injuries, requiring surgeons to expand the reconstructive armamentarium. Materials such as plaster, latex, leather, silver, and steel gained popularity and were used for several decades. Most of these options failed to maintain relevance due to their inherent characteristics. Issues with longevity, heat conduction, tensile strength, biocompatibility, and radio-opacity limited

D. A. Rengifo (✉) · R. Sawhney
Department of Otolaryngology, Head and Neck Surgery, University of Florida, Gainesville, FL, USA
e-mail: David.Rengifo@ent.ufl.edu

A. P. Simko
University of Florida School of Medicine, Gainesville, FL, USA
e-mail: ap.simko@ufl.edu



F. Sokoya, A. G. Vincent (eds.), *Manual of Head and Neck Reconstruction*,
https://doi.org/10.1007/978-3-031-65999-7_4

their long-term viability. Modern materials are increasingly clinically inert and can be molded, stretched, or color-matched to the defect being repaired. The development of osteointegration with titanium was another major step in implant development. Prior methods of implant retention included mechanical anchoring or adhesives which led to frequent dislocation and repetitive need for replacement.

Beyond the biomaterials, traditional methods of prostheses fabrication relied on highly skilled crafting that was both labor intensive and time consuming. The process relied on patients attending multiple clinic appointments and waiting weeks to months before a successful implant was created. Improvement in imaging modalities allows the rapid importation of patient data directly into the modeling environment. Technological advancements including computer-assisted presurgical planning and three-dimensional printing have made facial prosthetics more accessible and a wider variety of materials to be incorporated into the fabrication process.

## Fundamental Concepts of Prosthetics and Implants

In general, a *prosthetic* is a synthetic replacement which restores the cosmesis of the anatomical defect. An *implant* typically refers to an object that is osteointegrated and supportive in nature. That said, the terms are often used interchangeably, and further confounding the matter, some reconstructive materials can be both.

Multiple factors must be considered when determining the ideal reconstructive solution of an area. These include surgical requirements, limitations, and potential outcomes as well the patient's short-term and long-term desires. Reconstruction using an autograft is typically the ideal option for larger defects and advanced reconstructions; however, this option may not align with the patient's goals due to the extent of surgery, cost, or recovery time. Prosthetics and implants can often be a better reconstructive option by providing the patient with better cosmetic results while decreasing the operative risks. This may be especially true in certain patient populations including the elderly and those with significant comorbidities. Patients with highly nuanced anatomical defects which would require numerous reconstructive surgeries such as total nasal defects or those defects that are poorly mimicked by autografts including reconstruction after orbital exenteration often prefer prosthetics. Also, patients requiring long-term surveillance after cancer extirpation often benefit from a temporary prosthesis when interacting with society.

Successful implantation and prosthetic utilization rely heavily on their method for anchoring them in place and are impacted by anatomical, mechanical, and material variations. Early retention systems included eyeglasses, adhesives, or anatomical undercuts. Drawbacks to these systems included low durability, failure in patients with active lifestyles, skin irritations and allergic reactions, as well as difficult prosthetic positioning. Innovations in osteointegration have brought great advances in retention systems.

## Implant Materials

Several materials are used currently in facial reconstruction thanks in part to scientific and production advancements. Each has its advantages and limitations.

**Porous high-density polyethylene (PHDPE)** is made of simple carbon chains and commonly used for many soft tissue implants. Its favorable characteristics include ease of molding and radiolucency on imaging. Porous polyethylene is also highly biocompatible by inducing fibroblast ingrowth and eventual bony incorporation, which add to its stability. It has also been shown to have reduced risk of infections and increased vascular ingrowth. Porous polyethylene has been used extensively for the repair of orbital wall and lid defects, nasal implants, and auricular reconstruction. The material's ability to incorporate tissue can make it difficult to remove, if revisions are needed.

**Polyether ether ketone (PEEK)** is another polymer that is popular in both neurosurgical and facial reconstructions. It is quite strong, highly biocompatible, stable with temperature changes, and lightweight. PEEK is especially popular as a patient-specific implant (PSI) that is prefabricated using three-dimensional technology. The material can be altered intra-operatively allowing the correction of slight discrepancies between surgical plan and patient anatomy. PEEK can be used in conjunction with titanium and can tolerate the placement of plates in screws to hold it in place. Its biggest limitation is its lack of bio-integration which can increase the risk of dislodgement.

Lastly, **titanium** has long been a popular implant for a myriad of reasons. It is relatively inexpensive, and it is easy to alter its shape. It offers excellent tensile strength, especially against compressive forces. The implant has long been used in conjunction with other autografts and allografts and is usually the choice when placing free bone grafts or PEEK implants. It also limits heat conduction and is markedly more radiolucent when compared to other metals. Drawbacks to titanium include its reliance on surrounding bone stock for fixation. Titanium can also have a relatively high extrusion rate.

## Patient-Specific Implant Planning and Placement

Patient-specific implants (PSIs) created with CT imaging have gained a widespread acceptance. Improvements in product precision and manufacturing time as well as decreased cost have been at the heart of its spike in utilization. To create a PSI, the surgical team uploads the patient's CT scan data to the engineering team of the company producing the implant. Next, the surgeon and engineer review the imaging and discuss logistics. These include determining the best surgical approaches for placement as well as the material that will be chosen based on various merits. Next, the size and shape of the implant are determined. Smaller implants can be created as a single piece. Larger implants or those reconstructing several abutting anatomical subunits, maybe designed in multiple sections, can be united during implantation. This can be an incredibly important consideration when trying to navigate and place the PSI under the soft tissue. The placement of implants in the virtual space becomes exponentially more difficult once the constraints of soft tissue are in place. Beyond the creation of the implant, patient-specific cut guides can be designed and manufactured. These guides can be used to remove the unwanted bone and to pre-drill screw holes for the implant so that it sits exactly as planned. The guides can be placed and fixated intraoperatively and then removed after the desired cuts and holes are made. Additionally, the creation of a manufactured skeletal model can be beneficial. It can be used to reassess the defect area as well as to confirm correct implant position. The turnaround time for the production of the implants, once the plan is approved, is progressively becoming streamlined, though depending on multiple factors can still take a few weeks. There is also a learning curve when first using PSI intraoperatively, and extra surgical time for their incorporation should be worked into the equation. The addition of neuro-navigation, rigid endoscopy, and intra-operative imaging are valuable tools in verifying a proper placement of guides and implants which with practice can reduce surgical time significantly.

## Prosthetic Materials

The prosthetics of the early twentieth century were largely composed from latex rubber. As materials progressed, acrylic resin, silicone, methacrylate, and polyurethane elastomers were introduced [1]. As noted previously, the ideal prosthetic should be aesthetically pleasing, durable, nonirritating, and retentive. The most popular material utilized for prosthetics is **silicone** due to its clinically inert characteristics and soft texture. Silicone is the preferred choice for soft tissue implants due to its excellent color and texture match to surrounding tissues (Fig. 4.1). It retains body temperature without distortion, and it can be stretched so thin as to appear transparent.

## Prosthetic Placement

The choice for osteointegrated versus adhesive prosthetics depends on the patient-specific defect and site. Prosthetics that attach to an implant generally have better stability and show less skin irritation. Adhesive prosthesis may not last as long when compared to the implant-attached prosthetics. A larger defect is best reconstructed with osteointegrated implants, as they will hold the prosthetic more securely in place [2]. Issues with osteointegrated prosthetics include poor bone stock, extrusion, especially in radiated bone, and the need for more surgical procedures when compared to those prosthetics that are secured by adhesives [3]. They are also often expensive and may be uncovered by insurance.

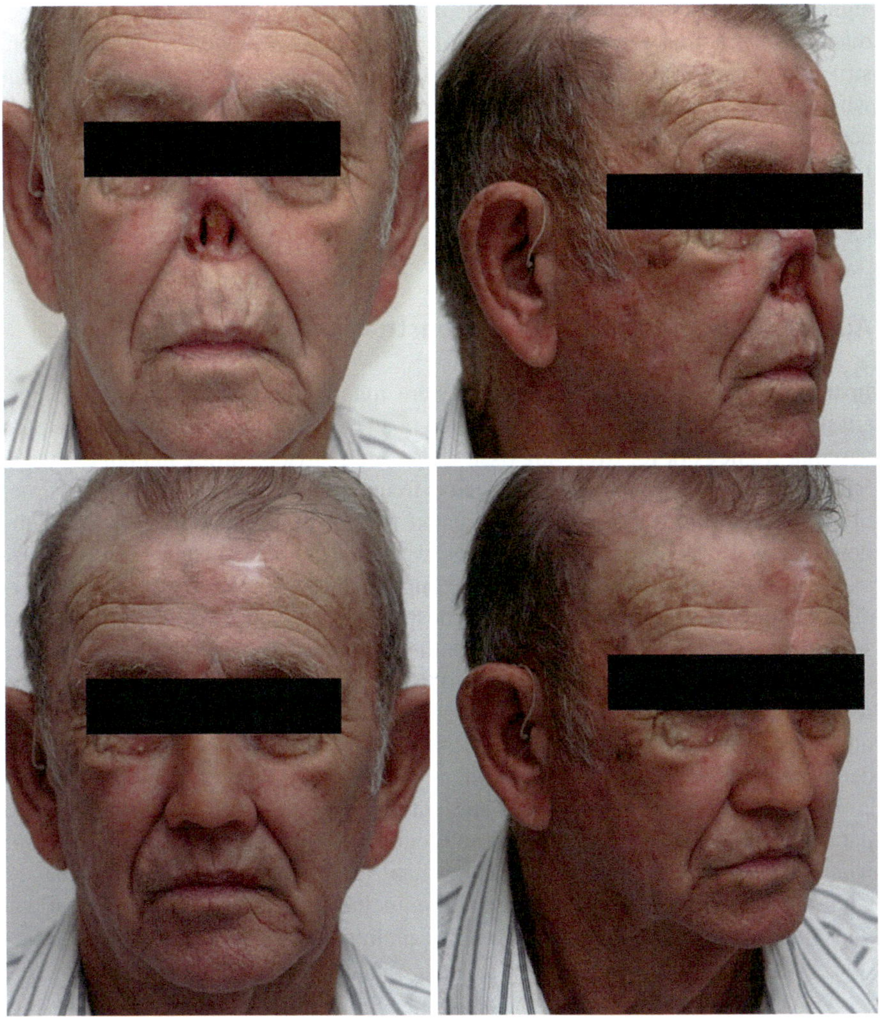

**Fig. 4.1** An example of a silicone nasal prosthetic in place. Note that the removal of the majority of the native nasal anatomy allows for the ideal size and placement of the prosthetic

## Site-Specific Considerations

### Auricular Reconstruction

Traditional auricular reconstruction can be achieved both with implants and prosthetics. Though not an absolute, most auricular implants occur in the pediatric population, while older patients tend to favor prosthetics. Several goals must be kept in mind when considering ear reconstruction. Cosmetic appearance and facial symmetry are the principal goals of reconstruction. Children with microtia often suffer significant psychological repercussions due to social ridicule, and therefore expedited reconstruction can be important [4]. For patients who wear glasses, a reconstruction of the auricle also provides a functional advantage for support. In situations where the hearing loss is associated with microtia, reconstruction serves to restore acoustic function. The literature pertaining to a two-stage porous polyethylene implant reconstruction combined with bone-anchored hearing aid notes better results in both aesthetics and hearing outcomes in comparison to autologous rib reconstruction and atresiaplasty [5].

## Auricular Alloplastic Implant Reconstruction

In the early 1990s, auricular implants were mainly fabricated from nonbiologic silastic ear implants. This material resulted in an early capsule formation and a poor vascular framework for overlying tissue flaps and grafts, resulting in high extrusion rates [5]. Currently, porous polyethylene is frequently used for auricular reconstruction, partially due to its reduced extrusion rates. The skeletal framework of the porous polyethylene implants is made of two parts: the helical rim and the ear base and is usually created as a PSI. It can be implanted as a single- or two-stage procedure and does not necessitate overnight hospital stay. When done in two stages, the second procedure occurs around 3 months after the initial surgery and involves minor revisions including improving auricle projection, lobule transposition, tragal reconstruction, or deepening of the concha. Successful implantation heavily relies on the recipient tissues. A large, well-vascularized soft tissue envelope is the main determinant of successful implantation..

Indications for porous polyethylene auricular reconstruction include microtia patients, especially those who failed autologous reconstruction, as well as patients who have suffered from auricular trauma or resection due to malignancy. Contraindications to implant reconstruction include compromised temporoparietal flaps due to congenital anomalies, trauma, malignancy, history of radiation, infection, or previous harvest.

As part of the preoperative planning, the contralateral ear is typically used as a guide to shape the implant. If a normal contralateral ear is not available, as may be the case for microtia, the implant can be constructed from a template of a parent's ear. Positioning of the implant in relation to the lateral canthus and nasal ala is important and varies depending on patient age.

The description that follows focuses on younger pediatric patients and should be supplemented with other sources based on individual patient parameters. Perioperatively, patients usually receive prophylactic intravenous antibiotics. Most surgeons will elect for the patients to receive a weight-appropriate dose of cephalexin or clindamycin; however, it is important to note that several large clinical trials have not shown results to confirm clinical advantage to prophylactic antibiotics in auricular reconstruction [4]. It is also recommended to soak the implant in an antibiotic solution prior to placement. Prior to making incisions, the superficial temporal artery branches can be traced using Doppler to prepare for the temporoparietal fascial (TPF) flap. It is also important to mark the path of the frontal branch of the facial nerve.

The TPF flap is then raised initially by making a Y-incision, where the bottom tail sits at the superior edge of the intended helix and the anterior extent placed 10 cm superior to the intended helical rim. The posterior tail of this incision is made at 5 cm posterior to the intended helical rim. The flap is then raised, beginning anteriorly, with dissection carried just superficial to the deep temporalis fascia. The anterior border is separated from the deep temporal fascia to the anterior branch of the superficial temporal artery. If the anterior aspect of the flap is encroaching into the path of the frontal branch of the facial nerve, only the lower portion fed by the anterior branch of the superficial temporal artery is included. The posterior border of the flap is then incised and raised with the intent to include subgaleal fascia, as this will add bulkier soft tissue coverage and decrease the risk of implant extrusion. Lastly, the raised flap is delivered through the inferior temporal incision by transecting the remaining anterior, posterior, and distal edges. After harvesting the flap, vestigial cartilage should be removed to maximize the fit of the implant; however, a portion can be banked subcutaneously and be used later for a second-stage procedure that includes tragal reconstruction [5]. Then, two bulb suction drains are inserted in the lateral neck.

At this point of the surgery, the surgeon may make last-minute adjustments to the implant if necessary. Ear assembly is started by delivering the TPF flap, and then the construct is placed in the ideal position. The TPF flap is laid over, and suction is applied. The flap should shrink wrap over the implant to achieve contour. Sutures may not be necessary to fix the framework into place as soft tissue suction is usually enough. At this point, a full thickness skin graft may be harvested to provide further coverage. Usually, the contralateral non-hair bearing retro auricular skin is used for the anterior and lateral surfaces of the implant. Other full thickness graft donor sites may include the abdominal wall or groin; however, the darker pigmentation in these areas can be a disadvantage, unless placed posteriorly to the implant, to provide a natural shadow [5]. Absorbable sutures are then used to fix the skin grafts over the TPF flap. Molded silicone putty, or prep sponges, are placed to prevent swelling without excessive compression on the reconstruction, and a protective cup is placed over the reconstructed ear.

Suction drains should be removed 5 to 7 days postoperatively. If used, the silicone mold or sponges are generally removed 7 to 10 days postoperatively. The plastic ear protective cup should be kept on for 2 to 4 weeks after surgery [5].

Postoperative complications pertaining to porous-polyethene auricular reconstruction are generally divided by time frame after surgery. The most common acute complications are the formation of hematoma and flap loss. A hematoma can be drained in the clinic setting as needed. Flap loss most commonly happens in the first 5 to 7 days after surgery and may be first noticed at the first postoperative dressing change in clinic [4]. The accepted treatment course for this flap loss is returning to the operating room for the removal of the implant and debridement. After allowing for appropriate healing, an ipsilateral occipital fascial flap or contralateral free TPF flap can be used as salvage options [3].

Subacute postoperative complications include implant extrusion and infection [6]. If the exposure or extrusion is limited without any evidence of infection, local tissue can be raised to maintain a good seal. If the implant exposure is less than 1 cm, this defect may heal by secondary intention. In cases of subtotal extrusions, the implant should be removed, and granulation tissue should be debrided. A new implant should be placed as soon as possible to take advantage of the preserved ear and soft tissue architecture constructed in the initial surgery [7]. Risk of implant extrusions and exposure may increase in patients with prior atresiaplasty, as this can lead to increased scarring and poorly perfused periauricular skin [6].

Postoperative implant infections are usually due to implant extrusion or exposure. The infected site is treated on the basis of severity. If the infection is mild or limited, antibiotic treatment and close observation of any implant exposure are recommended. In more severe infection, aggressive debridement and surgical site washouts are necessary. If frank purulence is encountered, complete removal of the implant is recommended [6].

Long-term complications of alloplastic auricular reconstruction are usually due to fracture of the implant. Treatment recommendations include removal of the damaged implant and immediate replacement with a newly constructed framework [6]. Trauma experienced in the long-term setting can also damage the overlying TPF flap and skin grafts. Additional complications include hair growth of the skin enveloping the implant, local alopecia at the donor site, as well as poor texture and color match of tissue coverage. Recent literature shows overall implantation exposure rates to be less than 10%, fractures rate of 3%, and overall complication rate of 6% [6].

Alloplastic reconstruction provides a reasonable size match with the contralateral ear and good definition of the conchal bowl, helical rim, and antihelical fold. Validated questionnaires in the literature have shown over 75% improvement in quality of life in patients who underwent porous polyethylene implant reconstruction, with nearly 73% of adults and 85% of children noting satisfaction with their aesthetic results [6].

## Auricular Prosthetics

As previously discussed, auricular reconstruction is complex and difficult. Auricular prosthesis provides satisfactory results in most patients with several studies showing aesthetic satisfaction in nearly 90% of patients who have chosen this option [8].

Silicone continues to be the most used material for auricular prosthesis, as it is malleable, which results in anatomically precise framework, providing excellent color and texture matching (Fig. 4.2). While adhesive attachment remains popular, osteointegrated implants have gained significant popularity as this retention system requires less maintenance and provides more stability. In comparison to autologous reconstruction, alloplastic implant reconstruction has significantly less morbidity due to fewer surgeries as well as due to a lack of donor-site morbidity. Similar to

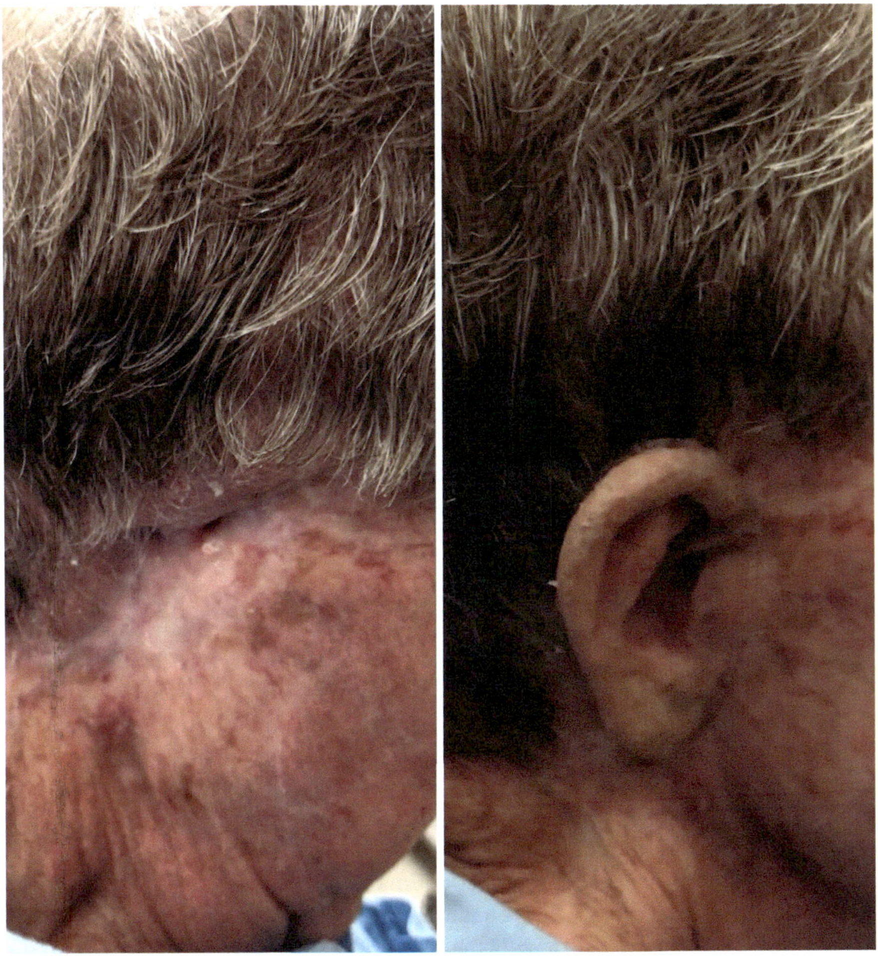

**Fig. 4.2** Example of the recipient site before and after placement of silicone auricular implant

alloplastic auricular reconstruction, reconstruction can be performed as early as 4 years of age.

The issues with auricular prosthetics are the same as with most facial prosthetics. Daily cleaning of the prosthetic-associated implants and the recipient site is necessary to maximize benefits and avoid infections. Additionally, daily activity exposes the prosthetic to general wear and tear and the risk of dislodgement [8].

In general, the major indications for the need of a prosthetic ear include auricular loss due to trauma, oncologic defects, and congenital abnormalities. Aggressive tumors involving the auricle require large resections and are frequently followed by radiotherapy, which will affect the local tissue vascularity and stability, thereby limiting the possibility for autologous or alloplastic reconstruction. While a history of radiation to the recipient site can increase complication risks in prosthetic reconstruction, it is not a contraindication for an ear prosthetic. Several studies have shown excellent outcomes in radiated patients when the implant placement of implant is delayed by 6 to 12 months after radiation therapy [9]. Congenital abnormalities such as microtia or partial auricular congenital abnormalities, especially relating to patients with prior reconstructive failures or lack of healthy tissue in the temporal bone region, have shown excellent aesthetic results after prosthesis reconstruction.

There are few absolute contraindications for a prosthetic. These include a compromised bony framework such as osteitis or osteomyelitis of the mastoid bone or a temporal bone that is thinner than 2.5 mm which will not support the construct. In this scenario, the use of adhesives may be an option. The discussion regarding the daily maintenance of the prosthetic and retention systems must be done with the patients and family, as a lack of hygiene can significantly increase the risk of infection of the implant, tissue reactions, and overall prosthetic failure. Lastly, some studies have shown significantly high risk of infection and extrusion of implants in patients who have been exposed to radiation and continue to use tobacco products.

Prior to the placement of bone-anchored prosthesis, a careful evaluation must be performed of the skin and subcutaneous tissue in the auriculotemporal area, with attention given to potential recurrent tumors, scars, and fibrosis. If hair is present, it must be permanently removed prior to surgery, as hair follicles may increase the risk of implant infection. Many surgeons opt for laser hair removal in these cases. Alternatively, hair roots may be removed while thinning the subcutaneous tissue in surgery. A dedicated CT scan of the temporal bones without contrast should be obtained preoperatively to evaluate for appropriate bone thickness and to evaluate any changes caused by prior therapies or congenital abnormalities. A team-based approach with the anaplastologist involved in manufacturing the prosthetic can be beneficial. They can assist the surgeon in determining which anatomic structures can assist or hinder optimal implant placement. Often, to optimize prosthetic placement, it is beneficial to remove all remnants of the auricle except the tragus, as it helps with the skin-to-prosthetic match and soft tissue transition. Leaving excess tissue may not provide the patient with the best cosmetic outcome due to difficulty with color matching and a more visible transition from prosthetic to native auricle.

Most surgeons perform prosthetic reconstruction in two stages, often under local anesthesia. The first stage involves the placement of titanium bone implants which requires raising a skin flap in the auricular temporal area. Perioperative antibiotics are not indicated but may be considered in diabetic patients or those with radiated tissues. The skin is incised, and dissection is carried deep to the periosteum. A flap is raised in the subperiosteal plane until the adequate sites of implant placement are reached. The ideal site for implants is 20 mm from the center of the external auditory meatus at the 8 and 11 o'clock positions. Usually, two implants are placed into the bone; however, literature suggests placing a third "sleeper" implant in case of implant failure. The initial holes are drilled to a depth of 3 mm. If there is no dural contact at the initial depth, one can proceed to 4 mm of depth to maximize load support. The implants are then introduced at a torque speed of 40 to 50 newton meters

(Nm) in a healthy bone or at the speed of 20 to 30 Nm in a compromised bone. Cover screws are also placed to prevent tissue ingrowth inside the implant, and the skin flap is laid back into place. Multilayered closure is necessary for decreasing implant infection. The second stage involves uncovering the implants. This is usually done around 3 to 4 months after the initial surgery. Prior to this second stage, the patient can be seen in the clinic to access healing and palpate the location of the implant. If the location is difficult to access, a lateral plain film can be obtained. The overlying skin can be excised by a punch biopsy or skin excision. If needed, the skin surrounding the implant is thinned or hair can be removed. Some surgeons may elect to place a skin graft over the surrounding implant periosteum if a larger skin excision is done to limit tissue movement around the fixtures and thereby decreasing the risk of granulation tissue formation. Alternatively, iodoform gauze can be wrapped around the implants. After a 2-week period to allow for healing, the clip and bar are fixed to the implant, and the prosthetic is attached.

It is important to discuss the bar clip versus the magnet retention systems. For many years after the introduction of implants, the bar and clip retention systems were favored due to increased strength and stability of the prosthetic. Recently, magnetic retention systems have been manufactured with higher quality retention forces and show improved stability. Patient age, manual ability, and level of activity in their daily life should be considered when choosing the best option. A recent prospective study evaluating the satisfaction and outcomes of patients between these two retention systems concluded that nearly 59% of their participants favored the magnetic retention system due to less need for daily cleaning and aftercare [10]. The elderly population significantly favored the magnetic retention prosthesis due to its decreased difficulty of daily cleaning. The bar clip system showed increased stability overall and was favored by younger patients with more active lifestyles. Lastly, the surgeon must keep in mind jaw movements when discussing these options, as large jaw movements have been shown to dislocate the magnetic retention ear prosthetic.

Complications of prosthetic reconstruction include skin infections, granulation tissue overgrowth, and implant failure. Peri-fixture infections are seen in 15% to 20% of cases [9]. The incidence can increase due to skin mobility around the fixtures and poor hygiene. Usually, oral antibiotics lead to a resolution without complete loss of fixture. It is recommended to refrain from wearing the prosthesis until complete resolution of infection.

Granulation tissue and skin reaction around the implants can be seen in up to 33% of patients and can be exacerbated by poor hygiene, extensive daily use of the prosthetic, and exposure to humid weather. One potential way to treat this complication is by carefully thinning subcutaneous tissues around the implants during the second surgical stage. Providers usually prefer silver nitrate application with aggressive cleaning of the site and iodoform gauze placement around the implant, as this will dry the wound. The prosthetic should again not be worn until near-complete resolution of granulation tissue is achieved. Lastly, there are reports of failed osseointegration though the exact incidence rate of failure is unknown. However, bone-anchored hearing aid implant, which is a similar procedure, has a failure rate up to

29% [11]. Mitigation of risk can be achieved by implantation in favorable bone stock and diligent cleaning of the implant site by the patient. Failure of the implant does increase in patients with comorbidities such as diabetes and history of radiation exposure to the temporal bone. The surgeon should consider placing a "sleeper" implant in patients with a high risk of implant failure [11].

## Nasal Reconstruction

Reconstruction for large nasal defects is commonly performed with the use of regional tissue transfer such as the paramedian forehead flap. There are several scenarios where nasal prosthetics may be preferred. Difficulty recreating the intricacies of the nasal anatomy, morbidity associated with the multiple surgical revisions, and risk of delayed wound healing or flap failure with radiation are all scenarios where autologous tissue may not be the ideal choice. Anecdotal experience has found that in cases of total nasal reconstruction, the appearance of the prosthetic nose is far superior to local or free tissue. Prosthetic reconstruction also decreases the need for several staged procedures necessary in autologous reconstruction, which decreases overall operative and anesthetic complications.

Once the determination has been made to recreate the nasal defect with a prosthetic, there are several ways to improve the outcomes for the patient. If possible, the patient should meet with the anaplastologist prior to extirpation, so that a mold may be created of the patient's normal external nasal anatomy. This can help create a prosthetic that closely mimics the native anatomy. In cases where a subtotal nasal resection is performed, the surgeon should consider the resection of remnant nasal anatomy to improve prosthetic fit and color match. Salvaged tissue often does not aid in camouflaging the prosthesis and instead forces the anaplastologist to create a larger prosthetic than the native nose so that it fits over the remnant tissue. In cases of subtotal rhinectomy, the surgeon should consider removing both alas. Additionally, removing the anterior one-third of the cartilaginous septum and associated mucosa, columella, and distal bony nasal pyramid will also improve prosthetic fit. Lastly, the lateral surrounding skin of the defect should be thinned, if possible, to allow for improved prosthesis-to-skin transition and color match. In cases where resection extends beyond the natural nasal borders, extra care and deliberation should be taken regarding changes and reconstruction of the upper lip and melolabial creases. Changes to these anatomical landmarks affect how the prosthetic sits and are also difficult to mimic with the prosthetic. Ideally, these decisions are discussed with the anaplastologist prior to the case to help create the best skin-to-prosthetic transition, symmetry, and aesthetics possible.

Osteointegrated implants are increasingly popular retention systems for nasal prosthetics. This is true even in cases with prior nasal cavity radiation, though outcomes can vary depending on radiation dose and time from radiation completion. The attachment system between nasal implants and prosthetic can be either a bar-and-clip configuration or the more popular magnetic retention system. Nasal implant configuration can include both vertical and horizontal components. This increases the linking area between implant and prosthetic and improves overall stability and retention. Recipient bone for the implants should be well vascularized to limit risks of extrusion [12].

Two popular sites for implant placement are the bony nasal sill and glabella. The nasal sill of the premaxilla can be a difficult platform for osteointegrated implants due to being largely composed of cancellous bone. In cases of prior radiation, consider limiting implants to the glabellar region. A disadvantage of glabellar implants includes interference with prosthesis placement due to their more pronounced emergence profile. Thinning of the glabellar tissue may improve prosthetic fit.

## Maxillary/Midface Reconstruction

Maxillary and midface defects can be incredibly complex and intrinsically come with a wide variety of presentations, sizes, and complications. Large defects typically are repaired with free tissue due to the absence of adequate structures to provide support for prosthetics as well as constant movement of the area when the patient is talking or eating. Prosthetic use depends greatly on the case. Often, a better cosmetic result is achieved by supplementing an autologous tissue reconstruction with a limited facial prosthetic. Several goals for the reconstruction of this area must be met by the prosthetic and/or implant. These include the appropriate closure of the oral cavity and support of orbital contents and midface, as well as appropriate strength to withstand the forces of speech, swallowing, and mastication. Other factors to consider include the material to be used and its ability to support dentition and the near-normal return to contour and symmetry. Traditionally, prosthetic reconstruction is done with a prosthetic obturator to separate the oral cavity from the sinuses. The stability of the obturator greatly depends on the mechanical fit and the support of the surrounding tissue. The high functional demands of the oral cavity can cause frequent wear and slippage of the obturator, leading to potential compromise of the seal between the oral and nasal cavities. Osteointegration is dependent on the availability of viable bone around the defect, and multiple implant sites are generally required for full load support. The support recipients include the zygomatic buttresses, supraorbital rims, vomer, and remaining hard palate. Due to the multiple planes of force applied to the midface, the implant needs to be constructed with strong and stable materials such as titanium or PEEK.

## Orbital Reconstruction

Globe removal is separated into different classifications depending on the extent of resection. Evisceration involves removing the contents of the eye while keeping the sclera, optic nerve, and the associated extraocular muscles attached. Enucleation involves removing the entire globe while leaving the extraocular muscles and orbital contents intact, as well as maintaining periorbital fat, eyelids, and eyelashes. Orbital exenteration involves removing the entire contents of the orbit, including extraocular muscles, eyelashes, orbital fat, periorbita, and at least partial eyelid removal [13].

Evisceration is more commonly employed after localized trauma to the globe in which the globe itself and eyesight cannot be preserved, but the surrounding orbital structures maintain viability. Small intraocular tumors are also a common cause of evisceration, and this resection may be performed if the malignancy does not invade past the sclera. If the oncological resection achieves negative margins via enucleation, the surgeon should not continue further into exenteration, as the cosmesis for an orbital prosthetic is improved with a patient's remnant eyelids and periorbital fat due to the maintained orbital volume. Additionally, the option to spare extraocular muscles in enucleation is a significant advantage, as the orbital implant can be attached to these muscles and result in mimicry and movement of the contralateral eye, which vastly improves cosmetic outcomes [13].

The orbital prosthetic is a synthetic replacement of the eye, which restores the orbit, eyelids, immobile eye, and periorbita. A prosthetic is the standard choice in cases of orbital exenteration. An orbital implant is usually an osteointegrated structure, such as a post, that acts to support this prosthetic. An ocular implant is a spherical synthetic replacement of the iris, pupil, and sclera that provides movement to an ocular prosthesis, if extraocular muscles are spared during resection [14].

## Ocular Implants

The ideal ocular implant replaces lost volume, maximizes mobility when possible, and is aesthetically pleasing. In cases of evisceration, the implant is placed within the remaining scleral envelope to which the muscles remain attached, allowing for natural movement. In cases of enucleation, the implant must be attached to the extraocular muscles to allow movement. Today, ocular implants are usually classified as being made of porous or nonporous materials, shape, and wrapped implants versus non-wrapped. Wrapping refers to these implants being literally wrapped with a polyglycolic mesh or autogenous tissue such as auricular muscle or sclera to suture the extraocular muscles to the implant and prevent extrusion. Porous implants are constructed with materials such as hydroxyapatite or high-density porous polyethylene. Porous options are also known as integrated implants because they allow ingrowth of vasculature [14]. Nonporous implants, otherwise known as nonintegrated, are made from materials such as polymethyl methacrylate, acrylic, and silicone, which typically require wrapping.

Advantages of integrated implants include reduced infection, migration, and extrusion rates, as well as being lightweight which may minimize lower lid lag over time. They are noted to improve motility due to their ability to be held by a post or a peg [14]. A noted disadvantage is the additional procedure to place a peg and the added costs of the implant. The peg is placed on the anterior aspect of the defect and attaches to the ocular implant. A peg can be placed to help secure a porous orbital implant, but nonporous implants cannot be pegged. Recent surveys showed that 90% of patients preferred unpegged implants due to their lower costs and avoidance of additional surgery, while still imparting acceptable motility [15]. Complications are rare in nonporous implants; however, common issues of unpegged implants include exposure, infection, and pyogenic granuloma. In pegged implants, common complications include exposure, discharge, and pyogenic granulomas. It is important to note that the risk of pyogenic granulomas is significantly increased in porous implants that utilize a peg system due to the risk of peg displacement [15].

## Orbital Prosthesis

While partial defects of orbital contents, such as eyelid defects, can be reconstructed with autologous flaps, prosthetic reconstruction is a cost-effective option that will reduce the need for several procedures, while resulting in an improved aesthetic appearance. Today, acrylic resin, methacrylate, and elastomers are frequently used to fabricate orbital prosthetics. Silicone continues to be the most popular material. There are implant-associated prostheses, as well as free prostheses that are secured with adhesives or to glasses. Implant-attached prosthetics typically have greater stability, less skin irritation, and less need for maintenance [16]. Additionally, literature notes that bone-anchored prosthetics tend to last longer than adhesive prosthetics. Bone-anchored retention systems can be stabilized on the orbital rims, nasal bones, and zygomatic arch. Issues with osteointegrated implants arise due to poor bone stock and radiated bone, and therefore adhesive retention may be better suited for patients who exhibit compromised surrounding tissues.

Exenteration defects can be approached via several reconstructive options. The creation of a barrier between the outside and persistent naso-orbito-maxillary tissues is vital to making a safe cavity for further reconstruction [16]. At a minimum, a split thickness skin graft can be used to create this barrier. Autologous free tissue can provide vascularized tissue coverage of the defect to help mitigate the risk of osteoradionecrosis in patients requiring adjuvant radiation therapy after exenteration. While a bulky flap may be ideal for limiting post-radiation complications, it can hinder optimal cosmetic results upon the placement of the prosthetic. Debulking of a thick flap may be necessary to allow for adequate prosthetic wear or to assist with implant placement.

There are several techniques that will maximize results when placing implants. Fixture placement is initiated by making two semicircular incisions at the external edge of the orbital rim along the superior and inferior border down to the bone. After raising the tissue flaps, fixture holes into planned sites of retention are made, using a drill at a speed of 1500 to 3000 RPMs, with copious irrigation. A tap wrench may also be used on hard osseous tissues. The holes are generally 3.75 mm in diameter, with a depth of roughly 3.8 mm. The fixtures are then placed and covered over the cutaneous flap, which should be thinned of subcutaneous fat. This is necessary to obtain optimal adherence between the skin and bone, while decreasing any excessive movement of the soft tissues around the implant, which may lead to excess inflammation and failure. Transcutaneous titanium cylinders are then connected to the fixtures. The skin flap is reapproximated in a multilayered fashion. Vaseline gauze and antibiotic ointment are usually placed around the implants. Lastly, a compression bandage is applied around the implants. The bandage should be removed by the patient the next day, to increase flap adherence. Patients are then seen 7 to 10 days after surgery to evaluate wound healing. A visit with the anaplastologist around this time should also be arranged.

## Conclusion

Facial prosthetic and implant reconstructions often provide a reasonable treatment option for patients who have undergone reconstruction for trauma, malignancy, and congenital deformities. While not the ideal option in all cases, the ability to utilize and maximize their use can be beneficial in improving the outcomes for many patients.

## References

1. Futran ND, Mendez E. Developments in reconstruction of midface and maxilla. Lancet Oncol. 2006;7(3):249–58. https://doi.org/10.1016/S1470-2045(06)70616-7.
2. Sophie Yi JY, Dierks EJ, Over LM, Hauck MJ. Prosthetic reconstruction of the orbit/globe. Oral Maxillofac Surg Clin North Am. 2012;24(04):697–712.
3. Toljanic JA, Eckert SE, Roumanas E, et al. Osseointegrated craniofacial implants in the rehabilitation of orbital defects: an update of a retrospective experience in the United States. J Prosthet Dent. 2005;94(02):177–82.
4. Ali K, Trost JG, Truong TA, Harshbarger RJ 3rd. Total ear reconstruction using porous polyethylene. Semin Plast Surg. 2017;31(3):161–72. https://doi.org/10.1055/s-0037-1604261.
5. McKinnon BJ, Jahrsdoerfer RA. Congenital auricular atresia: update on options for intervention and timing of repair. Otolaryngol Clin N Am. 2002;35(4):877–90. https://doi.org/10.1016/s0030-6665(02)00058-0.
6. Braun T, Gratza S, Becker S, et al. Auricular reconstruction with porous polyethylene frameworks: outcome and patient benefit in 65 children and adults. Plast Reconstr Surg. 2010;126(04):1201–12.
7. Al Kadah B, Naumann A, Schneider M, Schick B, Linxweiler M, Papaspyrou G. Auricular reconstruction with polyethylene implants or silicone prosthesis: a single institution experience. J Craniomaxillofac Surg. 2018;46(12):2150–6. https://doi.org/10.1016/j.jcms.2018.10.005.
8. Younis I, Gault D, Sabbagh W, Kang NV. Patient satisfaction and aesthetic outcomes after ear reconstruction with a Branemark-type, bone-anchored, ear prosthesis: a 16 year review. J Plast Reconstr Aesthet Surg. 2010;63(10):1650–5. https://doi.org/10.1016/j.bjps.2009.10.004.
9. Giot JP, Labbé D, Soubeyrand E, et al. Prosthetic reconstruction of the auricle: indications, techniques, and results. Semin Plast Surg. 2011;25(4):265–72. https://doi.org/10.1055/s-0031-1288918.
10. Visser A, Noorda WD, Linde A, Raghoebar GM, Vissink A. Bar-clip versus magnet-retained auricular prostheses: a prospective clinical study with a 3-year follow-up. J Prosthet Dent. 2020;124(2):240–7. https://doi.org/10.1016/j.prosdent.2019.05.033.
11. Hamming KK, Lund TW, Lander TA, Sidman JD. Complications and satisfaction with pediatric osseointegrated external ear prostheses. Laryngoscope. 2009;119(7):1270–3. https://doi.org/10.1002/lary.20305.
12. Granström G, et al. A detailed analysis of titanium implants lost in irradiated tissues. Int J Oral Maxillofac Implants. 1994;9:6.

13. Kesting MR, Koerdt S, Rommel N, Mücke T, Wolff KD, Nobis CP, Ringel F, Frohwitter G. Classification of orbital exenteration and reconstruction. J Craniomaxillofac Surg. 2017;45(4):467–73. https://doi.org/10.1016/j.jcms.2017.01.003.
14. Su GW, Yen MT. Current trends in managing the anophthalmic socket after primary enucleation and evisceration. Ophthal Plast Reconstr Surg. 2004;20(04):274–80.
15. Lin CJ, Liao SL, Jou JR, Kao SC, Hou PK, Chen MS, Complications of motility peg placement for porous hydroxyapatite orbital implants. Br J Ophthalmol. 2002;86:394–6.
16. Cervelli V, Bottini DJ, Arpino A, Colicchia GM, Mugnaini F, Trimarco A, Gentile P, Grimaldi M. Orbital reconstruction. J Craniofac Surg. 2006;17(5):848–53. https://doi.org/10.1097/01.scs.0000229556.04953.fa.

# Reconstruction of the Lip

# 5

Scott Kohlert

## Introduction

Lip defects are commonly encountered by facial reconstructive surgeons. Common causes include congenital abnormalities [1], facial trauma [2], and neoplastic disease. Carcinoma of the lip is one of the most frequently encountered malignancies in the head and neck [3]. Surgical resection is the primary treatment modality of lip cancer and can result in significant defects of the lips and surrounding tissues.

## Anatomy

While excellent outcomes are often easily achieved for small defects, large labial defects can be challenging to reconstruct, given the anatomical complexity in this location. The lip is a complex multilayered structure consisting of mucosa, submucosa, muscle, subcutaneous tissue, and skin. A detailed understanding of the underlying anatomy is critical in order to successfully restore form and function after a major lip reconstruction.

### Surface Anatomy of the Lip

The outer surface of the lip is divided into visibly distinct parts: the mucosal lip (also known as the vermillion or the red lip) and the cutaneous lip (sometimes referred to as the white lip). Each should be reconstructed with similar tissue if the surgeon wishes to obtain the best possible result. The transition point between the

S. Kohlert (✉)
CHRISTUS Health, Tyler, TX, USA


F. Sokoya, A. G. Vincent (eds.), *Manual of Head and Neck Reconstruction*,
https://doi.org/10.1007/978-3-031-65999-7_5

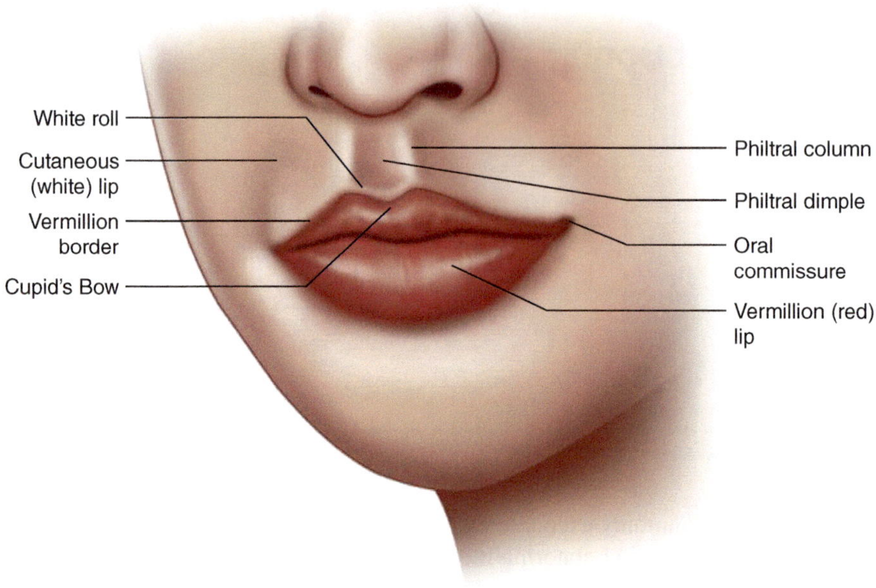


**Fig. 5.1** Surface anatomy of the lip

vermillion and the cutaneous lip is known as the vermillion border (Fig. 5.1). This border reflects light and has been shown to be a common gaze fixation point in eye-tracking studies [4]. Accordingly, careful reapproximation of this area is paramount in lip reconstruction [5] as any deformity or disruption of the border is easily perceived by both professionals and laypeople alike [6].

## Anatomical Subunits of the Lip

As with other aesthetic units of the face, the lips can be further divided into unique topographical subunits. While the lower lip is often considered as a single unit, Burget and Menick [7] long ago described the upper lip as having multiple subunits: a central philtrum, along with paired lateral subunits (Fig. 5.2). The philtrum is located centrally in the upper lip and is bound superiorly by the columella and part of the nasal sill, laterally by the philtral columns and inferiorly by Cupid's Bow. Each lateral subunit is divided into two separate components. The medial component is the part that sits inferior to the nasal sill and measures approximately one half of the width of the philtrum. The philtrum and the medial component of the lateral subunit are similar in so far as they are relatively more fixed to the surrounding structures (such as the maxilla and the nose) and are thus less mobile than the lateral component of the lateral subunit [8]. The lateral component extends

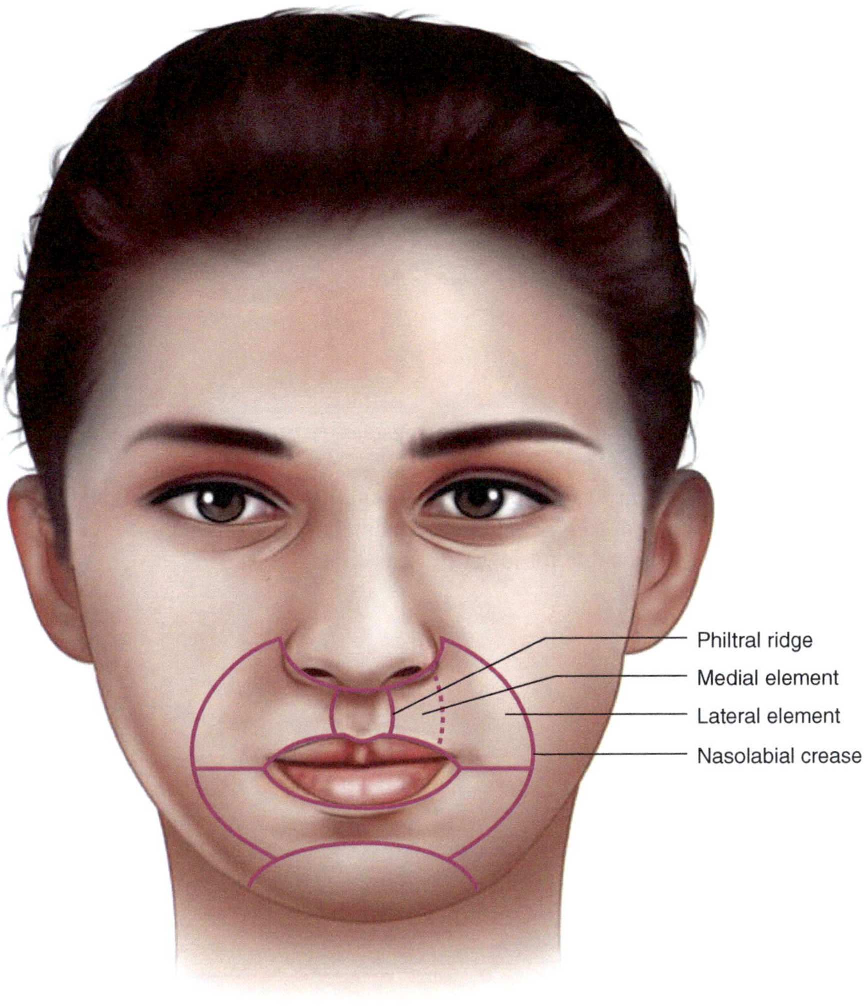


**Fig. 5.2** Subunits of the upper lip

superiorly along the alar-facial groove and laterally to the nasolabial fold. As with any other facial reconstruction, careful attention must be paid to the involved subunits, and, if possible, each involved subunit should be managed individually to improve the cosmetic outcome. Additionally, when the majority of a subunit has been resected, one will often obtain a superior result if the remainder of the subunit is resected prior to reconstruction [7].

## Musculature

There are multiple muscles involved in the movement of the upper lip including the levator labii superioris, the levator labii superioris alaeque nasi, levator anguli oris, and the zygomaticus major and minor muscles (Fig. 5.3). These muscles converge at the modiolus (a fibromuscular structure at the corner of the mouth). Muscles that retract the lower lip include the depressor labii inferioris, the depressor anguli oris, the platysma, the risorius, and the mentalis. Sphincteric action is achieved by the orbicularis oris muscle [9] (Table 5.1).

## Innervation

Motor innervation for all of the above muscles is provided by branches of the facial nerve.

Sensory innervation of the upper lip is primarily from the labial branch of the infraorbital nerve (from CN V2), while the mental nerve (from the inferior alveolar branch of V3) is responsible for lower lip sensation.

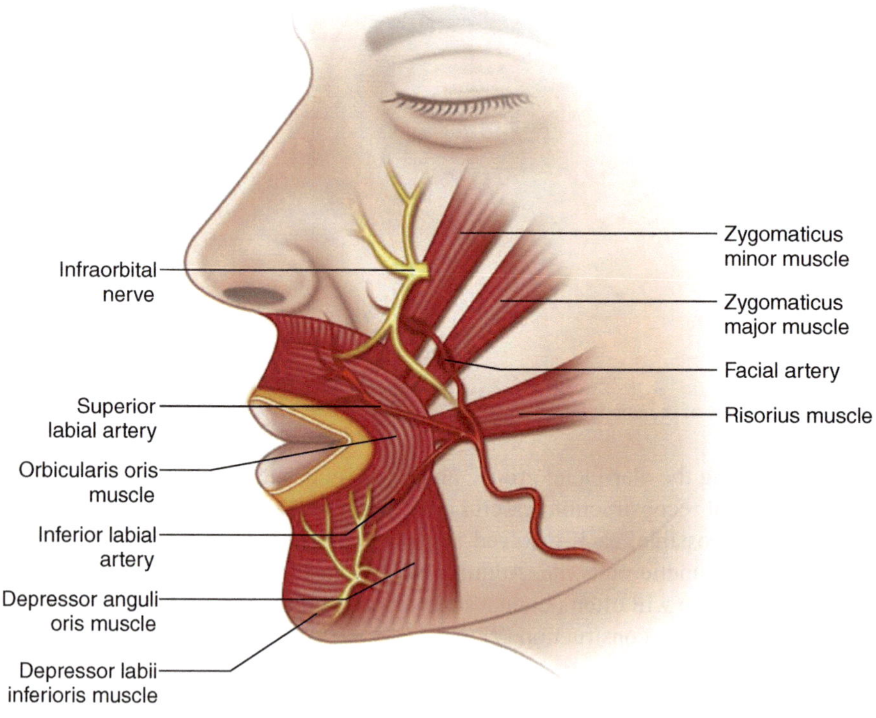


**Fig. 5.3** Relevant muscular and neurovascular anatomy

**Table 5.1** Relevant muscular anatomy of the lip

| Muscle | Origin | Insertion | Action |
|---|---|---|---|
| Orbicularis oris | *Upper lip:* alveolar border of maxilla<br>*Lower lip:* mandible (lateral to mentalis) | Modiolus | Sphincteric action, lip protrusion |
| Levator labii superioris | Orbit | Modiolus | Elevates the upper lip |
| Levator labii superioris alaeque nasi | Frontal process of maxilla | *Nasal component:* alar cartilage and nasal skin<br>*Lip component:* modiolus | Elevates the upper lip and dilates the nostril |
| Levator anguli oris | Canine fossa (maxilla) | Modiolus | Elevates the upper lip at the angle of the mouth, deepens nasolabial fold |
| Zygomaticus major | Zygoma, anterior to zygomaticotemporal suture | Modiolus | Elevation and posterior retraction of upper lip |
| Zygomaticus minor | Zygoma, posterior to zygomaticomaxillary suture | Modiolus | Elevates upper lip |
| Depressor labii inferioris | Oblique line of the mandible | | |
| Depressor anguli oris | Oblique line of the mandible | Modiolus | |
| Platysma | Skin/subcutaneous tissue of neck | Multiple areas including modiolus | Depresses lower lip (among other non-lip-related actions) |
| Risorius muscle | Parotid fascia | Skin at angle of mouth | Stretches lower lip, depresses lower lip, pulls lower lip laterally |
| Mentalis | Incisor fossa (mandible) | Skin of the chin | Elevates and protrudes the lower lip |

## Arterial Supply

The upper lip is supplied by the superior labial branch of the facial artery, as well as the superior labial branch of the infraorbital artery. The lower lip is supplied by the inferior labial artery (also a branch of the facial artery).

## Basic Considerations and Reconstructive Approach

### Form and Function

Restoration of normal form and function is the fundamental goal of the reconstructive surgeon. Impairment of either (or both) can have significant psychosocial implications for the patient. Primary functions of the lips include facial expression, speech and articulation, oral competence, and swallowing. Impairment of motor function can prevent a patient from smiling, kissing, or sucking through a straw [10]. Major lip reconstruction can impair a patient's ability to articulate certain sounds, and poor oral competence can lead to drooling. Adequate lip closure is also an important part of the swallowing mechanism, permitting pressure formation within the oropharynx that facilitates bolus propagation [11]. Furthermore, patients with poor lip function and/or microstomia may no longer be able to wear dentures as a result, limiting their ability to enjoy many solid foods.

Achieving a satisfactory cosmetic outcome should also be of absolute importance for the surgeon. Patients with central postoperative facial defects are perceived more negatively by others, even more so than those with peripheral facial defects [12]. It is therefore understandable that patients undergoing facial skin cancer surgery report being self-conscious and avoid socialization after surgery [13]. Lip cancer patients were found to be among a subgroup of oral cancer patients who reported poorer psychosocial adjustment scores in post-treatment surveys [14].

Lip reconstruction can be highly challenging, especially for larger defects. Extremely careful analysis of the defect including the size, depth, involved anatomical subunits, and quality and availability of the surrounding tissue (especially in patients with prior surgery or disease) is paramount in obtaining satisfactory cosmetic and functional results. Furthermore, full thickness defects require a meticulous multilayer closure. A proper reapproximation of the muscle layer is critical for the restoration of lip function and oral competence. When closing the external layer, it is also critical to properly align the vermillion border in order to prevent highly visible step deformities. We recommend that the first suture placed typically be a single tacking suture to precisely reapproximate vermillion border. While suture selection varies from surgeon to surgeon, we typically will use 5-0 chromic gut sutures for mucosal closure, vicryl sutures for the reapproximation of the muscular layer and deep dermis, and 6-0 Prolene for superficial closure of the skin.

## Reconstructive Ladder Approach

The reconstructive ladder is a well-known, incremental approach to the defect reconstruction (Fig. 5.4). It can be helpful to use this model as a framework for determining the best reconstructive option for the patient. As a general rule of thumb, the reconstructive surgeon should aim to use the least complex (i.e., lowest on the ladder) option that can reasonably be expected to provide the return of satisfactory form and function. For example, while certain small lip defects can be closed primarily or even left to heal by secondary intention, more advanced defects will require free flap reconstruction. A multitude of options for reconstruction spanning the length of the reconstructive ladder will be discussed in this chapter.

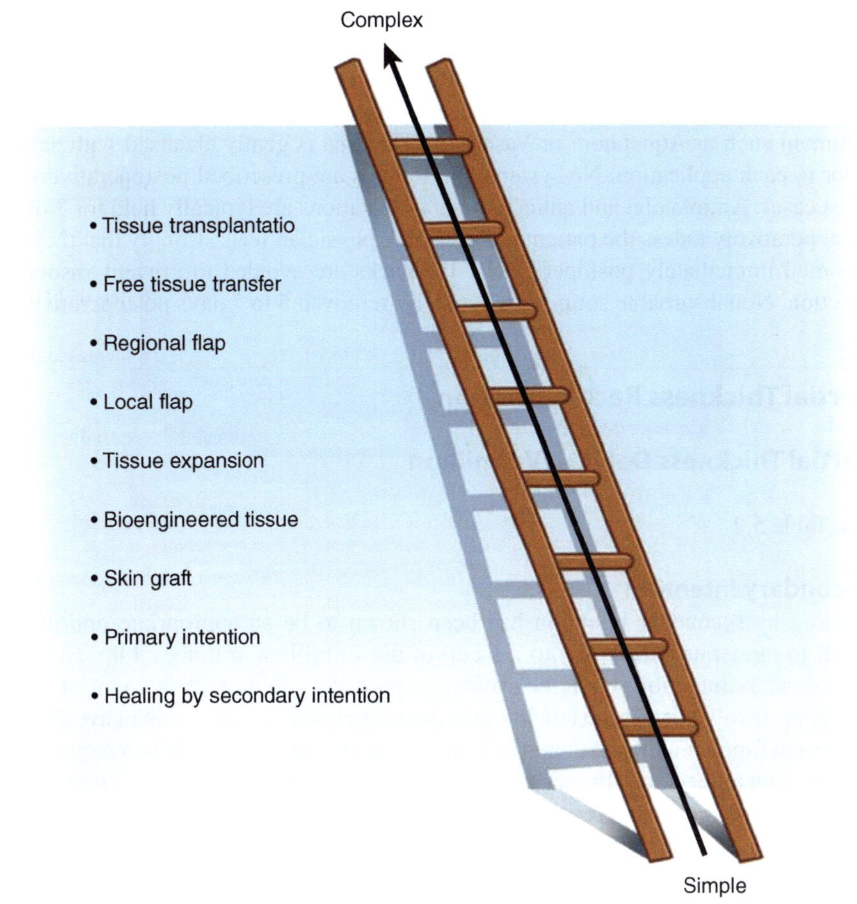


**Fig. 5.4** The reconstructive ladder

## Perioperative Care

### Intraoperative Setup

When feasible, we elect for nasotracheal intubation for patients undergoing surgical lip reconstruction in order to facilitate exposure and prevent distortion of the soft tissue related to the tube. The oral cavity and oropharynx are is cleansed with 0.12% chlorhexidine and the face prepped with Betadine paint. A single dose of IV cephalexin is administered within 30 min prior to the incision (for patients with an anaphylactic penicillin allergy, clindamycin is a suitable alternative).

## Postoperative Care

Antibiotic ointment (e.g., bacitracin ointment) is applied to the surgical site three times daily for the first week and is subsequently transitioned to a petroleum-based ointment such as Aquaphor® or Vaseline®. The area is gently cleansed with saline prior to each application. No systemic antibiotics are prescribed postoperatively in most cases. Antiplatelet and anticoagulant medications are typically held for 3 days postoperatively unless the patient's prescribing physician feels strongly that they be resumed immediately postoperatively. Ice packs are avoided to prevent vasoconstriction. Nonabsorbable sutures are typically removed 5 to 7 days postoperatively.

## Partial Thickness Reconstruction

## Partial Thickness Defects: Vermillion

See Table 5.2.

### Secondary Intention

Healing by secondary intention has been shown to be an appropriate option for small-to-moderate defects (up to 2.5 cm) of the vermillion or mucosal lip. Healing by secondary intention should be avoided in patients with more than 2 mm of cutaneous lip involvement or extension into the underlying muscle so as to avoid cosmetic and functional impairments including wound contracture with scar depression and oral incompetence. Proper wound care is essential for obtaining satisfactory cosmetic and functional results. Reepithelialization typically occurs within 3 to 5 weeks. Caution should be taken in employing this approach in poorly compliant patients or for those on antiplatelet/anticoagulant therapy [15].

Some authors also advocate for the use of acellular dermal matrix (e.g., AlloDerm®, Cytal Wound Matrix) to assist as a scaffold for healing by secondary intention and have demonstrated satisfactory cosmetic and functional results even with large defects involving much of the length of the vermillion lip [16].

### Vermillion Advancement Flap

Even very large defects limited to the vermillion can be repaired with vermillion advancement flaps. Wide undermining of the surrounding labial mucosa is performed in a plane just superficial to the orbicularis oris. The mucosa is then advanced and secured to the remaining vermillion or cutaneous lip. Potential drawbacks of this procedure include persistent hypoesthesia, apparent loss of lower lip fullness, and distortion of the vermillion border.

**Table 5.2** Reconstructive options for partial thickness defects (vermillion only)

| |
|---|
| – Healing by secondary intention |
| – Primary closure |
| – Vermillion advancement flap |
| – FAMM flap |

### FAMM Flap [17]

The facial artery musculomucosal (FAMM) flap is an axial flap based on the facial artery. It is harvested from the cheek and has multiple uses in oral cavity and oropharyngeal reconstruction. Pribaz and colleagues described its use to restore a normal appearing vermillion for patients with large defects [17].

## Partial Thickness Defects: Cutaneous

See Table 5.3.

### Primary Closure

Small cutaneous defects can be closed by primary closure alone. Primary closure should not be attempted for large defects as this can lead to poor scarring and distortion of the normal anatomy.

### Skin Grafting

Skin grafts often have poor color and texture matching with the lip and come with the risk of pincushioning [18]. While skin grafting is not commonly performed in the reconstruction of cutaneous lip defects, it can play a role in carefully selected patients. Luce recommends that full thickness skin grafts (FTSGs) only be used for small defects of the superior lip at the nasal sill [8], while others have reported satisfactory results after using the same for the defects of the philtrum as well [16]. FTSGs have been used for the repair of major upper lip defects in burn victims [19, 20], and split thickness skin grafts are used to cover functional gracilis muscle flaps for large full thickness lip defects (as discussed later in this chapter). Given the mobile nature of the lips, a bolster dressing is of utmost importance if a skin graft is to be used in order to prevent graft shear.

### Local Flaps

A wide array of local flaps can be employed including the ergotrid flap, V-Y advancement flap, alar-crescent flap, nasolabial flap, and the Karapandzic flap. Each of these flaps are discussed below (see the Full Thickness Reconstruction section for a discussion on the alar-crescent and Karapandzic flaps).

**Table 5.3** Reconstructive options for partial thickness defects (skin only)

| |
|---|
| – Primary closure |
| – Skin graft |
| – Ergotrid flap |
| – V-Y advancement flap |
| – Alar crescent flap |
| – Nasolabial flap |
| – Free tissue transfer |

## Ergotrid Flap

The term "ergotrid" is used to describe the cutaneous upper lip (i.e., the skin between the base of the nose and the vermillion border of the upper lip, marked laterally by the nasolabial fold on either side). Described in 2011, the ergotrid flap is a rotation-advancement flap based on branches of the superior labial artery [18]. This flap is well suited for small-to-moderate sized skin defects on the upper lip. It is especially useful in older patients with an increased laxity of the surrounding skin and deep nasolabial folds for scar camouflage.

The incision is designed to start at the lateral aspect of the defect and extend into the nasolabial fold. The surrounding skin is then widely undermined superficial to the orbicularis oris muscle. The flap is then advanced, and a standing cone is typically excised superomedially. The flap is then inset in the usual fashion (Fig. 5.5).

In the event that the ergotrid flap cannot be rotated sufficiently to fill the defect, it can be converted into a V-Y advancement flap (based on perforators from the facial artery) by extending a separate incision inferiorly.

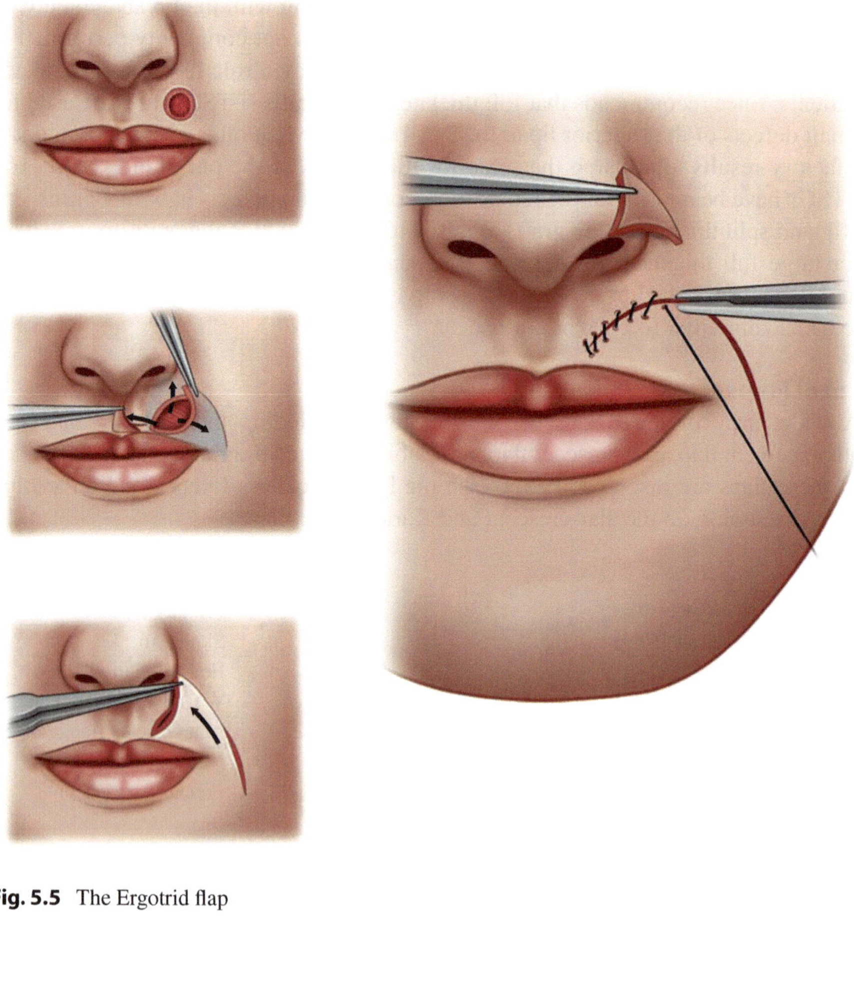

**Fig. 5.5** The Ergotrid flap

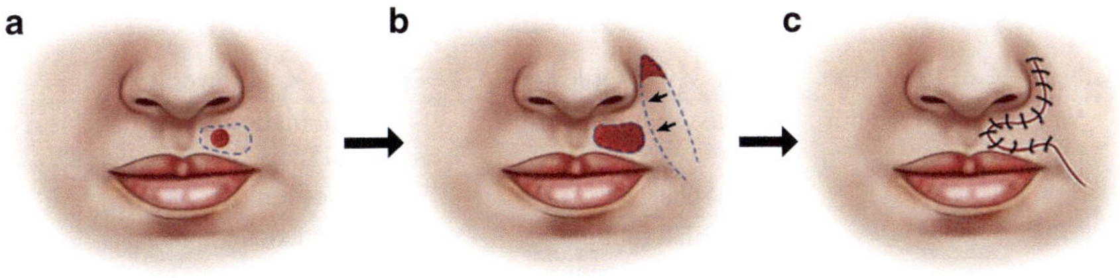


**Fig. 5.6** Melolabial flap for upper lip reconstruction

### Melolabial Flap

A melolabial flap (Fig. 5.6) can be used for cutaneous defects of both the upper and lower lips. Both superior and inferiorly based melolabial flaps can be used for lip reconstruction. A full description of this flap is provided in an earlier chapter of this book.

## Full Thickness Reconstruction

As previously discussed, the unique anatomical considerations of the upper lip render upper lip reconstruction more complex than lower lip reconstruction. Given the special considerations required for these cases, upper and lower lip reconstructions will be discussed separately.

## Special Considerations: Lower Lip

Lower lip defects are more common than upper lip defects due to the higher incidence of malignancy on the lower lip [21]. Fortunately, as previously discussed, the anatomy of the lower lip is less complex than the upper lip, and defects are thus typically easier to reconstruct. Available reconstructive options differ based on the length of the defect (Table 5.4).

### Small Defects

Primary closure can be achieved in defects measuring up to 40% to 50% of the lip length, especially in elderly patients with increased lip laxity [22, 23]. Surgical techniques include wedge resection (Fig. 5.7) and W-plasty (Fig. 5.8).

### Larger Defects

Larger defects require more complex reconstruction. Defects measuring less than two-thirds of the lip can typically be corrected in a satisfactory manner with local tissue rearrangement. Options for correction of medium-to-large-sized central lip defects include bilateral lip advancement flaps, stair-step advancement flaps, and cross-lip flaps such as the Abbe flap. For defects involving the oral commissure, the

**Table 5.4** Reconstructive options for full thickness lower lip defects

| Defect < $\frac{1}{3}$ of lower lip | Defect $\frac{1}{3}$–$\frac{2}{3}$ of lower lip | Defect > $\frac{2}{3}$ of lower lip |
|---|---|---|
| – Wedge (V or W) with primary closure | *Commissure not involved* | – Combination (synergistic use) of local flaps, see table below |
| | – Abbe | – Gillies fan flap |
| | – Bilateral lip advancement | – Extended Karapandzic |
| | *Commissure involved* | – Bernard–von Burow |
| | – Estlander | – Webster |
| | – Karapandzic | – Regional flaps |
| | | – Free flaps |

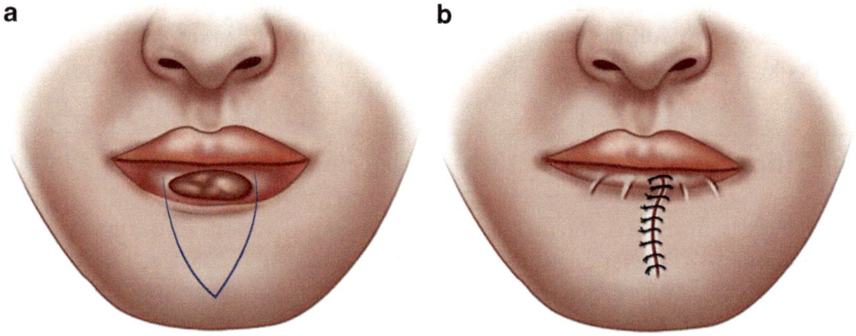


**Fig. 5.7** Wedge resection with primary closure

Estlander flap (another cross-lip flap) and the Karapandzic flap are commonly employed.

Very large defects (including subtotal and total defects) can be approached with complex local flaps such as the Gillies fan flap, the extended Karapandzic flap, the Bernard–von Burow flap, as well as its subsequent Webster modification. Surgeons can also be creative in combining the use of multiple different local flaps in order to obtain a satisfactory reconstruction of these major defects (Table 5.5).

Regional tissue transfer has been reported for major lip reconstruction. Potential donor sites include the radial forearm, ALT, gracilis, and more. Osteocutaneous flaps including the fibula, scapula, and osteocutaneous forearm have also been used for complex defects which also involve the mandible.

## Special Considerations: Upper Lip

As previously discussed, the upper lip can be broken down into multiple anatomical subunits, and an accurate reconstruction of the upper lip is more challenging as a result. One of the most challenging areas in the upper lip to reconstruct is the

**Fig. 5.8** W-plasty

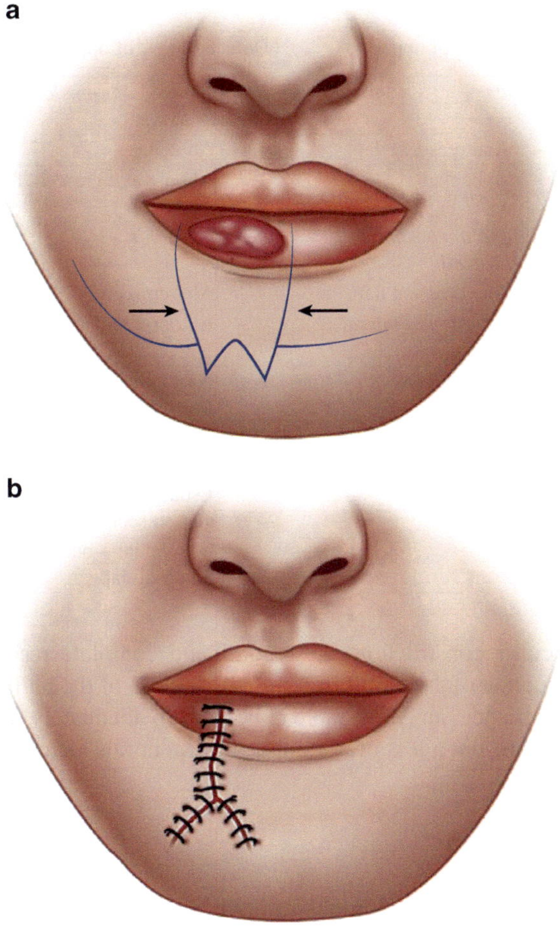


**Table 5.5** Published examples of synergistic local flaps for the reconstruction of large/complex defects

| |
|---|
| – Karapandzic + bilateral cross-lip flaps [24] |
| – Abbe + bilateral stair-step flaps [25] |
| – Double rhomboid with Estlander [23] |
| – Combined Karapandzic + Webster [26] |
| – Lip switch + composite modiolus [27] |
| – Bilateral nasolabial + pedicled submental flap [28] |
| – Bernard–von Burow + Abbe [29] |

philtrum, along with the lateral philtral columns. A careful consideration to the specific reconstruction of the philtral configuration is fundamental for defects involving the central upper lip, as the loss of definition in this area tends to result in an eye-catching cosmetic deformity. Similar to the basic principles of other subsites of

**Table 5.6** Reconstructive options for full thickness upper lip defects

| Defect < $\frac{1}{3}$ of upper lip | Defect $\frac{1}{3}$–$\frac{2}{3}$ of upper lip | Defect > $\frac{2}{3}$ of upper lip |
|---|---|---|
| *Philtrum* | *Philtrum +/– alar portion of lateral subunit* | – Abbe + bilateral alar crescent flaps |
| – Alar crescent flap | – Abbe flap | – Abbe + nasolabial flap |
| – Abbe flap | – Abbe + alar crescent flap | – Nasolabial + buccal mucosal flap |
| *Medial (alar) portion of lateral subunit* | *Lateral subunit* | – McGregor flap |
| – Alar crescent flap | – Alar crescent | – Free flap |
| *Lateral portion of lateral subunit* | – Alar crescent + cheek flap | |
| – Primary closure | – Nasolabial + buccal mucosal flap | |
| – Nasolabial flap (if vermillion is intact) | *Philtrum, lateral subunit, and commissure* | |
| | – Estlander + contralateral alar crescent flap | |
| | – Nasolabial + buccal mucosal flap | |

facial reconstruction, we recommend complete resection and subsequent reconstruction of the philtrum if more than 50% of the philtral subunit is involved. In our experience, an Abbe flap can be used to adequately reconstruct the philtral subunit and prevent a loss of normal definition in this area (Table 5.6).

## Local Flaps

Local flaps are commonly employed in lip reconstruction. The basic principles of local and locoregional flaps have been discussed in earlier chapters. This section aims to focus on specific flaps described for lip reconstruction.

### Bilateral Lip Advancement Flap

Bilateral lip advancement flaps are useful for the reconstruction of full thickness defects of both upper and lower lip defects.

For lower lip defects, an incision is marked out in the mental crease. Undermining of the skin and muscle is performed prior to flap advancement. Partial thickness incisions (sparing the mucosal layer) are often possible, given the innate elasticity of the mucosa, but a full thickness incision can be carried out for larger defects. If necessary, Burow's triangles are excised at the lateral edge of the incision in the mental crease bilaterally to prevent standing cone deformities (Fig. 5.9). The flaps are then advanced, and multi-layer closure is then performed, adhering to the basic principles discussed earlier in this chapter.

Bilateral upper lip advancement is typically performed using the alar crescent flap technique, discussed in detail below.

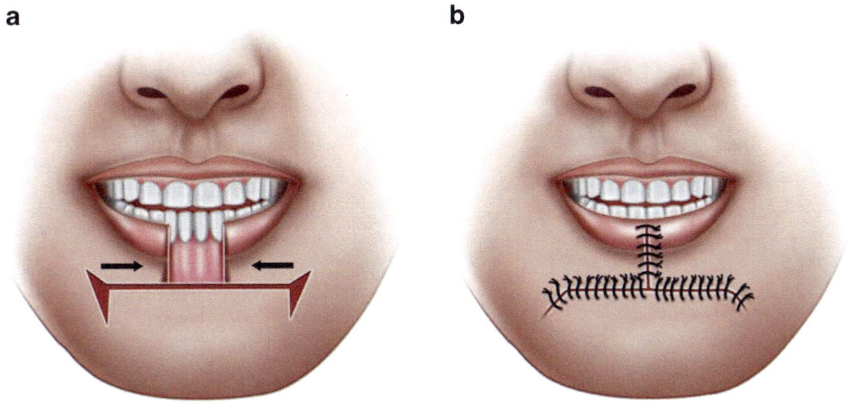


**Fig. 5.9** Bilateral lower lip advancement flap

### Stair-Step Advancement Flap

A variation of the lower lip advancement flap is the stair-step advancement flap, described in the 1970s by Johanson and colleagues [30]. They described this flap as a more functional and cosmetically appealing alternative to fan flaps for defects measuring up to two-thirds of the width of the lower lip.

The flap is designed for rectangular defects. Starting at the lateral edge of the defect bilaterally, stepwise incisions are designed inferiorly and laterally. Small squares of tissue are excised from the inferior aspect of the incision (under each step) until the final step, which is then excised as a triangle. The skin is undermined and the flaps are advanced, followed by a routine multilayer closure of the defect and donor site incisions (Fig. 5.10).

### Alar Crescent Flap

Designed for the reconstruction of central upper lip defects, the alar crescent flap is a single-stage procedure that permits the mobilization of skin and functional muscle (if needed) with an intact neurovascular supply. This helps preserve normal sphincteric activity while providing a reasonable cosmetic result. It can be used for the reconstruction of both partial and full thickness upper lip defects. The primary disadvantage to this procedure is the loss of philtral detail [31], especially in patients undergoing bilateral flaps for large central defects. For large upper lip defects, an Abbe flap can be performed in conjunction with alar crescent flaps, with the Abbe flap used for the reconstruction of the philtral subunit (allowing the recreation of this central anatomical detail).

The flap is designed by marking out an incision within the alar groove which is extended inferiorly to connect with the defect (Fig. 5.11). A second incision is designed lateral to this, creating a crescent shaped piece of tissue that is excised in order to prevent distortion of the perialar region with advancement of the flap. Wide subcutaneous undermining of the lip and cheek tissue is then performed. The flap is

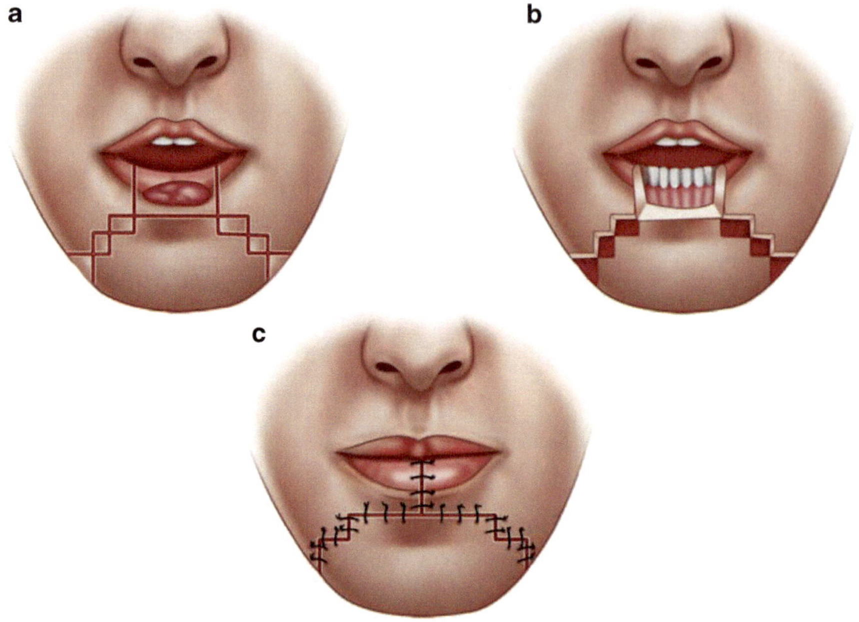


**Fig. 5.10** Stair-step flap

then rotated and advanced to fill the defect. Multilayer closure is performed. Bilateral flaps can be performed to repair large defects that cannot be repaired with a unilateral flap alone.

### Karapandzic Flap

Initially described in 1974, Karapandzic developed this flap as a surgical option for patients with poor vascular supply including radiated patients and the very elderly [32]. This circumoral flap design was unique compared to prior techniques (such as the Gillies fan flap discussed below) through the use of partial thickness incisions and blunt dissection for neurovascular preservation. It remains in use today as an option for the correction of upper or lower lip defects involving more than half of the lip. The major concern with this flap design is microstomia, with 22% (13/58) of patients in the original case report requiring later surgical correction of their significantly reduced oral circumference. Blunting of the external commissure is very common and may require subsequent commissuroplasty.

For lower lip defects, the inferior aspect of the incision is designed within the mental crease to improve cosmesis. It is extended bilaterally in a circumoral fashion and carried superiorly along the nasolabial fold, typically terminating just inferior and lateral to the nasal ala (Fig. 5.12). A similar incision is designed for upper lip defects, without the inferior incision through the mental crease. The incisions are then carried out in a partial thickness fashion. Blunt dissection is performed in the orientation of the vessels in order to mobilize the tissue while preserving the

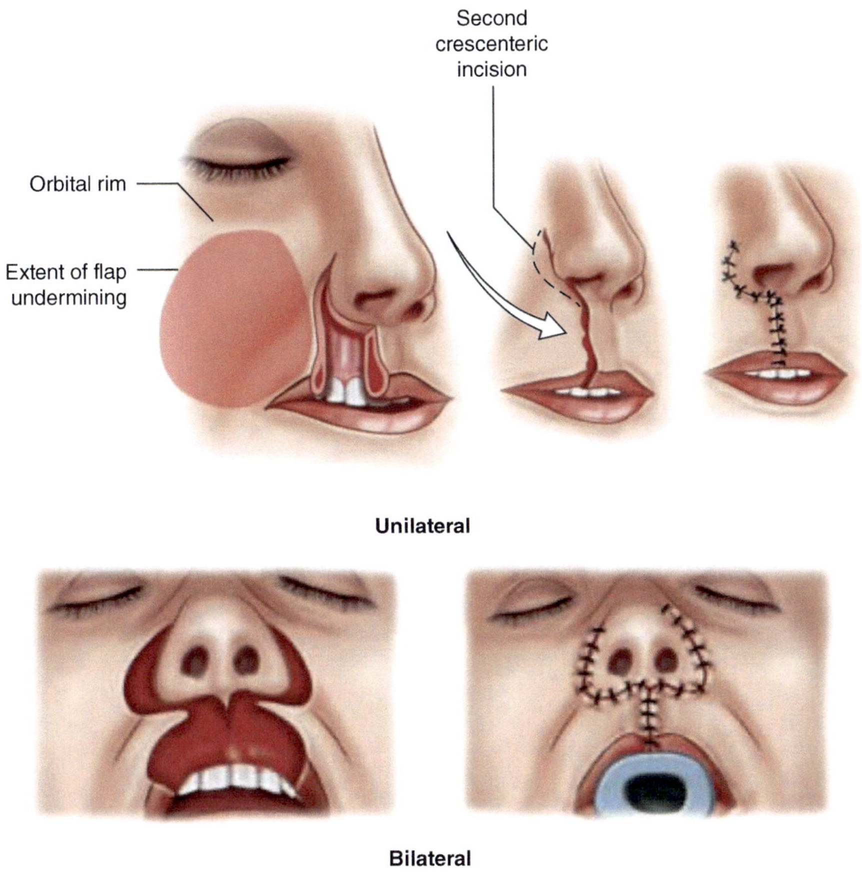


**Fig. 5.11** Alar crescent flaps (unilateral and bilateral)

neurovascular structures. Karapandzic described the flap without any long mucosal incisions, although separate mucosal incisions can be carried out if there is not enough elasticity of the mucosa to permit sufficient flap mobilization after complete dissection. Precise multilayer closure is then carried out. Postoperative microstomia can often be addressed with lip-stretching devices (as discussed in the complications section below).

Multiple modifications of the Karapandzic flap have recently been described for the successful reconstruction of even larger defects. Hanasono and Langstein described a modification which recruits perioral cheek tissue to help reconstruct these large defects while maintaining normal or near normal mouth opening [33]. A subsequent series of 21 patients by Dediol and colleagues went further, using extensions of the flap to the medial canthus bilaterally to successfully reconstruct near total defects of the lip and chin [34].

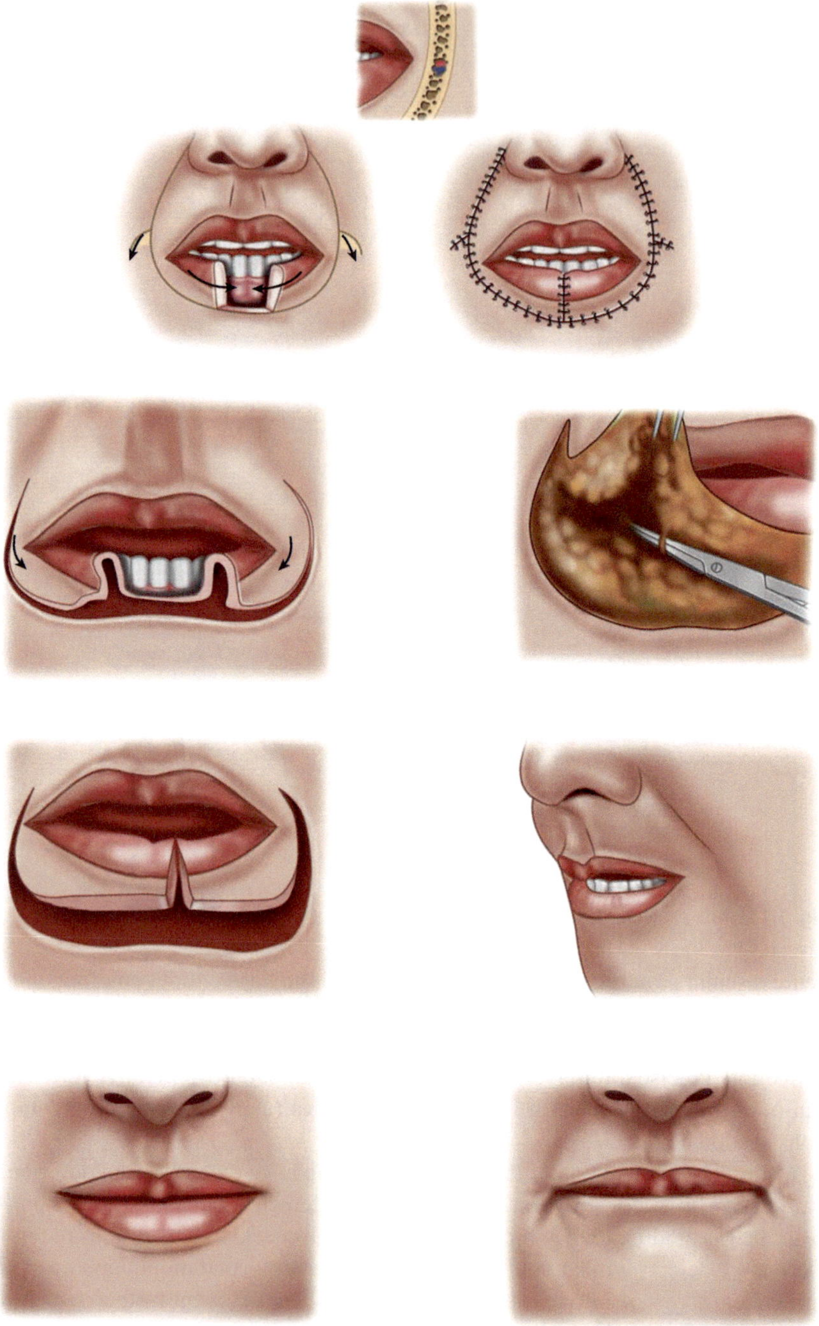

**Fig. 5.12** Karapandzic flap

### Gillies Fan Flap

The Gillies fan flap was designed in the early-to-mid-twentieth century as an option for the reconstruction of full thickness lower lip defects [35].

Flap design is relatively simple. A full thickness incision is carried laterally from the inferior aspect of the incision around the oral commissure and extended superiorly along the nasolabial fold. A 60-degree back cut is then performed medially towards the ipsilateral oral commissure. The flap is rotated, and multilayer closure is performed in the usual fashion (Fig. 5.13).

Given that this technique involves full thickness incisions through the skin of the lower lip and part of the upper lip and can consequently result in prolonged anesthesia of the lip, it also tends to lead to the distortion of the commissure, often requiring additional surgical intervention in the future. Bilateral Gillies flaps can be performed but tend to result in significant microstomia [36].

### Bernard–von Burow (and Webster Modification)

In the mid-nineteenth century, Bernard [37] and von Burow [38] separately described a flap involving bilateral full thickness cheek advancement flaps. Multiple triangles of skin and subcutaneous tissue ("Burow's triangles") are excised, two for lower lip reconstruction (three including the defect) and four for upper lip reconstruction (Figs. 5.14 and 5.15) to prevent standing cone deformities. Full thickness advancement of the cheek skin is then performed bilaterally.

In 1960, Webster and colleagues described a modification of the Bernard–von Burrow flap for total lower lip reconstruction [39]. The Webster modification of this flap provides an improved aesthetic outcome by altering the shape and orientation of the superior Burow's triangles to better place the scars within natural skin creases (the nasolabial folds). Furthermore, while the Bernard–von Burow technique for lower lip reconstruction involves a third Burow's triangle through the aesthetic

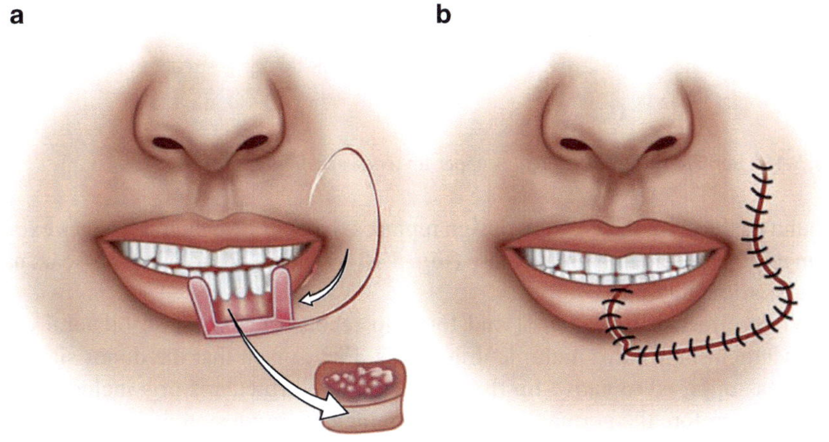


**Fig. 5.13** Gilles fan flap

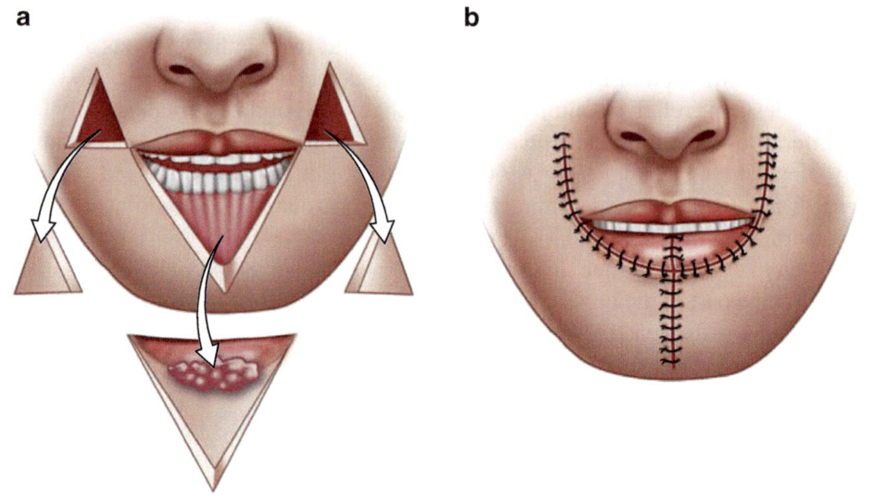


**Fig. 5.14** Bernard–von Burow flap for lower lip reconstruction

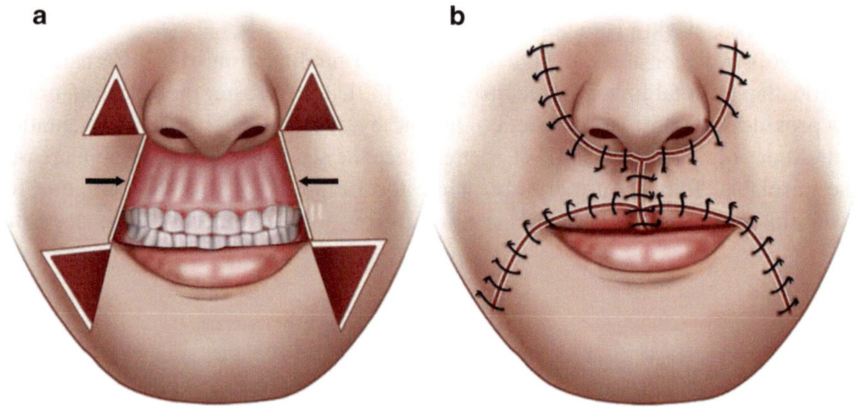


**Fig. 5.15** Bernard–von Burow flap for upper lip reconstruction

subunit of the chin, the Webster design replaces this with two lateral wedges excised from around the cicummental crease (Fig. 5.16), which tends to place the scars near/at the marionette lines.

While effective for subtotal and total lip reconstruction, these bilateral cheek advancement flaps have multiple drawbacks. First, given that the donor site is the cheek (as opposed to native lip tissue), there is no orbicularis oris included in the flap and therefore the normal orbicularis sphincter is not restored. Additionally, the full thickness incisions described in the above techniques can result in neurovascular compromise, and significant postoperative sensory disturbance in the

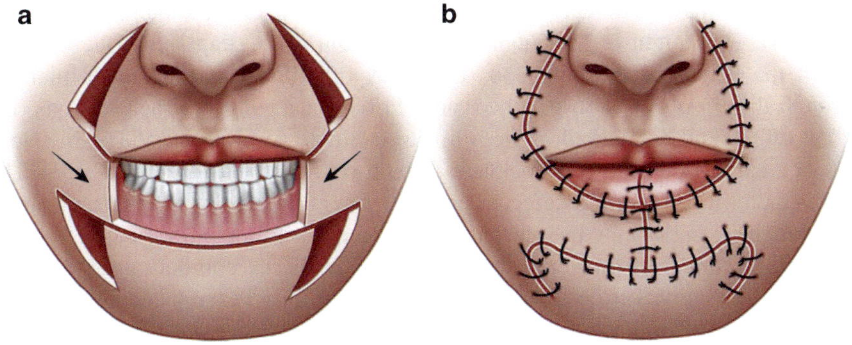


**Fig. 5.16** Webster modification

surrounding area may ensue. A more challenging technique involving partial thickness incisions through skin and subcutaneous tissue with meticulous subcutaneous dissection can mitigate this risk [40].

## Local Flaps: Cross-Lip Flaps

Early descriptions of cross-lip flaps (by Sabattini and subsequently by Stein) date back to the mid-nineteenth century [41–43]. Further modifications of this flap were subsequently published by Estlander and Abbe in 1872 [44] and 1898 [45], respectively, and have remained critical options in the facial reconstructive surgeon's arsenal ever since. Cross-lip flaps can be employed (alone, or in conjunction with other local flaps) for the reconstruction of large defects that would result in significant transverse lip tightness and microstomia if repaired via other techniques. Furthermore, the Estlander cross-lip flap design is the workhorse flap for the reconstruction of medium-to-large defects involving the oral commissure.

### Abbe Flap

The Abbe flap is commonly used for the reconstruction of medium-to-large defects of either lip where the commissure is spared. It is based on the labial artery (with venous drainage through its venae comitantes) and can be pedicled either medially or laterally. The flap typically includes a vermillion lip and cutaneous lip component. A classic Abbe flap can be used for lip defects measuring up to 60% of the total lip length upper lip length [46] and in our experience has been successfully used for even larger defects of the lower lip. Sensory and motor deficits do occur initially in the transferred lip. Early recovery begins within 2 to 3 months of the procedure, with near normal recovery expected by 12 to 18 months [47–49].

The width of the designed flap is typically designed to measure 50% of the width of the defect, ensuring that the widths of the upper and lower lips remain proportional after flap division. Exceptions do exist; for example, we will elevate a flap of the same width as the defect for the reconstruction of an entire subunit (such as the philtrum). The height of the cutaneous component of the flap should be made to match the height of the cutaneous defect. A full thickness incision is planned through the lip on the non-pedicled side. Prior to carrying out the incisions, the white roll should be marked on both lips to facilitate accurate inset. The incisions are then carried out in a full thickness fashion (except for the pedicled side). The flap is then rotated into the defect (Fig. 5.17). On rare occasions, it is necessary to make an incision through the inferior aspect of the vermillion of the pedicled side to facilitate rotation. This maneuver is safe as long as the surgeon does not breach the orbicularis oris muscle (the pedicle runs between the muscle and the labial mucosa). After satisfactory rotation, the flap is then inset into the defect site, ensuring to carefully repair the muscular layer and align the previously marked white roll.

Division and inset are typically performed 2 to 3 weeks after the initial procedure. We prefer to delay the division of the flap for up to 4 to 6 weeks in cigarette smokers to reduce the risk of vascular compromise.

#### Extended Abbe Flap

The extended Abbe flap was described by Kriet and colleagues in 1995 as a method of addressing large upper lip defects. Thanks to the course of the vertical labiomental branch of the labial artery, this flap can be designed to extend into the submental area and can provide both a wider and longer flap [46] (Fig. 5.18). It has been employed for the reconstruction of defects measuring more than 60% of the horizontal lip length, as well as taller upper lip defects extending into the medial cheek.

#### Estlander Flap

First described by Estlander in 1872 [44], this flap is an excellent choice for the reconstruction of significant defects (typically those impacting one-third to two-third of the lip) with the involvement of the oral commissure. It can be used for defects involving either lip.

The flap is designed on the opposite ipsilateral lip. The width of the flap on the donor vermillion lip is designed to measure half of the width of the defect. A wedge of cutaneous lip is also included for the reconstruction of any skin defect on the involved lip. The incisions are then carried out in a full thickness fashion. Medially, the incision is carried down to the white roll which facilitates mobilization and rotation of the flap while minimizing the risk of injury to the contralateral labial artery (upon which this flap is pedicled). If additional dissection must be done beyond the white roll/vermillion border to allow for adequate rotation, it should be done meticulously and without the use of cautery to avoid inadvertent vascular injury. Once the opposite ipsilateral lip has been adequately mobilized, it is then rotated by 180 degrees and inset into the defect in a multilayer fashion as discussed above.

Blunting of the oral commissure is a common sequela of this procedure, and many patients will require secondary commissuroplasty (which is further discussed in the Complications of Lip Reconstruction section below).

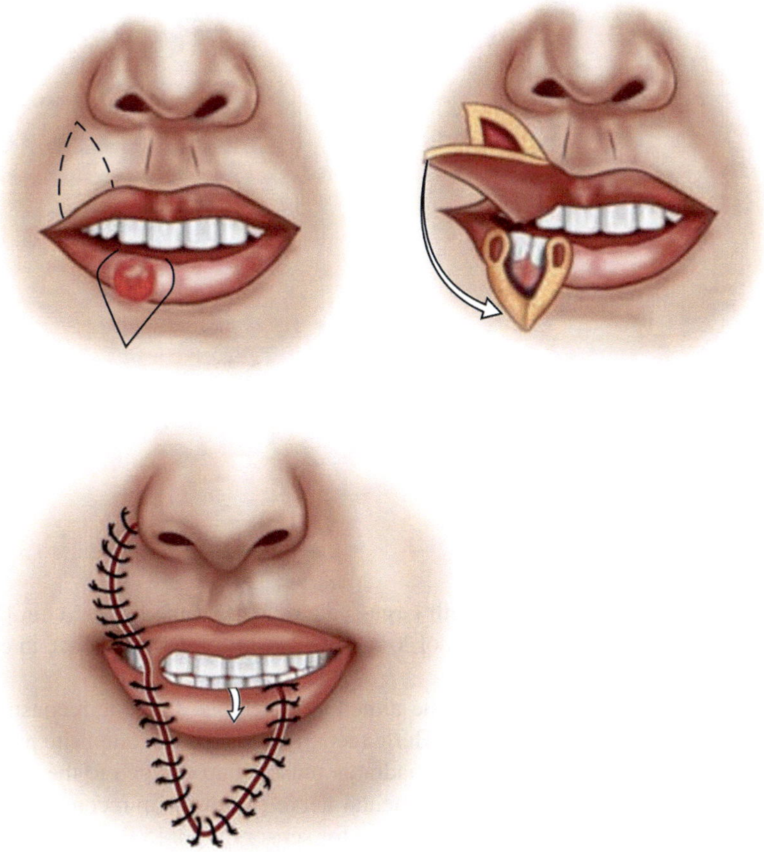

**Fig. 5.17** Abbe flap

## Free Tissue Transfer

### Radial Forearm Free Flap

Very large defects (especially those involving the majority portion of the lip as well as the surrounding tissue) can be challenging, if not impossible, to reconstruct with the use of local/logo-regional flaps. In these cases, microvascular reconstruction can be a valuable tool. Thanks to its pliability, versatility, and reliable blood supply with a long vascular pedicle, the radial forearm free flap (RFFF; see chapter ___ in this text) is the most commonly employed free flap in lip reconstruction. A composite flap consisting of the skin paddle along with the palmaris longus may be harvested to help achieve a static suspension of lip, assisting with oral competence. First described in 1989 [50], this modification of the RFFF provides improved cosmetic

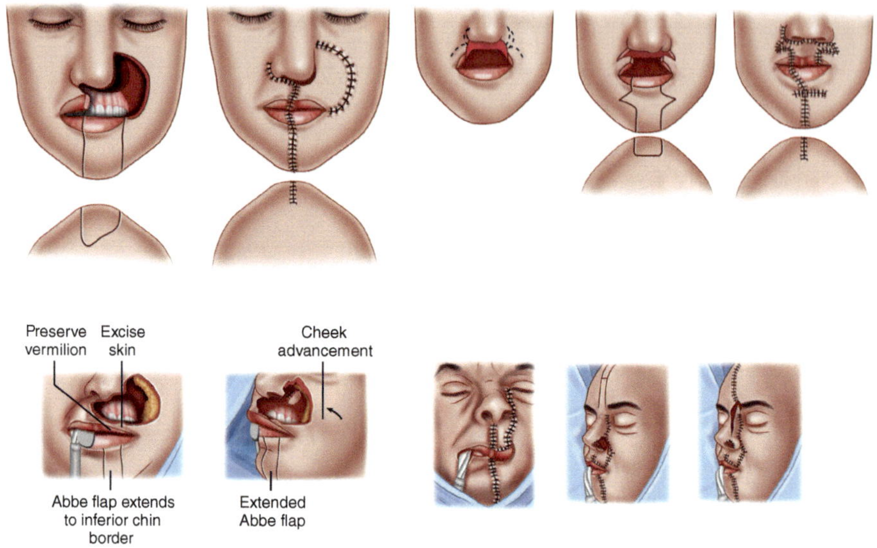


**Fig. 5.18** Extended Abbe flap

and functional results for patients with large-scale defects of the lip and chin [51, 52], although there have been reports of long-term loss of oral competence in certain patients [16].

Modifications to the RFFF technique aimed at providing dynamic reconstructions of major lip defects. Grinsell and Herle recently described a composite procedure including an innervated pronator quadratus muscle flap coapted to the buccal branch for motor innervation and to the mental nerve (in lower lip reconstruction) or infraorbital nerve (upper lip reconstruction) for sensory input [53].

## Alternative Donor Sites for Free Tissue Transfer

While the RFFF is the workhorse for total lip and chin defects, other donor sites are occasionally used for free tissue transfer as well. Functional gracilis muscle flaps (covered by split thickness skin grafts) can be employed for total lip defects. Studies have demonstrated satisfactory cosmetic and functional outcomes (with clinical recovery of sensation to the flap as well as normal pattern motor unit potentials in the muscle on postoperative needle electromyography studies with this technique) [54]. Composite defects of the lip and mandible can be reconstructed with osteocutaneous flaps from a wide array of donor sites including the radial forearm, fibula [55], scapula [56], and latissimus dorsi with rib [57, 58]. While anterolateral thigh flaps have traditionally been felt to be too bulky for lip reconstruction, "super-thin" ALT flaps have been successfully employed for large lower lip and skin defects with good success [59]. Details regarding the harvest of many of these flaps can be found in the later chapters of this text.

## Complications of Lip Reconstruction

Complications of lip reconstruction can be divided into short-term and long-term complications. Short-term complications include pain, infection, wound dehiscence, difficulty tolerating a normal diet, flap failure, numbness of the surrounding area (temporary or permanent), and need for additional surgery. Long-term complications include poor cosmetic result, microstomia (which may impair the patient's ability to wear dentures or eat certain foods), abnormal mobility of the lips/facial muscles, dysarthria, and permanent loss of oral competence (and associated drooling). The risk of many of these complications is mitigated by a proper choice of reconstructive method and meticulous operative technique, although not all can be avoided completely (especially in patients presenting with very large and complicated defects).

## Managing Microstomia

While the risk can be mitigated, microstomia is a somewhat common complication of major lip reconstruction, especially in patients with large defects. In our practice, significant improvement is often seen when following therapy with a combination of manual massage techniques, orofacial exercises, as well as the use of formal oral stretching devices. A wide array of oral appliances have been developed throughout the years [60]. We employ the Therabite® rehabilitation system (Atos Medical; New Berlin, WI) for our patients with microstomia and trismus. Unfortunately, the Therabite® can be prohibitively expensive for many patients, and we often employ a modification of the thermoplastic mouth stretcher described by Dougherty [60, 61] for home-based exercises in this population.

## Commissuroplasty

Blunting of the oral commissure is a potential complication of lip reconstruction, especially when the defect involves the oral commissure. Given the nature of the Estlander and Karapandzic flaps, blunting is frequently observed after these procedures. Oral commissuroplasty can be performed secondarily to improve the cosmetic result.

There are two primary techniques for commmissuroplasty: buccal mucosal advancement and myomucosal advancement (of the labial mucosa and the underlying orbicularis oris). Both approaches begin with a triangular-shaped resection of the skin lateral to the blunted oral commissure, with the apex of the triangle in the location of the expected position of a normal commissure.

The simpler of the two techniques (and our preferred approach) is the buccal mucosal advancement flap technique. After wedge resection of the skin lateral to the blunted commissure, the vermillion over the commissure is excised, and the underlying orbicularis oris is divided horizontally through the commissure. The upper

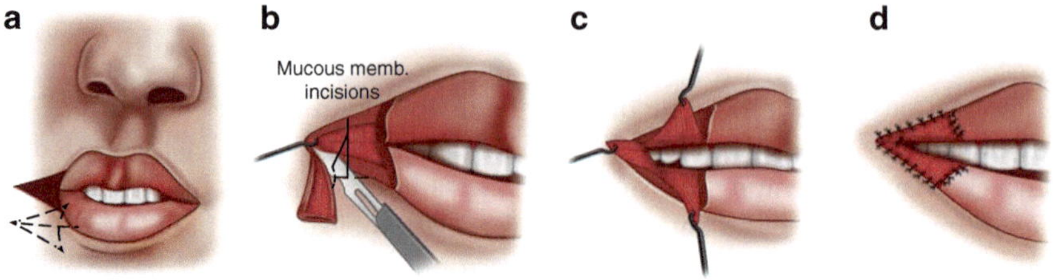


**Fig. 5.19** Oral commissuroplasty

and lower muscle edges are then advanced and attached to the skin at the apex of the previously excised triangular wedge (Fig. 5.19). Buccal mucosa is then advanced over the top of the muscle and secured to the skin with resorbable suture.

A full description of both approaches has been well described in an excellent review article by Parsel and Winters [62].

## Summary

Lip defects are commonly encountered by the head and neck reconstructive surgeons. Neoplasia, trauma, and congenital abnormalities are the most common causes.

There are a wide array of reconstructive options available for upper and lower lip reconstructions that span the length of the reconstructive ladder. The surgeon should carefully assess the defect (including which subsites are involved) and select the least complex reconstructive option available that will result in a satisfactory cosmetic and functional result. Complications of reconstruction include poor cosmetic result, temporary and/or permanent loss of sensation, impaired motor function and loss of oral competence, dysarthria, and microstomia. A careful flap selection and meticulous surgical technique can mitigate the risk of these complications.

## References

1. Gatti GL, Freda N, Giacomina A, Montemagni M, Sisti A. Cleft lip and palate repair. J Craniofac Surg. 2017;28:1918–24.
2. Grunebaum LD, Smith JE, Hoosien GE. Lip and perioral trauma. Facial Plast Surg. 2010;26:433–44.
3. Zitsch RP 3rd, Park CW, Renner GJ, Rea JL. Outcome analysis for lip carcinoma. Otolaryngol Head Neck Surg. 1995;113:589–96.
4. Peterson DJ, Azad AD, Gkorila A, Patel AA, Boudreault MS, Nazerali RS. Assessing gaze patterns in common cosmetic procedures with eye-tracking technology. Ann Plast Surg. 2020;84:S268–72.
5. Sebben JE. Wedge resection of the lip: minimizing problems. J Dermatol Surg Oncol. 1985;11:60–4.

6. Tan RA, Mulder FJ, Schwirtz RMF, Mosmuller DGM, De Vet HCW, Griot JPWD. Atypical outcomes of nasal and lip appearance after unilateral cleft lip repair: judgment by professionals, patients, and laypeople. Cleft Palate Craniofac J. 2021;58:1226–35.
7. Burget GC, Menick FJ. Aesthetic restoration of one-half the upper lip. Plast Reconstr Surg. 1986;78:583–93.
8. Luce EA. Upper lip reconstruction. Plast Reconstr Surg. 2017;140:999–1007.
9. Janfaza P. Surgical anatomy of the head and neck. Harvard University Press; 2011.
10. Vanison C, Beckmann N, Smith A. Recent advances in lip reconstruction. Curr Opin Otolaryngol Head Neck Surg. 2019;27:219–26.
11. Ono T, Hori K, Masuda Y, Hayashi T. Recent advances in sensing oropharyngeal swallowing function in Japan. Sensors. 2010;10:176–202.
12. Dey JK, Ishii M, Boahene KDO, Byrne P, Ishii LE. Impact of facial defect reconstruction on attractiveness and negative facial perception. Laryngoscope. 2015;125:1316–21.
13. Lee EH, Klassen AF, Lawson JL, Cano SJ, Scott AM, Pusic AL. Patient experiences and outcomes following facial skin cancer surgery: a qualitative study. Australas J Dermatol. 2016;57:e100–4.
14. Wang T-J, Lu M-H, Kuo P-L, Chen Y-W, Lee S-C, Liang S-Y. Influences of facial disfigurement and social support for psychosocial adjustment among patients with oral cancer in Taiwan: a cross-sectional study. BMJ Open. 2018;8:e023670.
15. Gloster HM Jr. The use of second-intention healing for partial-thickness Mohs defects involving the vermilion and/or mucosal surfaces of the lip. J Am Acad Dermatol. 2002;47:893–7.
16. Sanniec K, Harirah M, Thornton JF. Lip reconstruction after Mohs cancer excision: lessons learned from 615 consecutive cases. Plast Reconstr Surg. 2020;145:533–42.
17. Pribaz JJ, Meara JG, Wright S, Smith JD, Stephens W, Breuing KH. Lip and vermilion reconstruction with the facial artery musculomucosal flap. Plast Reconstr Surg. 2000;105:864–72.
18. Becker S, Lee MR, Thornton JF. Ergotrid flap: a local flap for cutaneous defects of the upper lateral lip. Plast Reconstr Surg. 2011;128:460e–4e.
19. Roh DS, Bojovic B, Woolard AC, Donelan MB. Triangular fossa graft for philtral reconstruction after facial burns: a 34-year experience. Ann Plast Surg. 2020;84:144–8.
20. Yen C-I, Chen H-C, Hsiao Y-C, Chang S-Y, Chuang S-S. Upper lip reconstruction with modification for creating a philtrum with single-stage full-thickness skin graft in burned face injury. Ann Plast Surg. 2019;83:513–7.
21. Baumann D, Robb G. Lip reconstruction. Semin Plast Surg. 2008;22:269–80.
22. Gómez A, Pomares A. Primary W-plasty closure for surgical repair of the injured lip. J Craniofac Surg. 2016;27:e57–8.
23. Harris L, Higgins K, Enepekides D. Local flap reconstruction of acquired lip defects. Curr Opin Otolaryngol Head Neck Surg. 2012;20:254–61.
24. Uglesic V, Amin K, Dediol E, Kosutic D. Combined Karapandzic-Abbé/Estlander/Stein flap for subtotal and total lower lip reconstruction. J Plast Reconstr Aesthet Surg. 2019;72:484–90.
25. Salgarelli AC, Bellini P, Magnoni C, Anesi A, Collini M. Synergistic use of local flaps for total lower lip reconstruction. Dermatol Surg. 2011;37:1666–70.
26. Campos MA, Varela P, Marques C. Near-total lower lip reconstruction: combined Karapandzic and Bernard-Burrow-Webster flap. Acta Dermatovenerol Alp Pannonica Adriat. 2017;26:19–20.
27. Gunnarsson GL, Demmissie MB, Havemann I, Topstad TK, Thomsen JB. Complete lower lip reconstruction with a large lip switch flap and a composite modiolus advancement flap. Plast Reconstr Surg Glob Open. 2017;5:e1607.
28. Oseni OG, Fadare AE, Majaro MO, Olaitan PB. Total reconstruction of the upper lip using bilateral nasolabial flaps, submental flap, and mucosa graft following complete resection for squamous cell carcinoma. Case Rep Surg. 2015;2015:782151.
29. Williams EF 3rd, Setzen G, Mulvaney MJ. Modified Bernard-Burow cheek advancement and cross-lip flap for total lip reconstruction. Arch Otolaryngol Head Neck Surg. 1996;122:1253–8.

30. Johanson B, Aspelund E, Breine U, Holmström H. Surgical treatment of non-traumatic lower lip lesions with special reference to the step technique. A follow-up on 149 patients. Scand J Plast Reconstr Surg. 1974;8:232–40.
31. Spinelli HM, Tabatabai N, Muzaffar AR, Isenberg JS. Upper lip reconstruction with the alar crescent flap: a new approach. J Oral Maxillofac Surg. 2006;64:1566–70.
32. Karapandzic M. Reconstruction of lip defects by local arterial flaps. Br J Plast Surg. 1974;27:93–7.
33. Hanasono MM, Langstein HN. Extended karapandzic flaps for near-total and total lower lip defects. Plast Reconstr Surg. 2011;127:1199–205.
34. Dediol E, Čvrljević I, Dobranić M, Uglešić V. Extended karapandzic flap technique for reconstruction of lower lip and chin defect. J Oral Maxillofac Surg. 2018;76:213–20.
35. Gillies H, Millard DR. The principles and art of plastic surgery. Butterworth; 1957.
36. Bhama PK. Lip reconstruction using the gillies fan flap. Oper Tech Otolaryngol Head Neck Surg. 2020;31:18–20.
37. Bernard C. Cancer de la levre inferieure opere par un procede nouveau. Bull Mem Soc Chir Paris. 1853;3:357–64.
38. Von Burow CA. Beschreibung einer neuen Trasplantations-Method (Method der seitlichen Dreiecke) zum Wiederersatz verlorengegangener Teile des Gesichts. Berlin: Nauk; 1855.
39. Webster RC, Coffey RJ, Kelleher RE. Total and partial reconstruction of the lower lip with innervated muscle-bearing flaps. Plast Reconstr Surg. 1960;25:360.
40. Renner GJ. Reconstruction of the lip. In: Baker SR, editor. Local flaps in facial reconstruction. Elsevier; 2014. p. 481–529.
41. Renner GJ, Zitsch RP 3rd. Reconstruction of the lip. Otolaryngol Clin N Am. 1990;23:975–90.
42. Sabattini P (1838) Cenno storico dell'origine e progressi dela rinoplastica e cheiloplastica seguita dalla descrizione di queste operazioni Praticamente eseguite sopra un solo individuo.
43. Stein SA. Lip repair (cheiloplasty) performed by a new method. Hospitals-Meddelelser. 1848;1:212–6.
44. Estlander JA. Eine Methode aus der einen Lippe Substanzverluste der anderen zu ersetzen. Arch Klin Chir. 1872;14:622–31.
45. Abbe R. A new plastic operation for the relief of deformity due to double harelip. Med Rec. 1898;53:1866.
46. Kriet JD, Cupp CL, Sherris DA, Murakami CS. The extended Abbé flap. Laryngoscope. 1995;105:988–92.
47. Smith JW. The anatomical and physiologic acclimatization of tissue transplanted by the lip switch technique. Plast Reconstr Surg Transplant Bull. 1960;26:40–56.
48. Thompson N, Pollard AC. Motor function in Abbe flaps. A histochemical study of motor reinnervation in transplanted muscle tissue of the lips in man. Br J Plast Surg. 1961;14:66–75.
49. Rea JL, Davis WE, Rittenhouse LK. Reinnervation of an Abbe-Estlander and a Gillies fan flap of the lower lip: electromyographic comparison. Arch Otolaryngol. 1978;104:294–5.
50. Sakai S, Soeda S, Endo T, Ishii M, Uchiumi E. A compound radial artery forearm flap for the reconstruction of lip and chin defect. Br J Plast Surg. 1989;42:337–8.
51. Carroll CM, Pathak I, Irish J, Neligan PC, Gullane PJ. Reconstruction of total lower lip and chin defects using the composite radial forearm—palmaris longus tendon free flap. Arch Facial Plast Surg. 2000;2:53–6.
52. Jeng S-F, Kuo Y-R, Wei F-C, Su C-Y, Chien C-Y. Total lower lip reconstruction with a composite radial forearm-palmaris longus tendon flap: a clinical series. Plast Reconstr Surg. 2004;113:19–23.
53. Grinsell D, Herle P. Composite pronator quadratus: radial forearm free flap in functional lip reconstruction. ANZ J Surg. 2019;89:940–4.
54. Coskunfirat OK, Bektas G, Cinpolat A, Unal K, Coskunfirat N. Experiences with functional gracilis muscle flap in lower lip reconstruction. Microsurgery. 2017;37:487–93.
55. Godefroy WP, Klop WMC, Smeele LE, Lohuis PJFM. Free-flap reconstruction of large full-thickness lip and chin defects. Ann Otol Rhinol Laryngol. 2012;121:594–603.

56. Jacobson L, Dedhia R, Kokot N, Chalian A. Scapular osteocutaneous free flap for total lower lip and mandible reconstruction. Microsurgery. 2016;36:480–4.
57. Huang R, Blackwell KE. Microvascular reconstruction of composite defects of the mandible and lip: aesthetic and functional considerations. Laryngoscope. 2000;110:1066–9.
58. Trignano E, Fallico N, Nitto A, Chen H-C. The treatment of composite defect of bone and soft tissues with a combined latissimus dorsi and serratus anterior and rib free flap. Microsurgery. 2013;33:173–83.
59. Bali ZU, Ozkan B, Parspancı A, Kececi Y, Yoleri L. Reconstruction of lower lip defects with free super-thin anterolateral thigh flap. Microsurgery. 2021;41:216–22.
60. Dougherty ME, Warden GD. A thirty-year review of oral appliances used to manage microstomia, 1972 to 2002. J Burn Care Rehabil. 2003;24:418–31; discussion 410.
61. Dougherty ME, Schwanholt CA. Thermoplastic mouth stretcher. J Burn Care Rehabil. 2001;22:S151.
62. Parsel SM, Winters RD. Commissuroplasty. Oper Tech Otolaryngol Head Neck Surg. 2020;31:33–7.

# Part II

# Muscular and Musculocutaneous Flaps

# 6 Pectoralis Major Flap

Nima Vahidi, Kevin Quinn, Cheryl Yu, Seung Lee, and Thomas S. Lee

## Introduction

Reconstructive surgery with the pectoralis major myocutaneous flap was first described in 1968; however, it wasn't until Ariyan in 1979 that its application in head and neck reconstruction was well described [1–3]. It is now commonly used in the reconstruction of soft tissue defects of the oral cavity, oropharynx, hypopharynx, as well as external skin defects of the face and neck. The pectoralis flap offers both myocutaneous and myofascial flap options to support reconstruction needs.

Prior to wide-scale adoption of microvascular free tissue transfer in the 1980s, the pectoralis myocutaneous flap was used extensively for head and neck reconstruction. It still remains a popular reconstructive option in developing nations with a limited access to microvascular surgery and is now used selectively in developed nations, particularly in the setting of salvage surgery or in patients without adequate donor vessels for free flap reconstruction [4].

N. Vahidi · C. Yu · S. Lee · T. S. Lee (✉)
Department of Otolaryngology, Virginia Commonwealth University Medical Center, Richmond, VA, USA
e-mail: Nima.vahidi@vcuhealth.org; Cheryl.yu@vcuhealth.org; Seong.lee@vcu.edu; Thomas.Lee@vcuhealth.org

K. Quinn
Department of Otolaryngology, Ohio State University Medical Center, Columbus, OH, USA
e-mail: Kevin.quinn@osumc.edu


F. Sokoya, A. G. Vincent (eds.), *Manual of Head and Neck Reconstruction*, https://doi.org/10.1007/978-3-031-65999-7_6

## Anatomy

The pectoralis major muscle is situated in the upper chest and functions to rotate and adduct the arm. It has four sites of origin which include the anterior surface of the medial half of the clavicle, the anterior surface of the lateral half of the manubrium and sternum, the costal cartilage from the second to sixth ribs, and the aponeurosis of the external oblique muscle. From these points, the muscle fibers converge laterally toward their insertion on the humerus. The pectoralis minor muscle, which lies deep to the pectoralis major, originates from the anterior surface of the third and fifth ribs and inserts on the coracoid process of the scapula. It functions to draw the scapula downward and forward. Typically, there is an avascular, fatty tissue plane present between the pectoralis major and pectoralis minor within which the motor nerve to the pectoralis major muscle is found. Deep to the pectoralis muscles are the serratus anterior and intercostal muscles. Superolaterally, the pectoralis major muscle is bordered by the deltoid muscle.

## Neurovascular Supply

The pectoralis major flap is an axial flap based on the pectoral branch of the thoracoacromial artery and vein (Fig. 6.1). The thoracoacromial artery is a branch of the axillary artery which is itself a continuation of the subclavian artery and can be traced back to the aorta.

The thoracoacromial trunk arises from the second segment of the axillary artery associated with the pectoralis minor muscle and has four distal branches including the acromial, humeral, clavicular, and pectoral branches. The pectoral branch travels along the deep surface of the pectoralis major muscle (superficial to the pectoralis minor muscle) and provides the majority of its blood supply. The lateral thoracic artery, which also arises from the second segment of the axillary artery, provides a secondary blood supply but is often sacrificed to maximize flap reach which can be restricted by its lateral attachment. The pectoralis perforator vessels may also provide supplemental blood supply to the overlying skin.

The venous drainage of the pectoralis major mirrors the arterial supply, with pectoral veins draining directly to the axillary vein. The cephalic vein which provides venous drainage for the upper extremities also supports the drainage of portions of the skin overlying the pectoralis muscle.

The pectoralis major muscle is innervated by the medial and lateral pectoral nerves which arise from the brachial plexus. Additionally, the pectoralis major and minor receive innervation from the seventh and eight cervical and first thoracic nerves. Of note, the motor nerve that innervates the pectoralis major muscle is often sacrificed during the harvesting process. It will appear as a nerve structure that pierces the pectoralis minor muscle and enters the pectoralis major muscle from its deep aspect. The denervated pectoralis major muscle will often lose significant soft tissue volume as a result of muscle atrophy, which can be advantageous in certain scenarios where such loss of tissue bulk is desired. However, if this volume loss is undesirable, such as if the flap is being used for near total glossectomy

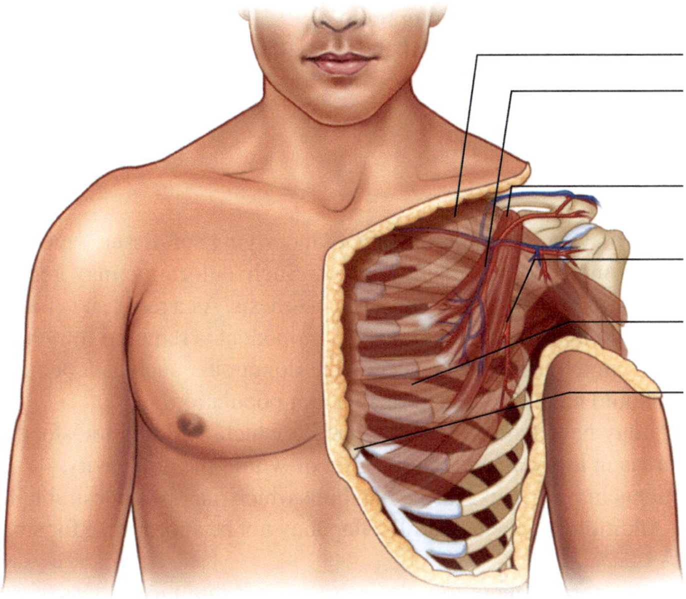


**Fig. 6.1** Anatomical depiction of the left chest, highlighting surgical landmarks for the pectoralis flap harvest. Halfway point along the clavicle marks the approximate location where the pectoral branch of thoracoacromial artery and vein is located immediately deep to the pectoralis major muscle. The pectoral branch of the thoracoacromial artery provides the primary blood supply for the pectoralis major, while the lateral thoracic is a secondary blood vessel and is often sacrificed during flap harvest

reconstruction, the surgeon should consider providing additional muscle and soft tissue bulk as in anticipation of these post-operative changes.

## Advantages

- The pectoralis flap offers a single-stage reconstructive option.
- It is a relatively easy flap to harvest and offers an abundance of soft tissue volume as well as a large skin flap for reconstruction.
- The vascular supply of the pectoralis flap is reliably identifiable within a well-established tissue plane located deep to the pectoralis major muscle.
- The tissue bulk and well-vascularized nature of the pectoralis major flap afford it a superior ability to withstand contamination with saliva, tissue infection, or radiation damage. It also typically lies outside the primary radiation fields for head and neck cancer and can provide healthy, non-radiated tissues in the previously irradiated patient. Thus, it is ideal for intraoral, pharyngeal mucosal defects in patients who are poor free flap candidates. Furthermore, it is the flap of choice in situations where there is a potential for carotid artery injury or exposure in the setting of a radical neck dissection with resection of sternocleidomastoid muscle.

- The patient remains supine during harvesting, which allows a two-team approach and increased efficiency in the operating room.
- Depending on the flap design, the distal end of the flap can reach up to 2–3 cm above the level of the zygoma.

### Disadvantages

- In women, the flap may include breast skin and underlying soft tissue which can result in breast asymmetry and disfigurement. Such deformity may require staged breast reconstruction to further optimize cosmesis. As a result, it is best to avoid using the pectoralis muscle flap if a skin component is required for young, female patients. A more cosmetically acceptable donor site, such as a pedicled latissimus flap, should be considered in this patient population.
- In men, the flap may have hair on the skin paddle which could be translocated into unsightly areas in the head and neck region or within the oral cavity.
- Overweight patients may have excessive flap bulk which may be undesirable for reconstruction. Additionally, the bulk of the flap may not be appropriate for small defects.
- Translation of the pectoralis major muscle can result in diminution or loss of arm abduction and/or rotation, which may require physical therapy to improve the strength and function of the remaining pectoralis minor muscle.
- The limited pedicle length can prevent flap rotation into defects superior to the zygomatic arch.
- Over time, it is common for patients to develop tethering of the neck associated with head turning. This can be addressed by transecting the pectoralis muscle at the level of the clavicle in a staged fashion, that is, at least 6 months out from the initial surgery, in order to give sufficient time for the skin flap to have sufficient peripheral vascular ingrowth.

## Preoperative Evaluation

Preoperative evaluation begins with a thorough history and physical examination, as is the standard prior to any surgery. The chest should be examined for any notable scars or defects that may interfere with flap harvest, and the presence and function of the pectoralis muscle should be assessed by adducting the arm and palpating the muscle. Congenital conditions such as Poland syndrome can result in the absence of this particular muscle.

Considerations should also be made depending on the sex of the patient. Males may have hairy chest walls which can obscure the surgical site and may require shaving to adequately expose surgical landmarks. For females, the thickness of the subcutaneous breast tissue or the presence of any breast implants should be noted. If a breast implant is present on the ipsilateral side where the reconstruction is required, the pectoralis major flap may be unreliable due to potentially compromised blood supply and also due to concern for damage to the breast implant. As such, if a breast implant is present, it is generally best to avoid using the ipsilateral pectoralis major flap.

The surgical site defect in the chest can result in postoperative chest pain and can significantly diminish forced vital capacity, which may negatively affect those patients with cardiac or pulmonary medical conditions. Additionally, the large donor site can present a challenge from a wound healing standpoint in those with severe diabetes, vasculopathy, cardiopulmonary disease, or chronic tobacco use.

## Flap Harvest

1. The patient is placed in a supine position, and the chest is prepared from the midline to the clavicle superiorly and the costal margin inferiorly. Surgical landmarks should be identified including the clavicle, ipsilateral sternum, xiphoid process, and inferior costal margin. The surgical site should be marked next. A line is drawn from the acromion to the xiphoid to mark the axis of the flap. A second line is then drawn vertically from the mid-clavicle, which marks the course of the vascular pedicle for planning purposes (Fig. 6.2).
2. The skin flap is then designed along the course of the vascular pedicle and may be designed as a curved ellipse to facilitate wound closure. The flap design can also be placed closer to or further away from the arc of rotation, depending on the length required to reach the tissue deficit. The skin flap is typically designed overlying the pectoralis major muscle while circumventing the nipple, though various modifications are possible (Fig. 6.2).
   (a) Medially Based—the placement of the skin flap medial to the nipple while overlying the pectoralis major muscle.
   (b) Laterally Based—the placement of the skin flap both superolateral and inferolateral to the nipple (while leaving the nipple blood supply to enter from its lateral aspect). This allows for a significant increase in the size of the skin flap that can be harvested. To preserve blood supply to the nipple while maximizing the size of the flap, the soft tissue bridging the nipple should be raised superficially to the underlying pectoralis major muscle fascia.
   (c) Maximal Reach—by designing the skin flap more inferiorly along the costal margin (but not extending past it), one can increase the flap reach/size. It is important to recognize that the distal portion of the skin flap will have a more tenuous blood supply than the portion of the skin flap that is located immediately superficial to the pectoralis major muscle. The deep tissue plane along the inferior extension will be the plane contiguous from the deep aspect of the pectoralis major muscle. This inferior extent can increase reach to 2–3 cm superior to the zygomatic arch.
   (d) In women, the skin paddle should ideally be placed to include the inframammary crease, if possible, to hide the scar and optimize cosmesis (Fig. 6.3).
3. Once the skin flap design has been finalized, the incision is made around the skin paddle with the dissection carried deep until the fascia of the pectoralis

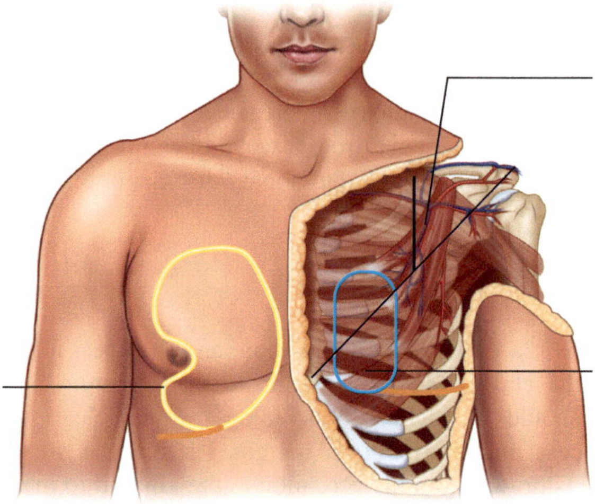


**Fig. 6.2** Variations of pectoralis major flap design depiction. The left chest (blue incision) depicts the surgical landmarks and course of the vascular pedicle. Also outlined are both the medial skin flap (blue/left chest) and larger (yellow/right chest) skin flap designs. An important consideration is that flap design can be placed closer or further away from the arc of rotation depending on the reach and the flap size required for reconstruction. Another important consideration is nipple location and ensuring the vascular supply is not compromised with flap design. The nipple blood supply can be left intact laterally while harvesting the skin flap located medial to the nipple. Orange line marks a releasing incision that is typically created to help with primary closure of the donor site defect by raising skin flap from the axilla and the superior rectus region

major muscle is identified. It is imperative to not violate the pectoralis major muscle fibers as the pedicle is located along the deep aspect of the muscle. Once the superficial pectoralis major muscle fascia is identified and the skin incision has been made circumferentially, the skin paddle can be secured to the underlying pectoralis major muscle with tacking sutures to minimize shearing injury to the perforator vessels.

4. A releasing incision is typically created along the inferolateral aspect of the skin flap to recruit axillary skin for the donor site closure as well as to improve exposure during the harvesting process. Through the lateral releasing incision, attention is turned to identifying the lateral border of the pectoralis major muscle.
5. Once the lateral border of the pectoralis major muscle is identified, a blunt dissection is performed to lift the pectoralis major muscle up while leaving the pectoralis minor muscle down. In patients with a very thin or underdeveloped pectoralis major muscle, the pectoralis minor muscle may be inadvertently raised instead. In such a case, the progression of rib exposure indicates that an incorrect plane has been employed. As the pectoralis major muscle is lifted, one

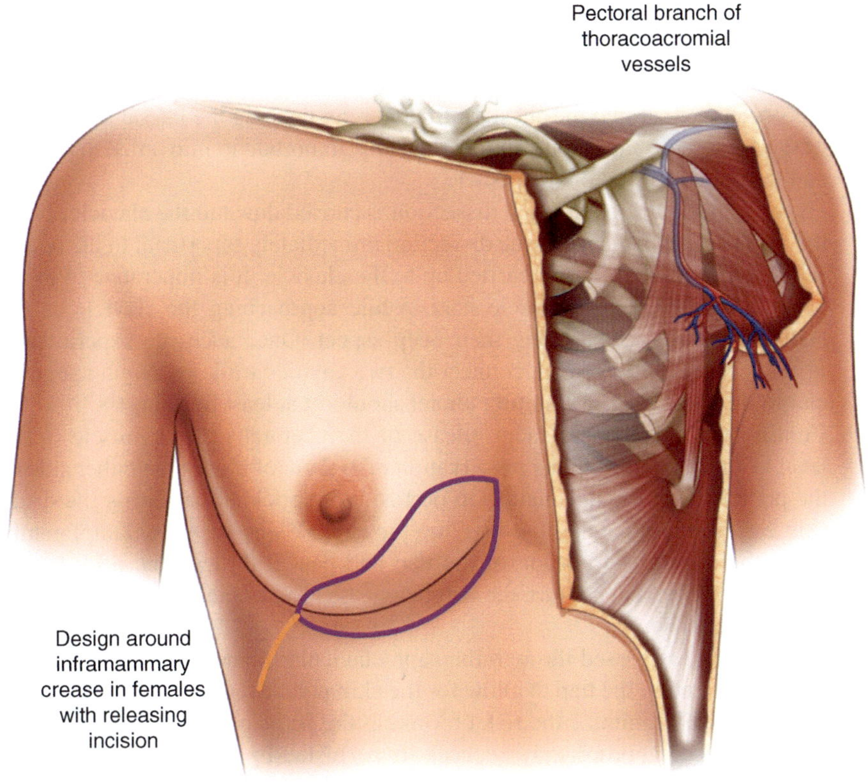


**Fig. 6.3** Flap design for female patients. The left chest demonstrates the vascular supply of the pectoralis major flap. The right chest illustrates the location of the skin paddle incision which should ideally be placed along the inframammary crease if possible to hide the scar and to optimize cosmesis when possible. In young females, it is best to avoid doing a pectoralis major flap as it can result in subjectively unacceptable breast deformity

can identify a fibrofatty tissue plane (appearing as "spider webs") overlying the pectoralis minor muscle.

In approaching the clavicle, blunt finger dissection and a long retractor can assist in identifying a prominent vascular pedicle—the thoracoacromial vessels—running along the undersurface of the pectoralis major muscle.

6. Once the vascular pedicle has been identified, the pectoralis major muscle should be divided with a 1–2 cm cuff located both medial and lateral to the vascular pedicle extending toward the clavicle. The pectoral branch of the thoracoacromial vessels, which runs the full length of the muscle, is preserved as it provides the main blood supply for the flap. While the preservation of the lateral thoracic artery allows for an additional vascular supply, it is often sacrificed to optimize the rotation and reach of the flap.

7. While dividing the pectoralis major muscle, one will encounter internal mammary perforators associated with the parasternal position of the ribs. These vessels should be clipped or tied to avoid a potential hemothorax that may occur if the vessels retract into the chest. Sufficient release along the lateral attachment of the pectoralis major to the humeral head is important to maximize flap reach and minimize tension on the pedicle.
8. From the neck, a subplatysmal dissection is carried down to the clavicle. From the chest, a subcutaneous tissue dissection immediately superficial to the pectoralis major muscle fascia is carried up to the clavicle. It is imperative to avoid penetrating through the muscle fibers while approaching the clavicle as the pedicle will be located along their deep aspect. Once adequate superior and inferior pockets are created, connect the two cavities while remaining superficial to the clavicle. The resulting tunnel should fit at least four fingers.
9. Confirm that there is sufficient release of the pectoralis major muscle to the level of the clavicle with the preservation of 1–2 cm of muscle on either side of the pedicle. Confirm adequate skin perfusion by pricking or cutting the distal skin edges before passing the flap into the neck. Using an Allis clamp, gently grasp the distal-most portion of the flap and pass it through the neck tunnel without twisting. Do not turn the flap below the level of the clavicle but instead flip it superiorly.
10. Once the flap is passed through the supraclavicular tunnel into the neck, start gently reorienting the flap to allow for the skin paddle to sit in the correct location. This will minimize the risk of kinking the pedicle in the chest. Once the flap is oriented appropriately, recheck its perfusion by pricking or cutting the distal skin edges. If there is a decrease in perfusion following positioning of the flap, ensure that the pedicle is not twisted and that the tunnel is adequately large to avoid pedicle compression.
11. Proceed with Flap inset with attention to achieving watertight closure wherever there is salivary exposure, as a salivary leak can lead to flap failure from infection. De-epithelialize any tissue that needs to be buried, as is commonly done for oral cavity, pharyngeal, or esophageal reconstruction. One or two Jackson–Pratt drains should be placed within the neck, with care taken to avoid pedicle compression.
12. The previously created lateral incision along the inferolateral aspect of the skin flap is used to recruit axillary skin, which will then be mobilized medially. The axillary skin flap is raised within the subcutaneous tissue plane while remaining superficial to underlying muscle fascia. An additional skin flap can also be raised from the inferior skin edge along the costal margin extending inferiorly and superficial to the rectus muscle.
13. The nipple is aligned to the contralateral nipple to optimize symmetry. Towel clamps are used to mobilize the remaining superolateral chest skin toward the medial incision. Simultaneously, the inferiorly located skin flaps from the costal margin and the ipsilateral axillary skin flaps are mobilized medially and superiorly to close off the donor site defect. The vast majority of the time, primary closure is possible with the recruitment of these skin flaps. If it is not

possible to achieve primary closure, one can consider the placement of a negative pressure dressing or other forms of delayed closure techniques along with skin grafting. One or two Jackson–Pratt drains are placed along the inferior aspect and the lateral (axillary region) aspect of the wound to minimize hematoma formation. The wound is then closed in two layers with absorbable buried sutures, followed by skin closure with sutures or staples.

## Important Considerations

- Generally, the superior most reach of a pectoralis major flap is the zygomatic arch. However, by designing a skin flap that extends more inferiorly along the costal margin and harvesting the skin flap within the same tissue plane as the deep aspect of the pectoralis major muscle, one can increase flap reach to 2–3 cm superior to the zygomatic arch pectoralis major flapzygomatic arch [5].
- When mobilizing the pectoralis major muscle from the chest to the neck, it is imperative to avoid twisting the pedicle. The skin tunnel should be sufficiently wide to accommodate at least three to four fingers at the level of the clavicle. More importantly, the senior author recommends flipping the pedicle vertically over the clavicle into the neck without twisting it below the level of the clavicle. Once the flap is in the neck (above the clavicle), create a gentle turn to the flap pedicle to reach the desired site of reconstruction. It is best to confirm adequate blood flow by pricking or superficially cutting the skin flap edges to ensure that there is no obstructive kinking of the pedicle once the gentle twisting of the pedicle has been introduced.
- It is important to consider soft tissue bulk shrinkage over time due to the denervation of the muscle and resulting muscle atrophy that will follow 6 to 12 months after the reconstruction process. As such, it is important to overcompensate for the skin flap size as well as the tissue bulk being used in reconstruction.
- The lower size limit of a skin island is considered to be 5 × 7 cm. However, depending on the body habitus and fatty tissue thickness, the minimal skin flap as well as the maximal skin flap size will vary greatly between patients.

### Muscle Dimensions

- Length: 15 cm (12–22 cm)
- Width: 24 cm (21–26 cm)
- Thickness: 1 cm (0.8–1.4 cm)

### Skin Island Dimensions

- Length: 12 cm (7–30 cm) [maximum size to close primarily 8 cm]
- Width: 8 cm (5–20 cm) [maximum size to close primarily 10 cm]
- Thickness: 1.4 cm (0.6–2.5 cm)

**Blood Supply:**

- Thoracoacromial Artery
  - Clavicular branch: length ~1 cm, diameter ~2 mm
  - Pectoral branch: length ~4.5 cm, diameter ~2 mm
- Venae Comitantes
  - Primary venae comitantes accompanying artery: length ~4.5 cm, diameter ~2.1 mm

## Flap Usage

The pectoralis myocutaneous flap or muscle can be used to reconstruct defects of the head and neck as well as the chest in its pedicled form. The pectoralis major flap can also be harvested as a free flap or a pedicled flap with costal cartilage, although these reconstructive options are rarely used. The pectoralis pedicle flap described above can reach externally to the level of the zygomatic arch and internally to the level of the soft palate.

- Reconstruction of intraoral defects (partial glossectomy, floor of mouth or buccal mucosa resections)
- Reconstruction of partial pharyngeal or cervical esophageal defects or pharyngocutaneous fistula
- Coverage of facial or neck cutaneous defects
- Coverage of major vessels in the neck following extensive ablative surgery with missing sternocleidomastoid muscle with concern for great vessel exposure
- Providing skin and soft tissue coverage (without bone) in patients without adequate donor vessels for free flap reconstruction

## Case Examples

This patient had a left-sided squamous cell carcinoma of the ear with gross invasion into the surrounding temporal scalp and external auditory canal (Fig. 6.4). He required wide local excision of the temporal scalp, total auriculectomy with surrounding cheek and superior neck skin, superficial parotidectomy with facial nerve dissection, and a modified radical neck dissection (Fig. 6.5). This led to a large skin defect that was closed with a pectoralis myocutaneous flap modified to reach the superior margin of the defect, 3–4 cm superior to the level of the zygomatic arch (Figs. 6.6 and 6.7).

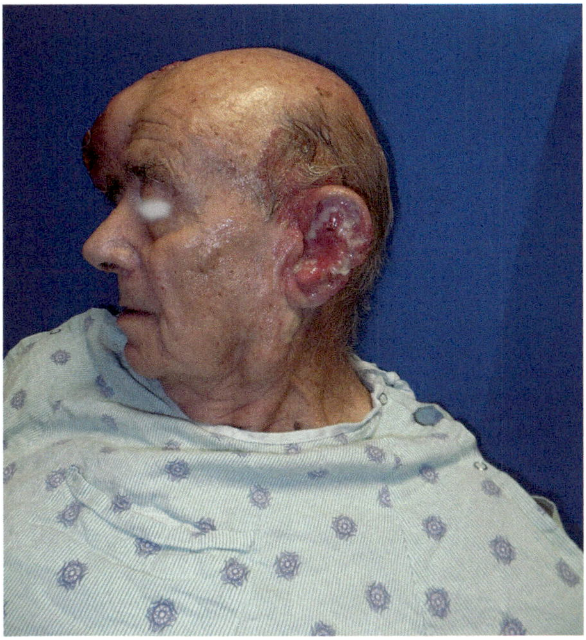

**Fig. 6.4** Patient case example: This patient had a left-sided squamous cell carcinoma of the ear with gross invasion into the surrounding temporal scalp and external auditory canal

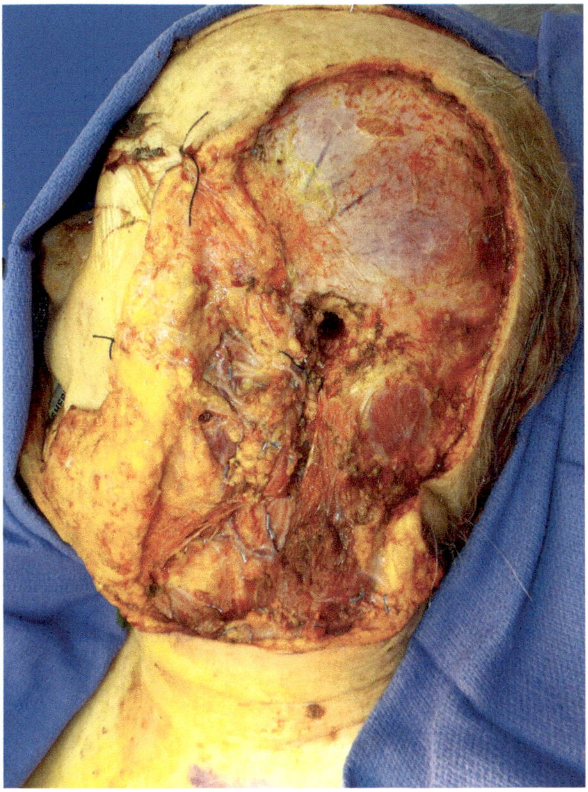

**Fig. 6.5** Patient required wide local excision of the temporal scalp, total auriculectomy with surrounding cheek and superior neck skin, superficial parotidectomy with facial nerve dissection, and a modified radical neck dissection

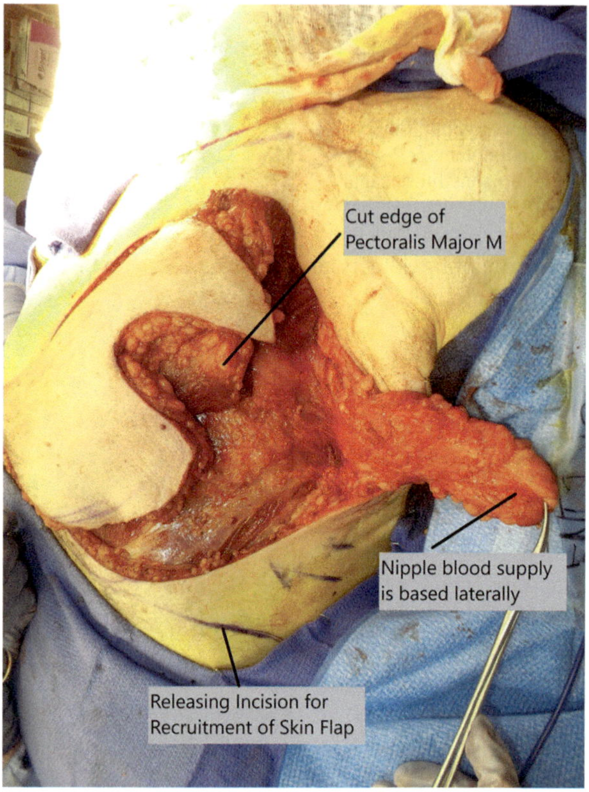


**Fig. 6.6** Large pectoralis myocutaneous flap with modification to reach above the zygomatic arch is obtained by raising the distal skin flap beyond the pectoralis major muscle by raising the skin flap deep to the pectoralis major muscle

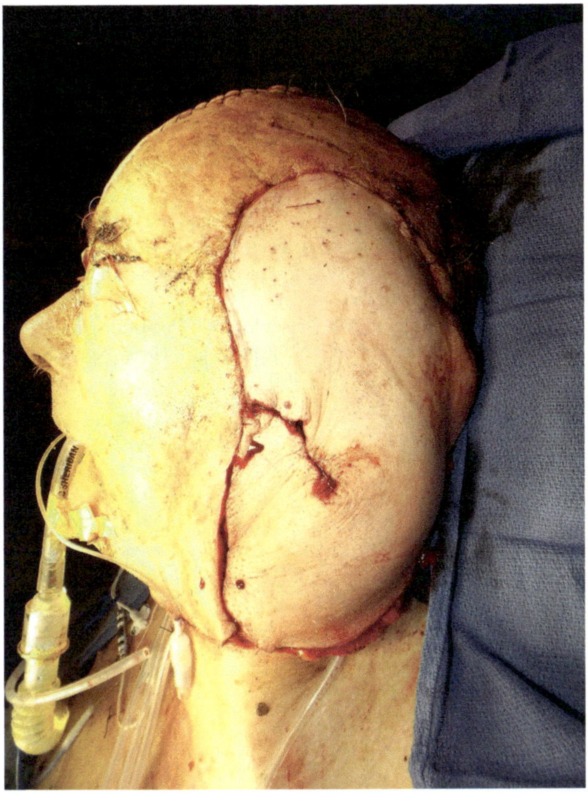

**Fig. 6.7** The pectoralis myocutaneous flap is rotated and inset to reach the superior margin of the defect, 3–4 cm superior to the level of the zygomatic arch

## Complications

The incidence of complete flap failure for pedicle pectoralis major flap is relatively low at 1–2%. The most common reason for failure is the occlusion of the pedicle, typically from inadvertent twisting during tunneling. In these instances, the pedicle should be untwisted or repositioned if the flap is salvageable. If the flap is not salvageable, it should be removed or aggressively debrided until bright red bleeding edges are encountered. A new flap will need to be placed to reconstruct the defect.

Occasionally, a partial necrosis of the skin paddle may occur, particularly in intraoral reconstructions from salivary exposure. As such, it is imperative to achieve watertight closure whenever the tissue is being placed within the oral cavity or pharynx in areas where salivary exposure is possible.

Donor-site complications are generally limited and can include scarring, keloid formation, diminished shoulder function, or hematoma occurrence. To minimize the risk of hematoma formation, the placement of two drains along the inferior most and lateral (axillary region) is recommended.

## References

1. Ariyan S. The pectoralis major myocutaneous flap. A versatile flap for reconstruction in the head and neck. Plast Reconstr Surg. 1979;63(1):73–81.
2. Erovic BM, Lercher P. Pectoralis major muscle flap. In: Manual of head and neck reconstruction using regional and free flaps. Vienna: Springer; 2015. p. 129–42. https://doi.org/10.1007/978-3-7091-1172-7_23.
3. Hueston JT, McConchie IH. A compound pectoral flap. Aust N Z J Surg. 1968;38(1):61–3.
4. Liu M, Liu W, Yang X, et al. Pectoralis major myocutaneous flap for head and neck defects in the era of free flaps: harvesting technique and indications. Sci Rep. 2017;7:46256. https://doi.org/10.1038/srep46256.
5. Resto VA, McKenna MJ, Deschler DG. Pectoralis major flap in composite lateral skull base defect reconstruction. Arch Otolaryngol Head Neck Surg. 2007;133(5):490–4. https://doi.org/10.1001/archotol.133.5.490.

# 7 Anterolateral Thigh Free Flap

Adrian A. Ong and Fiyin Sokoya

## Introduction/History

The anterolateral thigh (ALT) flap was first described by Song et al. and is based on branches of the descending branch of the lateral circumflex femoral artery (LCFA) [1]. Its original description was that of a fasciocutaneous flap supplied by septocutaneous perforators; however, it has since been described as a flap with predominantly musculocutaneous perforator vessels through the vastus lateralis muscle. The adoption of the ALT was initially slow due to concerns of unclear and unpredictable anatomy of the vascular pedicle. However, with a better understanding of the anatomy, it is now known as a flap with a long, large-caliber vascular pedicle; and due to the anatomic location, the ALT is amenable to a one- or two-team approach. The ALT has gained popularity since its initial introduction and has become a workhorse flap for the reconstruction of many types of head and neck defects, which can provide skin, fascia, muscle, or any combination of the above, with minimal donor site morbidity. The ability to harvest a large skin paddle, and use multiple pedicles, provides an additional advantage in reconstructing large skin defects of the face and scalp [2].

A. A. Ong
Otolaryngology and Facial Plastic Surgery Associates, Fort Worth, TX, USA

F. Sokoya (✉)
Wellstar Health Systems, Atlanta, GA, USA



F. Sokoya, A. G. Vincent (eds.), *Manual of Head and Neck Reconstruction*,
https://doi.org/10.1007/978-3-031-65999-7_7

# Anatomy

## Arterial Anatomy

In the majority of cases, the ALT flap is supplied by the descending branch of the LCFA, a branch of the profunda femoris artery, and travels between the rectus femoris and vastus lateralis muscles. Along its course, the descending branch of the LCFA provides intramuscular branches to the rectus femoris muscle as well as intramuscular branches to the vastus lateralis muscle, with one to three branches (the "ABC system") which then supply the skin in most cases. Figure 7.1 shows a cross-section of the thigh depicting the anatomy of the perforator vessels in the ALT flap.

There are three types of cutaneous perforators to the ALT flap as described in the literature [3]. In 90% of cases (type I), the cutaneous perforators originate from the intramuscular branches of the descending branch of the LCFA. The most common perforator ("perforator B") is located near the midpoint between the anterior superior iliac spine and supralateral corner of the patella with the other two cutaneous perforator vessels located approximately 5 cm proximal ("perforator A") and distal ("perforator C") to this point. In approximately 90% of cases, these are musculocutaneous perforators, with the remainder being septocutaneous perforators. In approximately 5–10% of cases, the type II cutaneous perforators arise from the transverse branch of the LCFA and have a long intramuscular course of up to 10 cm. Given the long intramuscular course, type II musculocutaneous perforators are onerous to dissect. In the remaining 1–5% of cases, type III cutaneous perforators

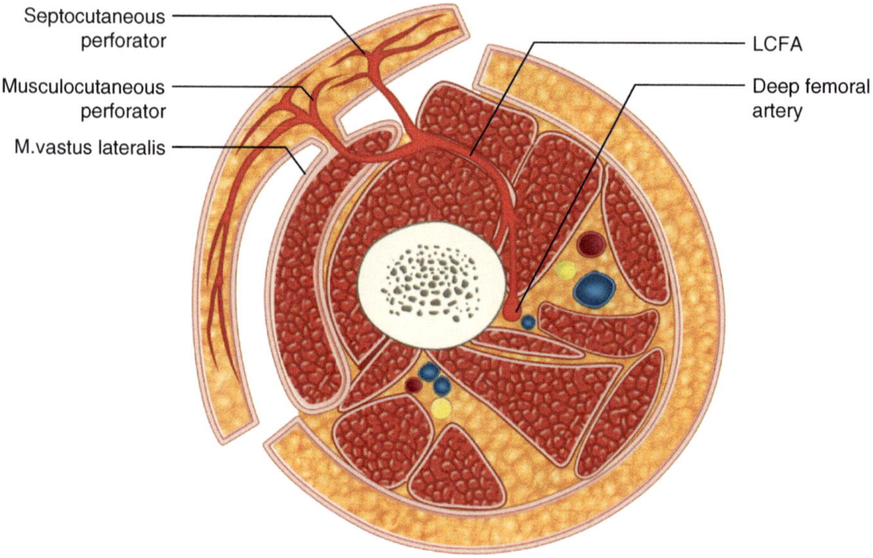


**Fig. 7.1** Location of septocutaneous and musculocutaneous perforators

arise directly from the profunda femoris artery and travel through the rectus femoris muscle before supplying the skin of the lateral thigh. The three types of vascular supply to the ALT flap can be seen in Fig. 7.2.

Depending on the perforator location, length of pedicle dissection, and location of recipient vessels, the vascular pedicle averages approximately 12 cm (range 8–16 cm) with a diameter of 2.1 mm (range 2–2.25 mm).

## Venous Anatomy

Two venae comitantes typically accompany the descending branch of the LCFA with an average diameter of 2.3 mm (range 1.8–3.3 mm). Due to the multiple H-type connections between the venae comitantes, one or both venae comitantes may be anastomosed to provide venous drainage.

## Neural Anatomy

The lateral femoral cutaneous nerve (L2–L3) provides the cutaneous innervation of the lateral thigh, and can be included with the flap for sensory reinnervation. This nerve arises approximately 10 cm below the inguinal ligament medial to the sensor

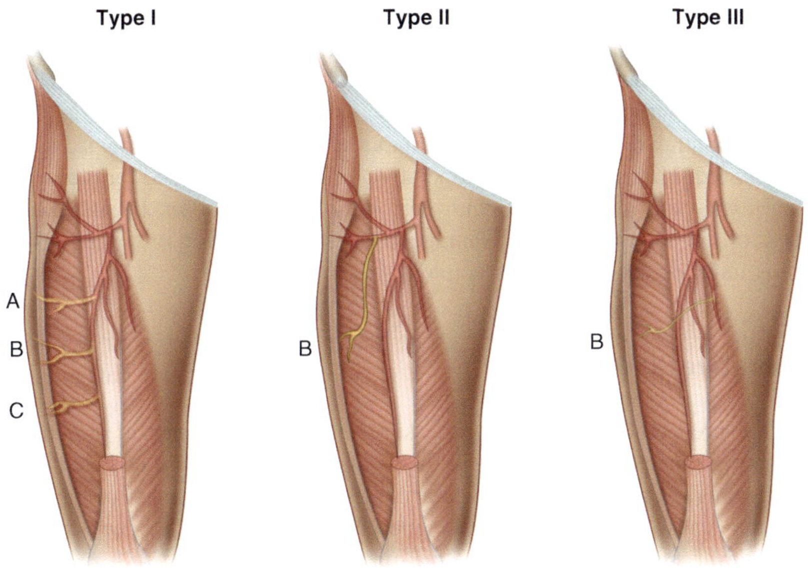


**Fig. 7.2** Three branching patterns of cutaneous perforators of the lateral circumference femoral artery

fascia lata, and branches into an anterior and posterior segment to supply the skin [4].

If the vastus lateralis muscle is to be included in the ALT flap, the motor nerve for the vastus lateralis muscle can be harvested as well for a functional reconstruction. The vastus lateralis muscle is innervated by a branch of the posterior division of the femoral nerve and travels in close proximity with the vascular pedicle. Prior to the descending branch of the LCFA enters the vastus lateralis muscle, the motor nerve turns laterally and sends branches to innervate the undersurface of the vastus lateralis.

## Indications/Contraindications

Due to the versality of donor site tissue, including skin, fascia, and/or muscle, the ALT flap lends itself to the reconstruction of a variety of head and neck defects. In the oral cavity, the ALT flap can be used for the full range of tongue reconstruction: as a thin cutaneous perforator flap for partial glossectomy defects or as a myocutaneous flap including the vastus lateralis muscle for the reconstruction of near-total or total glossectomy defects. In cases which require dead space obliteration such as orbital exenteration defects, the myocutaneous ALT flap with vastus lateralis muscle can also be used. For through-and-through defects requiring the reconstruction of intraoral lining and external fascial skin, the ALT can be harvested with multiple skin paddles with separate perforator vessels, or de-epithelialized to create separate skin islands with a single perforator vessel [5, 6]. Additionally, as a flap which can provide significant bulk, the ALT flap can be used in total parotidectomy defects to restore facial form and volume. Finally, the tubed ALT flap has been described for esophageal reconstruction.

Relative contraindications of the ALT flap include thick hair-bearing skin of the upper thigh requiring significant postoperative grooming when used for reconstruction intraorally and inexperience with perforator flap dissection. In addition, the thickness of the flap may be disadvantageous for reconstruction of certain defects, providing unnecessary bulk at the recipient site.

## Preoperative Planning

During the preoperative evaluation, the surgeon should pay careful attention to patient's knee range of motion. Due to the location of the vascular pedicle through the vastus lateralis muscle, intramuscular dissection or even harvest of the vastus lateralis may cause increased risk of functional impairment of the knee postoperatively; however, many regain preoperative functionality [7, 8].

Unlike the peroneal artery which supplies the fibula free flap, the LCFA is rarely affected by atherosclerotic disease, and angiography is seldom required preoperatively. However, angiography can be obtained if there is concern for significant atherosclerosis or previous injury or operations of the upper thigh.

The recipient site should be heavily considered when deciding on the use of the ALT flap. Male patients may have thick hair overlying the lateral thigh, which is not ideal for certain recipient sites such as the oral cavity. This can be addressed with laser removal of hair preoperatively, or frequent shaving of the flap after reconstruction. In addition, in obese patients, the ALT flap may be excessively thick requiring primary thinning or secondary debulking procedures to achieve optimal outcomes.

## Instrument/Equipment Set

A hand-held Doppler can be used preoperatively to identify the approximate location of the cutaneous perforators prior to the initial incision. A typical soft tissue instrument set can be used for the dissection. When beginning the initial dissection, skin hooks can be utilized to retract the rectus femoris medially and the flap laterally to provide better exposure to the intermuscular septum. Alternatively, Allis clamps can be placed on the fascia to provide counter traction for exposure of the intermuscular septum. During perforator dissection, surgical clips are used to isolate the cutaneous perforator as it is traced back to the lateral LCFA. Microvascular anastomosis is performed using an operative microscope. Arterial anastomosis is performed with 8.0 or 9.0 nylon sutures, while venous anastomosis is performed with an appropriately sized venous coupler. If there are concerns with the integrity of the flap intraoperatively, near-infrared angiography can be used to determine the quality of perfusion throughout the flap. Although no single monitoring technique is widely accepted, a handheld Doppler or an implantable Doppler can be used postoperatively to monitor flap perfusion on the floor.

## Flap Design/Surgical Technique/Ducic Pearls

In the operating room, the patient is generally placed in the supine position. The anterior superior iliac spine and superolateral aspect of the patella are identified, and a line is drawn connecting these points with the midpoint of the line being marked. Figure 7.3 illustrates these markings. A handheld Doppler can be used to identify the general location of the cutaneous perforators. Once the cutaneous perforator is identified, the flap is marked out based on the size of the recipient defect while centered on the cutaneous perforator. A flap measuring up to 8 cm in width allows for primary closure of the donor site. The length of the flap is determined by the recipient's defect size with a maximum length of 40 cm which can be harvested [9]. The flap design can also be modified after visualization of the size and quality of the cutaneous perforators intraoperatively.

After marking the flap, the medial incision is made first through the skin and subcutaneous tissue down to the fascia over the rectus femoris muscle. Depending on the recipient defect needs, the flap can be harvested in either a subfascial or a suprafascial plane. The subfascial dissection allows for easier identification of the intermuscular septum and the perforator vessels. The length of intermuscular

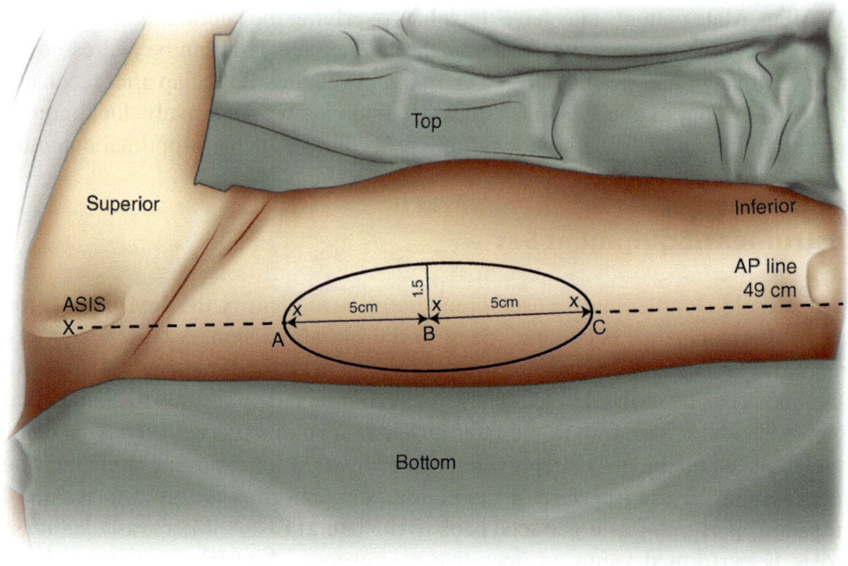


**Fig. 7.3** Position of the cutaneous perforators

septum is exposed, and the rectus femoris muscle is retracted medially to expose the descending branch of the LCFA. Septocutaneous perforators occur in approximately 10% of cases and can be traced back to the descending branch of the LCFA [10]. In cases with musculocutaneous perforator, an intramuscular dissection is executed and followed in a retrograde fashion to the descending branch of the LCFA. Fine tenotomy or Metzenbaum scissors are used to separate the muscle fibers from the perforator vessels. Any branching vessels that are identified are either cauterized with a fine bipolar tip or ligated. Once the descending branch of the LCFA is reached, the main pedicle is dissected until the adequate pedicle length is achieved. Care should be taken to identify and preserve the motor nerve to the vastus lateralis muscle along the course of the main pedicle. After confirmation of intact perforator vessels, the flap design is finalized. The posterior incision is made to complete flap harvest and taken to the vastus lateralis fascia if a subfascial dissection is performed. Carefully note the location of the pedicle as undue traction may injure the pedicle. The recipient vessels are prepared prior to pedicle division. Of note, a portion of, or the entire vastus lateralis musculature may be harvested with the free flap by dividing the muscle inferiorly and superiorly. This is helpful if additional bulk is needed at the recipient site. This technique also allows for expedited harvest of the ALT flap as time is saved by obviating the need for perforator dissection.

In most cases, the ALT donor site can be closed primarily as long as the width of the harvested flap is less than 8 cm. Defects that are wider require closure with a split-thickness skin graft. If a split-thickness skin graft is used, knee immobilization is preferred to allow for optimal skin graft take. Depending on the surgeon's preference, a closed-suction drain can be placed between the vastus lateralis and rectus femoris muscles to minimize seroma and hematoma formation.

## Postoperative Management

Flap monitoring to ensure flap viability is instituted immediately postoperatively and based on the surgeon's and institution's preference. Hourly flap monitoring is continued for the first 72 h postoperatively, either in the intensive care unit or in the specialized step-down unit. No specific pharmacologic therapies are required postoperatively; this is determined by the surgeon's preference. Our postoperative pharmacologic therapy includes the use of heparin and aspirin. For head and neck reconstruction, patients are positioned with the head of the bed elevated at 30°, and the neck is inspected to avoid compression by wires, intravenous lines, or tracheostomy straps, which may lead to pedicle compromise. If a closed-suction drain was placed, it can be removed once the output has decreased to ≤30 mL over 24 h.

The ALT flap has a low complication rate, which can include seroma, hematoma, wound dehiscence, infection, and neuroma [7]. The majority of patients regain their preoperative level of function, even with the division of the motor nerve to the vastus lateralis muscle or harvesting of the vastus lateralis muscle.

## References


1. Song YG, Chen GZ, Song YL. The free thigh flap: a new free flap concept based on the septocutaneous artery. Br J Plast Surg. 1984;37(2):149–59.
2. Sokoya M, Deleyiannis FW. A triple pedicle, near-total thigh flap supercharged with the flow-through technique. Eplasty. 2016;16:e4.
3. Yu P, Selber J. Perforator patterns of the anteromedial thigh flap. Plast Reconstr Surg. 2011;128(3):151e–7e.
4. Ribuffo D, Cigna E, Gargano F, Spalvieri C, Scuderi N. The innervated anterolateral thigh flap: anatomical study and clinical implications. Plast Reconstr Surg. 2005;115(2):464–70.
5. Lawson BR, Moreno MA. Head and neck reconstruction with chimeric anterolateral thigh free flap: indications, outcomes, and technical considerations. Otolaryngol Head Neck Surg. 2016;154(1):59–65.
6. Sun G, Lu M, Hu Q, Tang E. Reconstruction of extensive through-and-through cheek defects with free anterolateral thigh flap. J Craniofac Surg. 2014;25(1):e31–8.
7. Hanasono MM, Skoracki RJ, Yu P. A prospective study of donor-site morbidity after anterolateral thigh fasciocutaneous and myocutaneous free flap harvest in 220 patients. Plast Reconstr Surg. 2010;125(1):209–14.
8. Weise H, Naros A, Blumenstock G, Krimmel M, Hoefert S, Kluba S, et al. Donor site morbidity of the anterolateral thigh flap. J Craniomaxillofac Surg. 2017;45(12):2105–8.
9. Chen HC, Tang YB. Anterolateral thigh flap: an ideal soft tissue flap. Clin Plast Surg. 2003;30(3):383–401.
10. Wei FC, Jain V, Celik N, Chen HC, Chuang DC, Lin CH. Have we found an ideal soft-tissue flap? An experience with 672 anterolateral thigh flaps. Plast Reconstr Surg. 2002;109(7):2219–26; discussion 27–30.

# Free Rectus Flap Reconstruction

# 8

Aurora G. Vincent and Spenceer R. Anderson

## Introduction

The abdominal rectus free flap (ARFF) is a well-known vascularized free tissue flap utilized among reconstructive surgeons [1–4]. The ARFF was first described in 1980 [3] and later popularized by Hartrampf in 1982 [5], ultimately becoming a workhorse flap for a diverse array of reconstructive needs. The ARFF is often the head and neck reconstructive flap of choice for wounds that require bulky tissue for adequate reconstruction. The ARFF offers consistent flap anatomy, ease of technical elevation, up to 15 cm of pedicle length, as well as the opportunity for a well-hidden donor site scar [5, 6]. Herein, we review the ARFF including preoperative planning needs, patient candidacy, intraoperative technique, postoperative monitoring, and donor site management.

## Operative Steps

### Preoperative Considerations

The ARFF is a useful flap when a larger tissue bulk is needed for head and neck reconstruction. It is worth considering in patients with a normal or low BMI. However,

A. G. Vincent (✉)
Eisenhower Army Medical Center, Fort Gordon, GA, USA
e-mail: aurora.g.vincent.mil@health.mil

S. R. Anderson
Division of Plastic and Reconstructive Surgery, Wright State University Boonshoft School of Medicine, Dayton, OH, USA


F. Sokoya, A. G. Vincent (eds.), *Manual of Head and Neck Reconstruction*,
https://doi.org/10.1007/978-3-031-65999-7_8

it is often not appropriate in patients who are overweight or obese, as excess subcutaneous adiposity creates too much tissue bulk in those cases. The ARFF is ideal for reconstruction of total glossectomy defects and obliteration of deep wounds (such as maxillectomy defects that included overlying skin excision, exenteration defects, etc.) Patients should be queried about and examined for previous abdominal surgeries and scars. Ports for many laparoscopic procedures are often outside the dissection area for a rectus flap, so having had these procedures does not disqualify a patient from undergoing ARFF harvest. Previous open abdominal surgery, however, may have compromised the flap pedicle.

## Flap Features

1. Vascular Supply: The arterial supply is derived from the deep inferior epigastric artery and its perforators. The venous outflow is via the venae comitantes.
2. Bulk: Significant bulk suitable for total glossectomy defect reconstruction or deep wound obliteration. Flap includes muscle, subcutaneous adipose tissue, and overlying skin. If a thinner bulk is necessary and a thinner flap (such as a radial forearm flap) is not available, then the ARFF can be raised as a deep inferior epigastric perforator flap that includes only skin and subcutaneous tissue. This technique requires perforator dissection through the rectus muscle.
3. Innervation: Thoracoabdominal nerve. Harvested flap is insensate.

## Steps of Harvest

1. Prep the abdomen from the palpable inferior edge of the ribs to the iliac crest. Typically, prep can end, medially, just superior to where pubic hair begins; it should not need to be trimmed or prepped into the field.
2. Mark a box, roughly 6 × 6 cm, centered vertically at the umbilicus, with its medial edge just lateral to the umbilicus (Fig. 8.1). Releasing incisions can be marked extending superiorly and inferiorly, 2–3 cm lateral to the umbilicus. The superior extension should extend to the edge of the rectus muscle, just below the rib margin. The inferior incision should extend to where the anterior and posterior rectus fascia combine. Typically, this location can be visualized or palpated.
   (a) The shape of the flap can be altered from a square, as desired, given the wound location, function, and size. In general, a 6 × 6 cm square is a good starting point and is typically a sufficient size for a total glossectomy defect. The flap should not be made of a significantly smaller size, or there is an increased risk of damaging or excluding arterial perforators important for flap survival.
   (b) Note: There is no need to doppler out the location of perforating vessels. Arterial perforators are reliably located 2–3 cm lateral to the umbilicus.

**Fig. 8.1** Rectus free flap initial markings

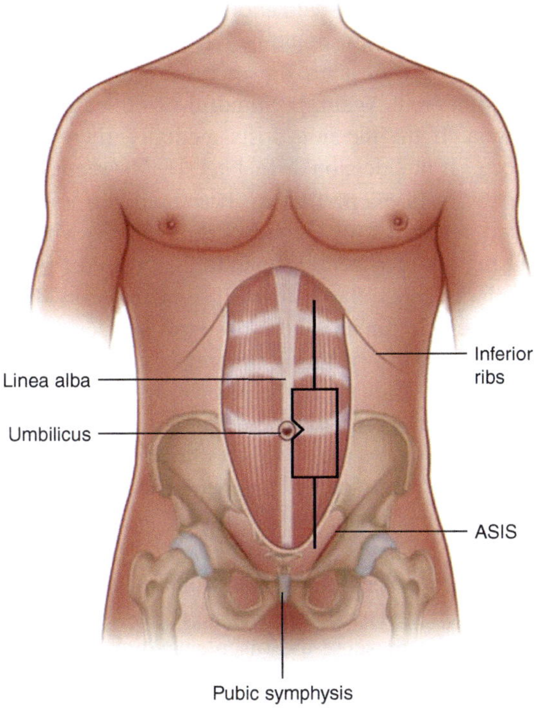


Thus, if making a 6 × 6-cm flap centered at the umbilicus, the perforating vessels will be in the center.

3. Incise along all markings; the authors prefer to make initial incisions with a #15, then carry incisions deeper with spatula-tipped insulated Bovie to the anterior surface of the anterior rectus sheath. Dissection should be carried deeply perpendicular to the anterior surface of the anterior rectus sheath. Of note, if the dissection drifts away from the perpendicular, it may risk damage to perforating arteries.
4. Laterally, dissection should extend along the superficial surface of the anterior rectus sheath until the rectus line is identified. This dissection can be completed rapidly with bovie, as it is not near any vascular structures of note.
5. Secure the skin paddle to the underlying anterior rectus sheath along the edges of the flap with multiple 3-0 vicryl sutures. This step is performed to prevent accidental shear of the skin paddle off the underlying muscle with future manipulation of the flap. Of note, if the flap is going to end up in the mouth or pharynx, then the sutures do not have to be buried. If the flap will end up on the skin, then the sutures should be buried.

6. Incise the anterior rectus fascia and rectus muscle at the lateral edge of the flap. If necessary for visualization, the superior cut can also be made, but the inferior aspect of the flap should be left along to preserve the pedicle. Extend this incision deeply through the rectus muscle until the posterior rectus sheath is encountered. Again, be mindful of dissection perpendicular to the abdominal fascia. If the incision drifts medially, then injury to the flap perforators can occur. If the incision drifts laterally, the rectus line may be encountered and the posterior fascia perforated. If a small perforation in the posterior fascia is created, repair it with 3-0 vicryl and oversew with 2-0 PDS.
7. Using a kitner, gently separate the posterior surface of the rectus muscle to be included in the flap from the posterior rectus sheath. Of note, the vascular pedicle vessels run along the posterior surface of the muscle, so it is important to be precise in separating the muscle from the fascia. Leaving muscular fascia down risks damage to the pedicle, whereas lifting posterior sheath into the flap risks sheath perforation and herniation of abdominal contents.
   (a) A kitner is a useful tool for sweeping along the face of the posterior sheath; it can neatly reveal the appropriate tissue plane, will not accidentally perforate the posterior sheath, and will not damage the pedicle vessels if it bumps them.
8. Visualize the pedicle vessels along the deep surface of the flap.
9. Complete incisions through the rectus muscle around all sides of the flap, taking care to preserve the vascular pedicle as it travels inferiorly and taking care not to separate the pedicle from the flap itself. Superiorly, the flap can be efficiently released by using monopolar cautery to cut through rectus muscle onto the surgeon's underlying finger. Take care medially not to enter the umbilicus. Inferior to the flap, the pedicle can be bluntly dissected away from overlying muscle with Metzenbaum scissors (in a cold fashion without cautery), then protected with a finger placed between the vessels and the overlying muscle while Bovie is used to rapidly separate that muscle.
   (a) A finger is a useful insulating tool in this dissection, as it will not conduct heat energy to the vessels. Monopolar cautery should be used cautiously or not at all when in close proximity to the flap vessels, as aberrant heat spread can injure vessels and compromise flap survival.
   (b) Metzenbaum scissors are useful for releasing the flap vessels from overlying muscle given their blunt tips. Appropriate spread will break weak, natural fascial attachments surrounding the vessels before breaking vessel walls or causing excessive muscular bleeding. Dissection with sharper scissors risks damage to vascular walls or bleeding from muscular tissue.
10. Dissect out the length of the pedicle inferiorly. Again, cold dissection with metzenbaum scissors allows efficient separation of tissue to proceed safely. After a sufficient length of the pedicle is achieved, the pedicle and flap can be separated. The authors prefer ligating the inferior aspect of the vessels with surgical clips, free silk ties, or a combination of the two. The pedicle vessels themselves

do not require clips or ties, and use of such may compromise the tip ends at the time of reanastomosis. The authors do not advocate the use of any cautery near the site of pedicle ligation, as it can cause vascular injury that may compromise flap survival. Figure 8.2 depicts a harvested ARFF before inset, and Fig. 8.3 depicts a total glossectomy wound (a) reconstructed with an ARFF (b).

## Steps of Closure

1. Irrigate the wound with copious amounts of saline. This is an important step before the closure of all surgical wounds, as it can greatly decrease the risk of surgical wound infections.
2. Dissect laterally along the anterior rectus sheath to allow primary closure of the wound.
3. Reapproximate the anterior rectus sheath. 2-0 pds can be used in a running fashion for this reapproximation. A wide ribbon retractor (3–4 cm width) should be placed over the posterior rectus sheath, beneath the anterior rectus fascia, during reapproximation to prevent accidental needle-violation of the posterior sheath.
4. Close the skin and subcutaneous tissue in layers. The skin can be tailored superiorly and inferiorly to where the flap was harvested to facilitate a straight-line closure.
   (a) The authors typically place two bulb-suction fully perforated 10F flat drains in the wound bed, to be removed 1 to 2 weeks postoperatively. At minimum, two layers of suture should be used.
   (b) The authors prefer closure of subcutaneous tissues with multiple 3-0 interrupted vicryl sutures, then skin closure with a running prolene as this allows efficient and cosmetically acceptable wound closure.
5. Cover the wound with antibacterial ointment, telfa, and an abdominal binder.

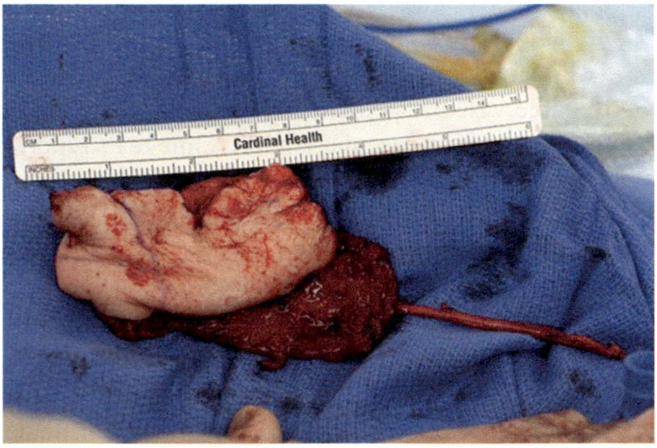


**Fig. 8.2** Harvested rectus free flap

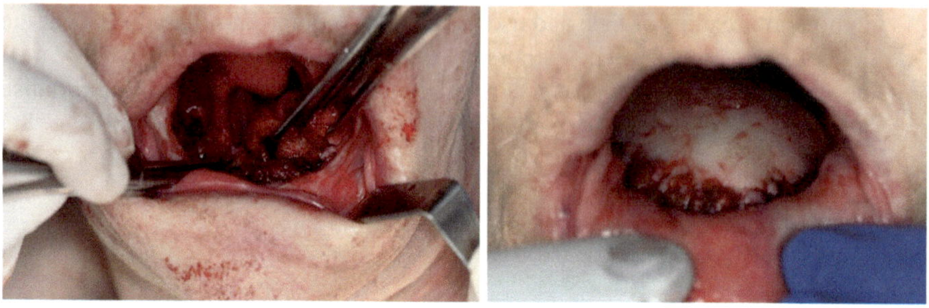

**Fig. 8.3** Glossectomy defect before and after rectus inset

## Postoperative Care and Complications

Rectus flaps should be monitored in a similar fashion to other free tissue transfers; flaps should be monitored very closely for vascular compromise in the initial 72 h after surgery, then closely but less intensively over the next 96 h. Drains are commonly left in the harvest site for one to 2 weeks, until the output is serous in quality and stable in quantity. Patients should wear an abdominal binder for 1 month after surgery and avoid abdominal exercise for 3 months. If permanent sutures are placed for skin closure, they should be removed 7 to 10 days after placement to avoid cosmetically unfavorable "train track" markings from forming. Light walking is acceptable the day after surgery and, if patients are capable, is encouraged to prevent venous thromboses.

## Pearls

1. Quick and easy harvest with no need for patient repositioning when combined with extirpation of the majority of head and neck cancers. Ultrasound identification of perforators is not necessary when muscle is harvested with appropriate initial markings.
2. Two-team approach (concurrent excision and flap harvest).
3. Reliable vascular pedicle anatomy, more so than from anterolateral thigh flaps, with a moderate vascular length. Some texts report that a vascular pedicle length of up to 15 cm can be harvested. The authors have observed a harvest length of 7 cm or so to be more typical, meaning, for a total glossectomy defect, the donor vessels in the neck need to be nearby (facial vessels, lingual artery, external carotid terminus, etc.) or vein grafts will be necessary to complete anastomosis.
4. Option for perforator flap harvest that does not include muscle and has less bulk and less recovery time.
5. Primary closure of the harvest site is standard.
6. If a small perforation of the posterior fascia is made, it can be repaired primarily with 3-0 vicryl, and the repair oversewn with 2-0 PDS. If this happens, surgeons should code for a hernia repair.

## Conclusion

The ARFF is an advantageous flap that can be employed in a diverse array of head and neck-based defects requiring skin, soft tissue bulk, and muscle. However, for a successful outcome, the prospective patient should be closely evaluated in effort to determine candidacy for an ARFF-based operation. Morbid obesity and prior abdominal procedures may preclude a patient from undergoing this specific flap procedure. For those patients who are candidates, the ARFF offers the opportunity for a two-team approach at both the donor and the recipient site, leading to overall operative efficiency. The ARFF technique displays consistent anatomy, ease of flap elevation, and vessel size similar to that of neck vessels without significant size to size mismatch. Additionally, pending patient body habitus, the ARFF provides a large cutaneous surface area in conjunction with fatty bulk and muscle not seen in other flap alternatives making this flap ideal for large, complex head and neck defect reconstruction. The ARFF is an established workhorse flap secondary to proven reproducible reliability and versatility and should be considered an effective tool within the reconstructive head and neck surgeon's armamentarium.

## References


1. Basaran B, Ünsaler S, Kesimli M, Aslan Î. Free flap reconstruction of the head and neck region: a series of 127 flaps performed by otolaryngologists. Turk Arch Otorhinolaryngol. 2021;59(2):103–10.
2. Low H, Lindsay A, Clark J, Chai F, Lewis R. Reconstruction of maxillary defect with musculo-adipose rectus free flap. Microsurgery. 2017;37:137–41.
3. Kozusko S, Liu X, Riccio C, et al. Selecting a free flap for soft tissue coverage in lower extremity reconstruction. Injury. 2019;50(S5):S32–9.
4. Pryor S, Moore E, Kasperbauer J. Orbital exenteration reconstruction with rectus abdominis microvascular free flap. Laryngoscope. 2005;115:1912–6.
5. Chung T, Wilson K, Patil Y. Double deep inferior epigastric arteries encountered during vertical rectus abdominis flap harvest: a case report and literature review. Ear Nose Throat J. 2013;92(6):E34–7.
6. Lee S, You H, Kim D. Dual vascular free transverse rectus abdominis myocutaneous flap for hemifacial reconstruction in a vessel-depleted neck. Arch Plast Surg. 2020;47:88–91.

# Part III

# Fasciocutaneous Flaps

# The Radial Forearm Free Flap

# 9

Sammy Othman and Jason Cohn

## Introduction/History

In 1970s, a concern for flap harvest involving reliable, thin, pliable skin became one of the forefront endeavors in regard to free tissue transfer. Subsequently, Song et al., a group hailing from China, described the earliest documented utilization of the radial forearm flap to address these concerns [1]. Subsequently, the radial forearm flap has become a workhorse as a pedicled, reverse-flow pedicled, and free flap for a variety of defects and lesions from head to toe [2–6]. The head and neck regions in particular have found great success in the re-surfacing of defects using various iterations of the radial forearm flap, with various components including fasciocutaneous, fascial, osteocutaneous, and neurotized flaps with several unique flap designs, owning to its consistent anatomy that allows for versatile tissue architecture [7–9].

## Anatomy

The radial forearm flap (RFF) is harvested as an axial flap based on the radial artery, which supplies the perforators to the radial forearm. The origin of the radial artery, stemming as a terminal branch of the brachial artery, can be palpated through the antecubital fossa, giving a large pedicle length between 15 and 22 cm, dependent on patient anatomy [2, 5, 7, 9–11]. The radial artery is accompanied by pairs of venae comitans, or alternatively, the cephalic or basilic veins can be harvested when larger source anastomoses are desired or when multiple venous anastomoses are desired.

S. Othman
Division of Plastic and Reconstructive Surgery, Department of Surgery, Northwell Health, New York, NY, USA

J. Cohn (✉)
Cohn Plastic Surgery, PC, Smithtown, NY, USA



F. Sokoya, A. G. Vincent (eds.), *Manual of Head and Neck Reconstruction*, https://doi.org/10.1007/978-3-031-65999-7_9

The perforators of the radial artery to this region are fasciocutaneous, piercing through the antebrachial fascia of the forearm. Rarely, the flap is raised as a perforator flap, and even more rarely in the context of free tissue transfer [11, 12]. Distally, the pedicle and radial artery runs just deep to the intermuscular septum between the brachioradialis and flexor capri radialis muscles.

The nerve supply to this region includes both the lateral and medial antecubital nerves, depending on desired dimensions of the flap and specific flap design [3, 7, 10]. Briefly, the lateral antecubital nerve is a branch of the musculocutaneous nerve, beginning near the antecubital fossa, and travels intimately with the cephalic vein where it divides into volar and dorsal branches. It is the volar branch that can be harvested for a sensate flap utilization. The medial antecubital nerve is a direct trunk from the branchial plexus, where in the middle third of the upper arm, descending along the ulnar half of the forearm distally [13–16].

When an osseous component is desired, a section of radius may be harvested. The exact dimensions are varied, but typically this ranges from the insertion of the pronator teres to proximal to the radial styloid, one-third in width or smaller, and up to 14 cm [6, 17–21].

Owning to this diversity in anatomy, this can be raised as fasciocutaenous flap (most common), fascial-only flap, or variations of osseous flap based on the radius. If desired, it can also include tendon and neurotization options [8, 22, 23]. There are many well-established flap designs, outlining the popularity and heterogeneity afforded by the radial forearm.

## Indication/Contraindications

The RFF is a versatile flap owning to its thin, pliable texture, ability to raise with or without hair, consistent blood supply, and options in raising fascial and osseous components. As such, it can be used for a range of defects for the head and neck, including nasal reconstruction, lip reconstruction, intraoral resurfacing, including tongue and buccal defects, ear reconstruction, scalp reconstruction, pharyngeal resurfacing, and neck resurfacing [2, 5, 8, 24–32].

Relative contraindications to harvest include general health concerns for major reconstruction and concerns for vascular compromise to the donor site. This includes poor perfusion to the digits and history or suspected clinical peripheral artery disease. If necessary, the radial artery may be reconstructed, most often with a saphenous vein graft, or an intact remaining cephalic and basilic vein, to keep an intact inflow to the palmar arch [33–37]. Furthermore, caution should be taken when considering an osseous component in the elderly or those prone to osteoporosis or other bony disease, given the donor site morbidity of radial bone harvest.

## Preoperative Planning

A commonly cited disadvantage of the RFF is what is often sacrifice of a major axial vessel in the radial artery. Clinically, this, along with the ulnar artery, is a main contributor to the palmer arch and subsequently blood supply to the hand. It is important to inquire about prior manipulation of the vessels, such as history of arterial lines, arteriovenous fistula formation, and intravenous catheters, particularly in the situation of cephalic vein harvest for venous egress. As such, evaluation of an intact palmer arch must be elucidated with the Allen's Test. At times, this exam may be equivocal, or patient history may dictate a requirement for further or more objective testing. This can necessitate computer tomography angiography (CTA) or ultrasound with an experienced sonographer [35–37].

Patients must also be counseled on donor site morbidity, as sensation may be lost the area. Additionally, an unsightly scar will be present in anatomically exposed area, particularly when a longer pedicle is required. When a bony component is planned, there will be a longer recovery period and a significantly increased risk of fracture, even patients are adherent to rehabilitation planning [12, 17, 19–21, 38]. This all includes the likelihood of requiring a skin graft to secondarily cover the donor site, which is always at risk and leads to skin mismatch, both at the skin graft donor and recipient site [12, 21]. Finally, the process of recovery after skin graft harvest is sometimes painful, and this should be discussed prior to the operation.

## Instrumentation

Standard operative instrumentation and microsurgical instrumentation are required. These include major plastic surgery/otolaryngology trays and biceps forceps trays. Specifically, necessary instruments include dissecting scissors, such as Stevens and Metzenbaum, hemoclip appliers, and nylon sutures. Additionally, Browns, Addison-browns, and jeweler forceps are also helpful during dissection. Iris and double skin hooks, Army-Navy, and Senn retractors all have a role in exposure. Finally, bovie cautery and various blade sizes are necessary for dissection dependent on surgeon preference and experience. The specific details of tool vary by surgeon preference and institutional tray setup. In most cases, a dermatome will be required for skin graft harvest, and a pneumatic tourniquet cuff will be utilized during flap dissection.

## Flap Design and Surgical Technique

### Flap Design and Preparation

The patient is placed in a supine position with the arm extended in anatomic volar-up positioning, prepped widely passed the antecubital fossa. Using a template for the defect to be reconstructed, this is traced over the volar distal forearm centered upon the radial artery with preference to the underlying cephalic vein. These markings can be extended ulnarly to the ulnar bone and radially to the lateral axial portion of the radius as necessary, and with desire to capture or spare hair-bearing regions as necessary. Length-wise, the flap can extend to near the takeoff the radial artery, resulting in a flap size of up to 30 × 15 $cm^2$, again dependent on patient habitus, though more commonly, significantly smaller flap dimensions are required. From the tip of skin paddle to the antecubital fossa, a lazy-S marking is created to minimize axial scar burden, contracture, and wound healing (Fig. 9.1). A pneumatic torniquet is placed proximal to the elbow joint and, when ready, elevated to 250 mmHg for up to 90 min. Only light exsanguination is recommended to facilitate identification of the vasculature during dissection.

## Dissection and Elevation

There are numerous described methods for approaches to dissection, including distal to proximal, proximal to distal, ulnar to radial, radial to ulnar, and combinations therein. One common approach involves dissecting in the ulnar to radial direction at the distal end of the flap. In this pattern, dissection begins from the ulnar border of the flap marking, elevating down to the deep fascia to reveal the palmaris longus tendon. Depending on flap design and goal, this can be left or dissected out to include within the flap. Dissection then continues until identification flexor capri radialis tendon. Superficial veins can be ligated throughout the process to prevent egress bleeding during dissection and later elevation. From the radial aspect of dissection, there is care to preserve two critical structures in the cephalic vein and superficial branch of the radial nerve, both of which run radial to the brachioradialis tendon. At this juncture, the superficial branch of the radial nerve, which runs closely to the cephalic vein and anteriorly to the brachioradialis tendon, is identified and protected to preserve sensation to distal dorsal forearm and hand. Additionally, the cephalic vein, which runs in the deep subcutaneous plane, should be protected if intended for harvest. Once adequate exposure is achieved, the deep fascia and

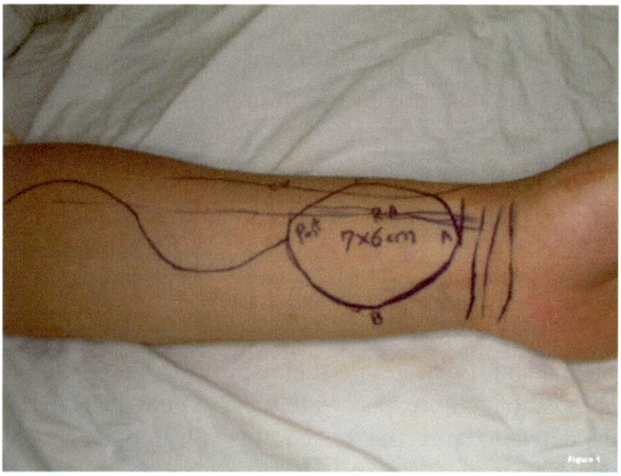


**Fig. 9.1** Preoperative markings for incision and flap design, with the presumptive pedicle path traced

intermuscular septum, which is located at the junction between the flexor carpi radialis and brachioradialis, is incised to reveal the radial artery and venae comitans.

As mentioned, the radial artery runs just deep to the intermuscular septum between the brachioradialis and flexor capri radialis muscles at the distal end. The distal edge of the flap can be incised at this point or prior towards radial dissection. Dividing the septum and fascia, with gentle muscular retraction, provides adequate exposure to the radial artery and its venae comitans as necessary (Fig. 9.2). Care must be taken to preserve the perforators to the flap. Additionally, care is taken to adequately dissect and elevate the vessels, with erroneous branches ligated. Additionally, the paratenon of surrounding tendons must be protected to ensure optimal skin graft take.

The distal edge of the vessels can be ligated and divided, and dissection continues with an incision of the proximal edge of the flap in order to dissect towards the source pedicle. An incision along the "Lazy-S" marking is made down to the muscular fascia. The vessels will then be traced distal to proximal. The radial artery tends to run under the brachioradialis muscle as it runs more proximally, and thus, the brachioradialis fascia must be incised with the muscle being released (Fig. 9.3). Gentle retraction is again necessary for complete exposure. Dissection is continued proximally to the source of the radial artery to its takeoff point from the brachial artery. At this point, there is debate of whether to preserve the deep and superficial venous systems if both were adequately preserved, though recent literature indicates that flap survival is not affected by either choice. Once elevated with adequate recipient site preparation, the proximal ends of the pedicle can be ligated, and the flap can be fully harvested for transfer.

## Donor Site Closure

If the width of the skin paddle is minimal, often 3 cm or less with good skin laxity, the donor site may be closed primarily. Often times, however, a split-thickness skin graft is required. The lateral thigh is the preferred donor site; meshing is often not required; however, fenestrations are recommended to maximize graft take. Dermatome setting is often to 0.0018 of an inch for harvest of the skin graft. The

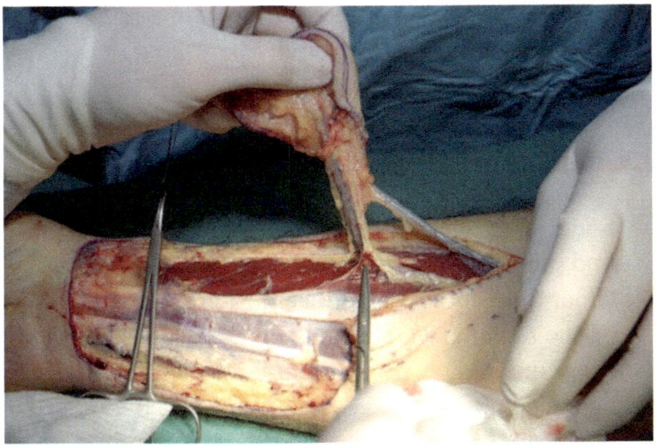

**Fig. 9.2** Radial forearm flap elevation with preservation of the accompanying venae comitans as well as the cephalic vein

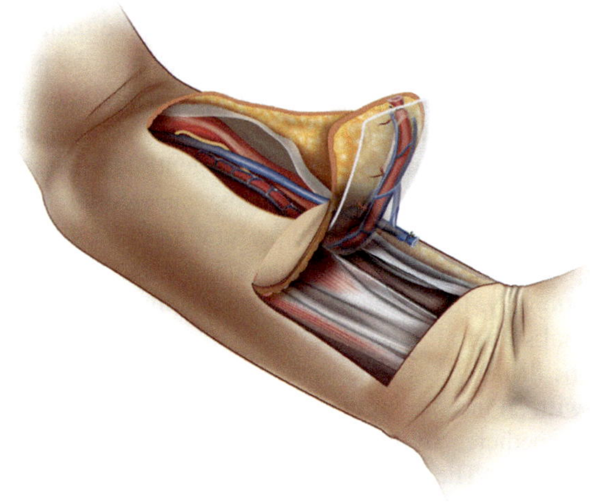

**Fig. 9.3** With the flap elevated, dissection of the pedicle commences. The radial artery enters deep to the brachioradialis muscle mid-way through the forearm, requiring gentle retraction of the muscle

graft should be adequately fitted placed, and ensuring of tendon exposure is critical. The authors recommend anchor sutures, followed by circumferential running sutures.

## Postoperative Management

Flap checks with a pencil Doppler are recommended every one to 2 h for the first 48 h postoperatively.

For the donor site, a splint or wound VAC can be used to expedite healing, optimize take, and minimize shear. Either is removed after 7 days. Patients may be allowed to the use the extremity as tolerated. However, care is taken to minimize postoperative pain and edema. These include elevation and appropriate use of multimodal pain control.

When an osseous component is removed, a minimum of 6 to 8 weeks of immobilization with splinting is required, with a restriction in usage of up to ten pounds, with a gradual increase in activity permitted.

## Pearls/Pitfalls

- Some surgeons advocate for proximal-to-distal dissection, though most surgeons find proximal to distal more intuitive and easier to learn.
- Ulnar dissection is safer, as most critical structures relevant to the operation are on the radial aspect (radial nerve branches and cephalic vein).
- Keep the goals of hair-bearing or hair-sparing regions in mind when planning flap design.

- Preoperative history and physical is paramount to optimizing vessel selection and minimizing postoperative complications.
- It is generally easier, and safer, to take a suprafascial approach until critical structures are identified, although some surgeons will pursue subfascial dissection due to experience, ease, and time efficiency.
- It is recommended to preserve both venous systems (i.e., both venae comitans and cephalic/basilic veins), even when not planned, due to unforeseen difficulties and to have "bailout" options.

## References

1. Song R, Gao Y, Song Y, Yu Y, Song Y. The forearm flap. Clin Plast Surg. 1982;9(1):21–6.
2. Soutar DS, Scheker LR, Tanner NS, McGregor IA. The radial forearm flap: a versatile method for intra-oral reconstruction. Br J Plast Surg. 1983;36(1):1–8.
3. Chicarilli ZN, Price GJ. Complete plantar foot coverage with the free neurosensory radial forearm flap. Plast Reconstr Surg. 1986;78(1):94–101.
4. Kelly KE, Anthony JP, Singer M. Pharyngoesophageal reconstruction using the radial forearm fasciocutaneous free flap: preliminary results. Otolaryngol Head Neck Surg. 1994;111(1):16–24.
5. Calhoun KH. Radial forearm free flap for head and neck reconstruction. Facial Plast Surg. 1996;12(1):29–33.
6. Harris PA, Butler PE, Takushima A. Radial forearm osteocutaneous flap for mandibular reconstruction. Plast Reconstr Surg. 2002;110(4):1196; author reply 1196.
7. Timmons MJ. The vascular basis of the radial forearm flap. Plast Reconstr Surg. 1986;77(1):80–92.
8. Petrolati M, Delaria G, Abbiati G, Tremolada C. Observations on the use of radial forearm (Chinese) and posterior interosseous reverse pedicled island flaps in hand surgery. Plast Reconstr Surg. 1991;88(1):175–7.
9. Moscoso JF, Urken ML. Radial forearm flaps. Otolaryngol Clin N Am. 1994;27(6):1119–40.
10. Demirkan F, Wei FC, Lutz BS, Cher TS, Chen IH. Reliability of the venae comitantes in venous drainage of the free radial forearm flaps. Plast Reconstr Surg. 1998;102(5):1544–8.
11. Chin KY. Dominant radial artery perforator in the proximal forearm. Plast Reconstr Surg. 2011;127(2):1013.
12. Chang EI, Liu J. Prospective comparison of donor-site morbidity following radial forearm and ulnar artery perforator flap harvest. Plast Reconstr Surg. 2020;145(5):1267–74.
13. Brown JM, Yablon CM, Morag Y, Brandon CJ, Jacobson JA. US of the peripheral nerves of the upper extremity: a landmark approach. Radiographics. 2016;36(2):452–63.
14. Anderson TB, Bordoni B. Anatomy, shoulder and upper limb, forearm nerves. In: StatPearls. Treasure Island: StatPearls Publishing; 2022.
15. Patel M, Varacallo M. Anatomy, shoulder and upper limb, arm nerves. In: StatPearls. Treasure Island: StatPearls Publishing; 2022.
16. Okwumabua E, Thompson JH. Anatomy, shoulder and upper limb, nerves. In: StatPearls. Treasure Island: StatPearls Publishing; 2022.
17. Yajima H, Tamai S, Yamauchi T, Mizumoto S. Osteocutaneous radial forearm flap for hand reconstruction. J Hand Surg Am. 1999;24(3):594–603.
18. Koshima I, Tsutsui T, Nanba Y, Takahashi Y, Akisada K. Free radial forearm osteocutaneous perforator flap for reconstruction of total nasal defects. J Reconstr Microsurg. 2002;18(7):585–8; discussion 589–90.

19. Villaret DB, Futran NA. The indications and outcomes in the use of osteocutaneous radial forearm free flap. Head Neck. 2003;25(6):475–81.
20. Arganbright JM, Tsue TT, Girod DA, et al. Outcomes of the osteocutaneous radial forearm free flap for mandibular reconstruction. JAMA Otolaryngol Head Neck Surg. 2013;139(2):168–72.
21. Dediol E, Uglesic V, Knezevic P, Lemac D. Donor-site outcomes for the osteocutaneous radial forearm free flap. J Reconstr Microsurg. 2017;33(8):e3–4.
22. Ciria-Llorens G, Gomez-Cia T, Talegon-Melendez A. Analysis of flow changes in forearm arteries after raising the radial forearm flap: a prospective study using colour duplex imaging. Br J Plast Surg. 1999;52(6):440–4.
23. Shuck J, Chang EI, Mericli AF, et al. Free lateral forearm flap in head and neck reconstruction: an attractive alternative to the radial forearm flap. Plast Reconstr Surg. 2020;146(4):446e–50e.
24. Chicarilli ZN, Ariyan S, Cuono CB. Single-stage repair of complex scalp and cranial defects with the free radial forearm flap. Plast Reconstr Surg. 1986;77(4):577–85.
25. McGregor AD. The free radial forearm flap—the management of the secondary defect. Br J Plast Surg. 1987;40(1):83–5.
26. Davidson J, Boyd B, Gullane P, et al. A comparison of the results following oromandibular reconstruction using a radial forearm flap with either radial bone or a reconstruction plate. Plast Reconstr Surg. 1991;88(2):201–8.
27. Cordeiro PG, Mastorakos DP, Shaha AR. The radial forearm fasciocutaneous free-tissue transfer for tracheostomy reconstruction. Plast Reconstr Surg. 1996;98(2):354–7.
28. Watanabe T, Furuta S, Hataya Y, Yuzuriha S, Otsuka Y. Reconstruction of the eyelids and nose after a burn injury using a radial forearm flap. Burns. 1997;23(4):360–5.
29. Zhou K, Luong JK, Clark JR, Ch'ng S. Coned radial forearm free flap for improved retention of orbital prosthesis following orbital exenteration. Plast Reconstr Surg. 2018;142(5):818e–9e.
30. Sokoya M, Bahrami A, Cohn J, Sahwney R, Kohlert S, Ducic Y. The radial forearm free flap for scalp and forehead reconstruction: a 20-year experience. Clin Otolaryngol. 2018;43(6):1611–3.
31. Salibian AH, Menick FJ, Talley J. Microvascular reconstruction of the nose with the radial forearm flap: a 17-year experience in 47 patients. Plast Reconstr Surg. 2019;144(1):199–210.
32. Sokoya M, Vincent A, Cohn JE, Kadakia S, Kohlert S, Ducic Y. Comparison of radial forearm free flap and gastric pull-up in pharyngo-oesophageal reconstruction. Clin Otolaryngol. 2019;44(3):405–7.
33. Kiehn M, Brooks D, Lee C, Kind G, Buntic R, Buncke G. Patency of radial arteries reconstructed after radial forearm flap harvest. J Reconstr Microsurg. 2007;23(6):347–9.
34. Knobloch K, Vogt PM. On "patency of radial arteries reconstructed after radial forearm flap harvest (J Reconstr Microsurg 2007;23:347–350)". J Reconstr Microsurg. 2009;25(1):77–8; author reply 79–80.
35. Kamienski RW, Barnes RW. Critique of the Allen test for continuity of the palmar arch assessed by Doppler ultrasound. Surg Gynecol Obstet. 1976;142(6):861–4.
36. Kaplanoglu H, Beton O. Evaluation of anatomy and variations of superficial palmar arch and upper extremity arteries with CT angiography. Surg Radiol Anat. 2017;39(4):419–26.
37. Krassnig R, Hohenberger GM, Schwarz AM, et al. The important relationship between the radial artery's course and the radius during Henry's anterior forearm surgical exposure. Clin Anat. 2020;33(7):983–7.
38. Deleyiannis FW, Sacks JM, McLean KM, Russavage JM. Patient self-report of disability of the upper extremity following osteocutaneous radial forearm free flap harvest. Plast Reconstr Surg. 2008;122(5):1479–84.

# Cervicodeltopectoral Flap

# 10

Nima Vahidi, Kevin Quinn, Cheryl Yu, Seung Lee, and Thomas S. Lee

## Introduction

The deltopectoral fasciocutaneous (DP) flap, also known as the Bakamjian flap, has been a widely used and described reconstructive option for head and neck surgery. In 1917, Aymard first described the use of the fasciocutaneous DP flap in a tubed fashion for staged nasal reconstruction. However, wide popularization of the DP flap did not come until the 1960s, when Bakamjian described the use of a medially-based DP flap for the reconstruction of laryngopharyngectomy defects and resurfacing of mucocutaneous defects of the head and neck [1]. A more recent modification to the original DP flap is the cervicodeltopectoral (CDP) flap which includes the cervical extension of the DP flap. The CDP flap is a pedicled fasciocutaneous flap that is based off of the first, second, and third internal mammary arteries. Along with its associated cervical skin and platysma, the CDP flap can be utilized to cover large anterolateral facial and neck skin defects. The CDP flap's unreliability with salivary exposure limits its usage in cases of intraoral mucosal and pharyngeal defects with extensive salivary exposure. Although it has been used successfully by Ducic and Smith to provide buccal mucosal lining as well as external cheek skin defect (by turning the skin flap on to itself and de-epithelializing the portion that will be buried), whenever it is being used around the oral cavity, it is imperative to avoid salivary exposure to the subdermal layers of the CDP flap as it will likely lead to skin flap infection and failure [2].

N. Vahidi · K. Quinn · C. Yu · S. Lee · T. S. Lee (✉)
Department of Otolaryngology, Virginia Commonwealth University Hospital, Richmond, VA, USA
e-mail: Nima.vahidi@vcuhealth.org; Kevin.quinn@vcuhealth.org; Cheryl.yu@vcuhealth.org; Seung.lee@vcu.edu; Thomas.Lee@vcuhealth.org


F. Sokoya, A. G. Vincent (eds.), *Manual of Head and Neck Reconstruction*,
https://doi.org/10.1007/978-3-031-65999-7_10

## Anatomy

The CDP flap includes superior extension of the fasciocutaneous DP flap that incorporates cervical skin and platysma located inferior to the site of the defect and anterior to the trapezius muscle. The CDP flap also includes the inferior neck and upper chest skin located medial to the cephalic vein and superior to the third intercostal space.

## Neurovascular Supply

The internal mammary artery (IMA), also known as the internal thoracic artery, is a branch of the subclavian artery that runs inferiorly along the inside of the rib cage, 1 cm lateral to the sternum (Fig. 10.1). The bilateral, paired arteries course deep to

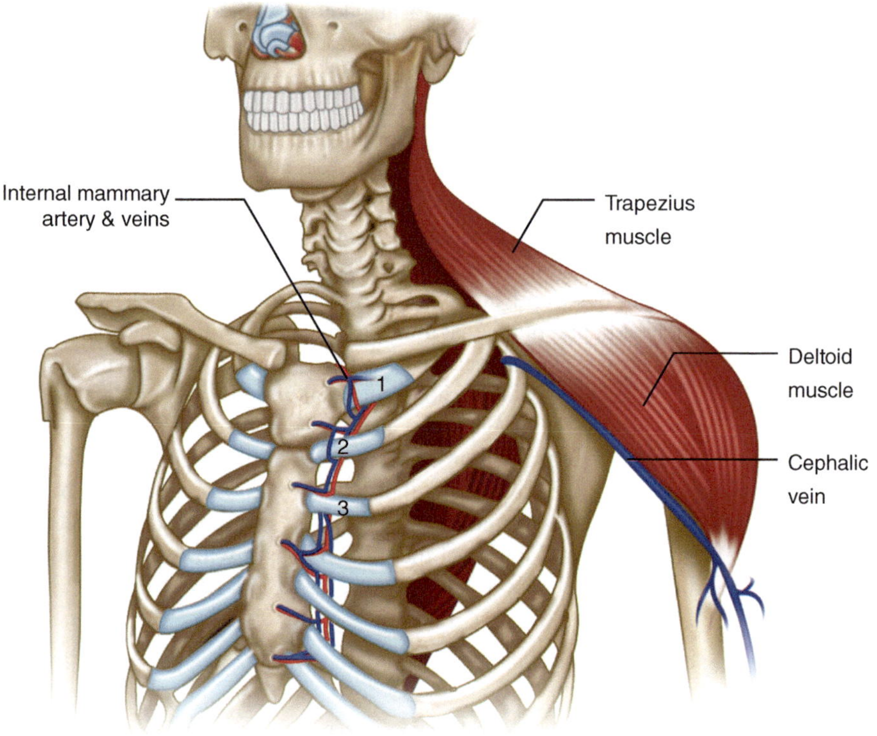


**Fig. 10.1** Trapezius muscle, deltoid muscle, pectoralis major muscle, deltopectoral groove, cephalic vein, internal mammary artery, clavicle, 1–4 intercostal space, and the area of blood supply where the skin flap should be left down

the clavicle but superficial to the pleura as they descend in the chest, providing perforating arteries through the intercostal spaces to supply the skin of the chest wall. Both the DP and CDP flaps are based on the first four perforators from the IMA, with the primary blood supply coming from the second and third perforators. These perforators run in a plane superficial to the pectoralis major fascia and deltoid muscles.

Understanding the angiosome model is essential in performing the flap harvest. The primary region and first angiosome supplied by the internal mammary perforators includes the skin from the sternum to the deltopectoral groove (medial to the cephalic vein). As one moves lateral to the cephalic vein and into the deltoid skin region, the risk of ischemia and tissue necrosis increases. In the context of the angiosome model, the DP is typically described as two distinct areas: a medial, arterial-based flap and a lateral, random cutaneous-based flap.

The CDP flap is a modification of the DP flap which includes cervical skin and platysma extending superiorly into the lower neck. As such, the primary blood supply remains based on the perforating branches of the IMAs. The original CDP flap illustrated by Ducic & Smith describes the skin flap being raised in subcutaneous tissue plane. However, the senior author (TL) recommends incorporating the platysma with the neck skin to further optimize blood supply to the skin and to provide additional tissue bulk, especially in situations where the donor neck skin was previous radiated. By raising in the subplatysmal plane, the skin flap has been noted to be more reliable, especially in radiated patients. The neck skin located anterior to the trapezius muscle and medial and superior to the cephalic vein are included to center around the third intercostal space.

The venous drainage of both the DP flap and CDP flaps is based on the venae comitantes that accompany the arteries in the region. These drain to the internal mammary vein (IMV), which can accompany the IMA as either a single or double vessel. The most common pattern is to have a single IMV that lies medial to the IMA.

The nerve supply to the deltopectoral skin arises from the supraclavicular nerves (C3 and C4) and the anterolateral intercostal nerves (T2, T3, and T4). The supraclavicular nerves of the cervical plexus supply the skin over the sternoclavicular joint to the upper deltoid muscle. The intercostal nerves supply the skin of the anterior chest wall and provide both sensory and motor function.

## Cervicodeltopectoral Flap Advantages

- Relatively easy flap to harvest and offers significant skin flap volume.
- Can be performed as a single-stage reconstruction.
- Offers a thin skin flap with ideal color match for face and neck skin reconstruction.
- Can be harvested even if the patient had a previous pectoralis myocutaneous flap, as long as the blood supply to the skin flap (medial chest along second and third intercostal space) has not been disrupted.

## Cervicodeltopectoral Flap Disadvantages

- May be raised in patients with previous radiation therapy (at least 6 months after radiation therapy) but there likely is an increased risk of poor wound healing. Radiated patients with neck skin that does not slide from underlying soft tissue (i.e., woody neck) is not a good candidate for CDP flap.
- Not as reliable for intraoral mucosal defects or pharyngeal mucosal defects where significant salivary exposure can occur.
- Less reliable in scenarios where the skin flap tents up from excess tension. Draping the CDP skin flap by following the underlying the contour of the facial and neck soft tissues without tension will optimize vascular ingrowth from the underlying wound bed, leading to highest chance of flap success.
- If the skin flap is closed with excessive tension that results in excess dead space between the CDP flap and the underlying soft tissue, there is an increased risk of poor wound healing or partial skin flap necrosis, especially in those who have undergone previous radiation to the area.
- Results in an unsightly donor site defect, particularly if skin grafting is required. Although the donor site defect can usually be closed primarily with undermining and mobilization of the posterior neck/deltoid skin and the lateral chest/axillary skin towards each other, skin grafting may be required near the deltopectoral groove or along the site of trifurcation in case of excess tissue tension (see Fig. 10.6).
- In women, distortions to breast symmetry and nipple positioning may occur.

## Preoperative Evaluation

Preoperative evaluation includes a thorough history and physical examination. Particular emphasis is placed on the history of prior head and neck surgeries and/or radiation therapy. The surgical site is evaluated for the presence of any scars or defects that may interfere with flap harvest. If the patient has had a previous pectoralis myocutaneous flap, the blood supply to the CDP flap may have been disturbed. Typically, additional imaging or vascular studies are not needed prior to surgical intervention. The patient's sex should be taken into consideration, as males may have excess chest hair which could compromise reconstruction where excess hair is less desirable while females are at risk for breast and nipple position asymmetry.

## Flap Harvest

1. The patient is placed in a supine position and the chest is prepped from the midline to the posterior neck and deltoid. The thigh is prepped and draped for potential skin grafting. Surgical landmarks are trapezius muscle, clavicle, sternum, and the second and third intercostal spaces.

2. One can think of the CDP flap with two large limbs similar to a large bilobed flap. One limb will be centered around the posterior neck extending into the deltoid while the second limb will be centered from the superolateral chest skin (located superolateral to the second and third intercostal spaces). The first limb will rotate to reconstruct the cervicofacial neck skin defect while the second limb will rotate to fill the donor site defect along the deltoid/posterior neck region.
   (a) From the deltopectoral groove, an incision is marked to include the posterior neck skin staying along the anterior border of the trapezius muscle and extending superiorly to reach the inferior aspect of the tissue defect located in the face or the neck. This will make up the first limb.
   (b) Next, the second limb is designed to fill the defect from the first limb. The second and third intercostal spaces are marked immediately lateral to the sternum, with the latter marking the inferomedial aspect of the CDP flap. The incision is made around 2–3 cm lateral to the sternal border in the third intercoastal space and extends obliquely toward the deltopectoral groove. This oblique, curvilinear line from the third intercostal space to the deltopectoral groove marks the inferior margin of the CDP flap. While designing the CDP flap, avoid including the skin flap region that would typically be included for a pectoralis myocutaneous flap (Figs. 10.2 and 10.3). In addition, while raising the skin flap, it is important to avoid raising the skin flap 2–3 cm lateral to the sternum in the second and third intercostal spaces to avoid injury to the CDP flap blood supply.
3. The size and anticipated reach of the flap are verified using an imaginary line extending from the inferoposterior aspect of the defect to second intercostal space. This line marks the axis of rotation required to reach the supero-anterior most aspect of the skin defect (Fig. 10.4).
4. The neck skin flap is raised in the subplatysmal tissue plane following the anterior border of the trapezius. Along the inferior border of the mandible, one should be mindful to avoid injury to the marginal mandibular nerve and resulting lower lip paralysis. The platysma is left attached to the skin flap as dissection is carried medially towards midline. It is important to remain superficial to the sternocleidomastoid muscle and leave the adjacent external jugular vein and greater auricular nerve down in the wound bed.
5. While dissecting over the deltoid and pectoralis major muscles, the CDP flap is raised immediately on top of the underlying deltoid and pectoralis muscle fascia. It is important to remain in a subplatysmal tissue plane as one dissects inferomedially over the clavicle as thinning the skin flap over the clavicular region may compromise blood supply. The flap is elevated medially up to a point 2–3 cm lateral to the sternum along the first, second and third intercostal spaces. This avoids injury to the perforating vessels of the IMA (Fig. 10.2).
6. Once the skin flap is raised, it is rotated superomedially to reach the site of the defect. After it is appropriately positioned, flap perfusion can be checked by making a superficial cut at the distal skin edges or by nicking the skin flap with a needle. While positioning, it is important to allow the skin flap to drape along

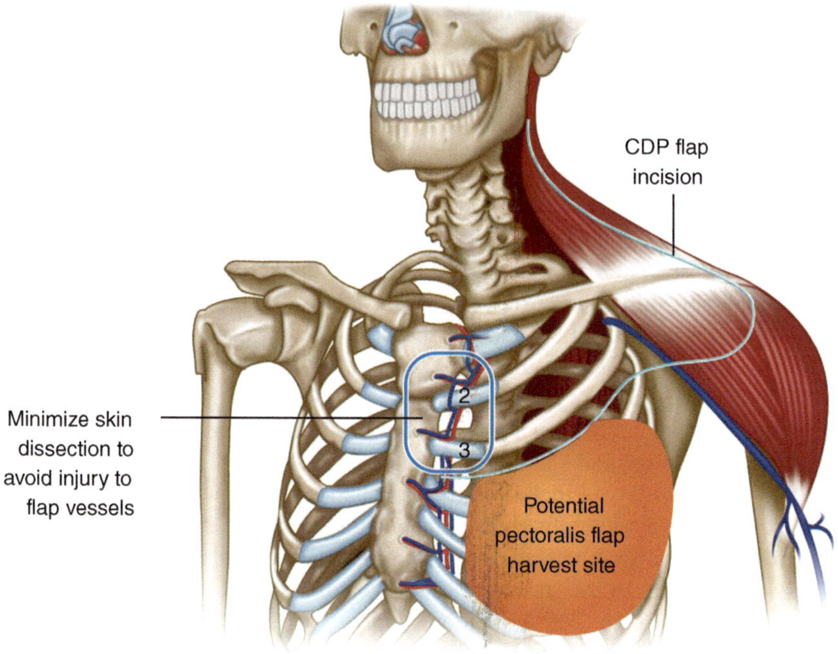


**Fig. 10.2** CDP flap incision is designed around second and third intercostal spaces. It is important to avoid injury to these flap vessels by minimizing dissection 2–3 cm immediately lateral to the sternal border within the second and third intercoastal spaces. In addition, in case of future reconstruction needs, avoid disturbing the skin that may be used for future pectoralis muscle flap which border the inferior aspect of the CDP flap design. Axis of rotation from posteroinferior corner of the defect to the second intercostal space that can rotate superomedially to meet the superoanterior aspect of the defect. Two limbs of the CDP flap

the contour of the underlying soft tissue of the neck and avoid tenting which can compromise perfusion and inhibit neovascularization.

7. Once the CDP flap is positioned into the desired location without tension, closure of the donor site is performed by advancing the surrounding local tissue. Two skin flaps are mobilized to achieve this (Figs. 10.5 and 10.6). The skin overlying the trapezius and deltoid muscles is raised immediately on top of the underlying muscle fascia towards the direction of the scapula, allowing for anterior mobilization of the posterior neck and posterior deltoid skin. At the same time, a secondary skin flap is raised along the superolateral chest, axilla, and anterior deltoid skin located lateral to the deltopectoral groove. The skin flap is

**Fig. 10.3** CDP flap is highlighted in light blue incision. Purple incision marks the expected skin defect after cancer resection. The CDP flap can be based on second and third intercoastal spaces (located inferior to the corresponding rib).

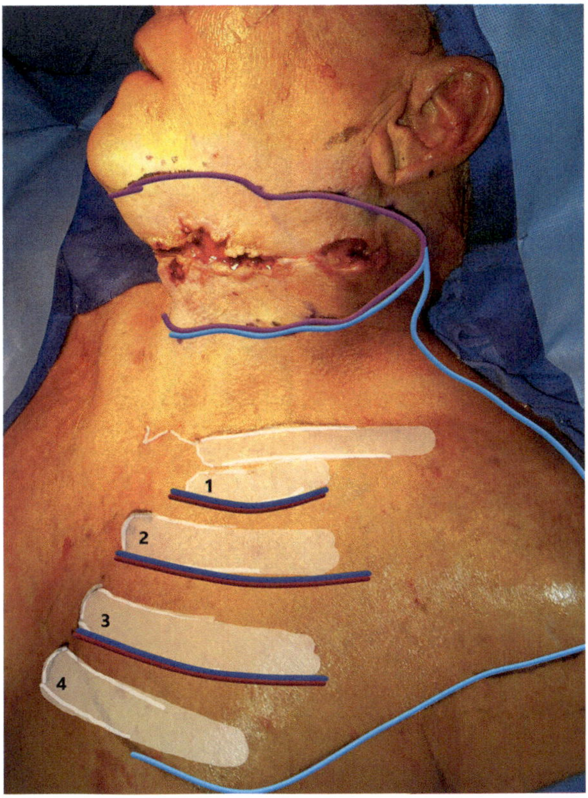


raised superficial to the pectoralis major muscle fascia and the deltoid muscle fascia, while paying attention to avoid sacrificing the pectoralis muscle skin flap in case the flap is needed in the future (skin medial and inferior to the nipple is left undisturbed). The superolateral chest, axilla, and anterior deltoid skin are recruited as a skin flap is then mobilized superiorly to meet the posterior neck/deltoid skin flap. Towel clamps can be used to help oppose the two skin flap edges that typically end up in a horizontal orientation near the clavicle. However, it is best to avoid placing the incision directly over the clavicle to minimize the risk of bone exposure. If there is excessive tension that prohibits primary closure, typically near the deltopectoral groove or at the site of skin flap trifurcation, either a split thickness or full thickness skin graft may be employed.

8. Two Jackson Pratt (JP) drains are placed into the neck. One JP drain is placed from the posterior neck/deltoid skin flap to sit along the posterior neck/inferior neck gutter. A second JP drain is placed through the superolateral chest/axilla/deltoid skin flap or from the opposite neck skin flap to sit along the anterior neck/inferior neck gutter. It is best to avoid placing any drain through the CDP flap as it can negatively affect the blood supply.

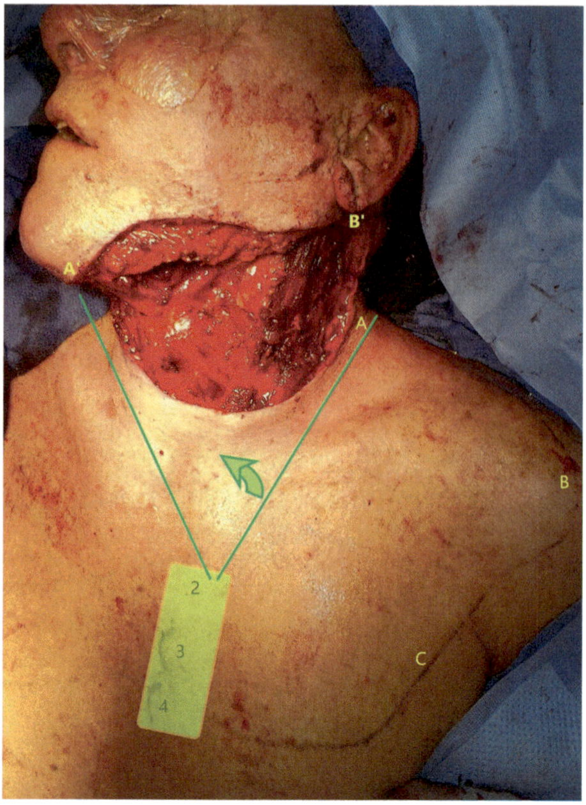


**Fig. 10.4** Ensure adequate flap reach by checking from the posteroinferior corner of the defect (A) to the second intercoastal space and attempting to reach the superoanterior most point of reconstruction (A′). This line marks the axis of rotation from posteroinferior corner of the defect to meet the superoanterior aspect of the defect. The second limb of the CDP flap (marked as point C) allows closure of the donor defect with local tissue advancement in vast majority of cases

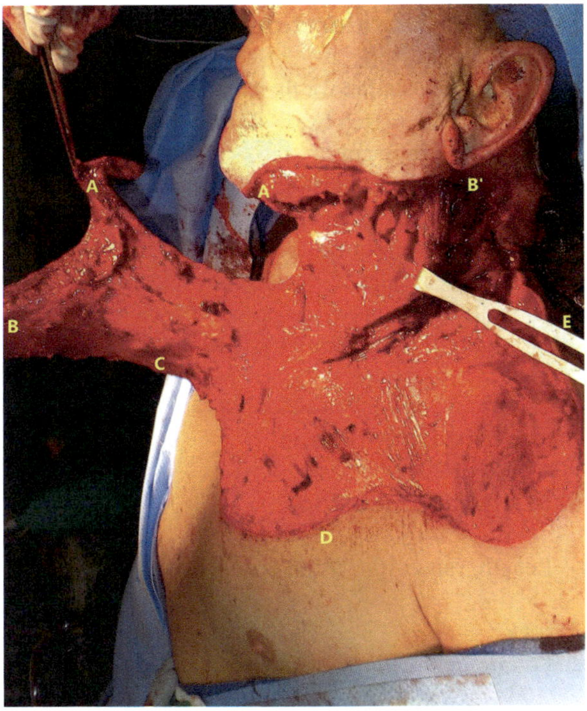


**Fig. 10.5** Donor site closure can be achieved by advancing the posterior neck/posterior deltoid skin flap (E) anteroinferiorly while moving the lateral chest/axillary skin/anterior deltoid skin flap (D) superiorly for the incision line to line up near the level of the clavicle. Be mindful of not disrupting the pectoralis myocutaneous muscle flap site in case of future reconstruction needs.

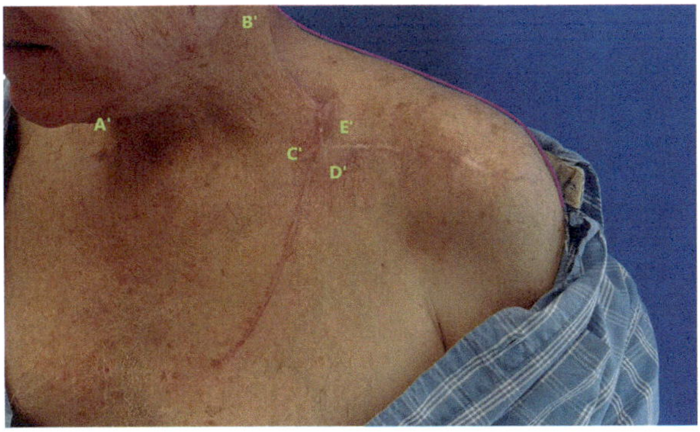


**Fig. 10.6** Maximal wound tension will commonly occur near the trifurcation (C′, D′, and E′) as well as along the length of the posterior neck/deltoid skin flap and superior chest/anterior deltoid skin flap (D′, E′). One should expect wound dehiscence, especially at the trifurcation, to avoid exposure of critical structures in case of lack of SCM. Best practice is to bring the posterior neck skin flaps (E′) anteriorly closer to the clavicle and along the anterior aspect of the deltoid muscle. If possible, avoid the flap incision coming together along the top aspect of the trapezius and deltoid (purple line) to minimize wound dehiscence that can occur from the skin flaps falling away from each other due to gravity

## Important Considerations

- The arch of rotation for the DP flap can limit its use in the head and neck region, but can be increased by dissecting out the perforators and freeing the parasternal skin with a back cut.
- If the sternocleidomastoid muscle has been sacrificed, one must be mindful of the potential for great vessel exposure in the event of wound dehiscence. In such a case, consideration should be taken to drape any remnant sternocleidomastoid muscle over the great vessels for protection. An alternative option is the pectoralis major flap to provide proper muscle bulk to sit on top of the great vessels, especially if postoperative radiation therapy is anticipated.

## Important Dimensions

### Skin Island Dimensions

- Length: range 10–30 cm.

#### Artery

2nd or 3rd perforating branches of internal mammary artery (dominant)

- Length ~1.5 cm, diameter ~1 mm.

  1st and 4th perforating branches of internal mammary artery (minor)

- Length ~1.5 cm, diameter ~0.7 mm.

  Direct cutaneous artery that arises from thoracoacromial system (minor)

- Provides the blood supply to skin lateral to the deltopectoral groove (this area is not typically included as part of the CDP flap but is typically used for donor site closure).

#### Vein

Vena comitans

- Primary vena comitans accompanying artery: length ~1.5 cm, diameter ~2.5 mm.

#### Nerve

Supraclavicular and intercostal nerves

- Sensory innervation comes from the supraclavicular nerves (C3 and C4) and the anterolateral intercostal nerves (T2, T3, and T4).
- There is no motor innervation for this flap.

## Cervicodeltopectoral Flap Usage

The CDP flap can be used to reconstruct defects of the face and neck up to the level of the zygoma. It offers a skin flap with appropriate color and thickness match for cutaneous cervicofacial defects.

- Reconstruction of facial or neck cutaneous defects.
- Reconstruction of intraoral defects (buccal mucosa, floor of mouth) or pharyngeal defects, although there is a higher risk of flap necrosis from salivary exposure. Thus, use of the CDP flap is generally discouraged where there is a potential for salivary exposure.

## Complications

There is an insufficient number of studies reporting complications after CDP flap usage. Ducic and Smith report that 2 out of 18 patients had partial flap necrosis which was managed successfully with conservative therapy (0.25% acetic acid wound dressing changes) [2]. In situations of wound dehiscence, conservative management with secondary healing and local wound care is appropriate in most situations. However, in such situations, it is essential to ensure that there is no risk of great vessel exposure located deep to the site of dehiscence. Donor site complications include postoperative hematoma, seroma, scarring, or wound dehiscence.

## Case Example

1. This patient had a large squamous cell carcinoma involving the inferior cheek and unilateral neck skin with concern for nodal and deep tissue plane involvement. A 2-cm margin around the cancer is marked out.
2. The anticipated CDP flap harvest with its landmarks is marked out. Again, the CDP flap is based on the second and third perforators from the internal mammary artery on the ipsilateral second and third intercostal spaces (inferior to the corresponding ribs). It extends obliquely to include the deltopectoral groove laterally and superiorly along the trapezius muscle border until the inferior margin of the skin defect is encountered (Fig. 10.3).
3. The patient underwent wide local excision of a malignancy resulting in a large skin defect ($17 \times 10$ cm$^2$) extending from the inferior border of the mandible to the clavicle and crossing midline. A neck dissection of levels 1–3 with preservation of the sternocleidomastoid muscle (SCM) was performed, with sacrifice of the greater auricular nerve and external jugular vein for oncologic reasons (Fig. 10.4). As the SCM was preserved, the great vessels remained protected.
4. A left-sided CDP flap was designed based off of the second and third perforating branches of the internal mammary artery. Point A marks the posterior/inferior most aspect of the defect which will be rotated towards the anterior/superior

most aspect of the defect (A′). Point B marks the lateral-most aspect of the CDP flap at the deltoid which will move towards the posterior/superior aspect of the defect (B′). Point C marks the half-way point along the curvilinear incision from the third intercostal space to the deltopectoral region. The green line marks the axis of rotation. Confirmation of adequate flap reach should be confirmed prior to proceeding with CDP flap incision. In this case, confirmation of adequate reach from point A to A' and from B to B′ while following the contour of the underlying soft tissue was performed. Dissection should not be carried 2–3 cm lateral from the sternum at the second and third intercostal spaces to ensure that the perforating branches from the internal mammary artery are preserved (Fig. 10.4).

5. After definitive cancer resection, the CDP flap was raised in the subplatysmal tissue plane immediately superficial to the deltoid and pectoralis muscle fascia below the level of the clavicle. Point D marks approximately the midpoint along the remaining chest skin flap, and Point E marks the posterior neck overlying the trapezius and posterior deltoid skin that will be advanced anteriorly to assist in closure of the donor site defect (Fig. 10.5).
6. The CDP flap is seen to be well healed at the 1-year postoperative visit. Local tissue advancement was performed allowing for primary closure using the superolateral chest/axilla/anterior deltoid skin flap (D′) and the posterior neck/posterior deltoid skin flap (E'). It is common for wound dehiscence to occur at the site of trifurcation where points C′, D′, and E' converge as this area is at risk for heightened tension. When closing the donor site defect, it is imperative to avoid applying tension on the CDP flap to optimize perfusion. Thus, skin graft placement can be considered in this location, if excess tension is present (Fig. 10.6).

## References

1. Bakamijam VY. A two-stage method for pharyngoesophageal reconstruction with a primary pectoral skin flap. Plast Reconstr Surg. 1965;36:173.
2. Ducic Y, Smith JE. The cervicodeltopectoral flap for single-stage resurfacing of anterolateral defects of the face and neck. Arch Facial Plast Surg. 2003;5(2):197–201. https://doi.org/10.1001/archfaci.5.2.197.

# Trapezius Flap for Head and Neck Reconstruction

11

Kathryn Bradburn Wie and Weitao Wang

## Introduction

The trapezius muscle flap can be used in primary and salvage settings to reconstruct a wide range of head and neck defects. Multiple variations of the trapezius muscle flap have been reported in the literature. These include multiple musculocutaneous flaps, osteocutaneous flap, free flap, and perforator flap.

Review of the literature is challenging due to lack of uniform and clinically applicable flap descriptions. Furthermore, early reports of trapezius flap complications related to poor vascularization raised concern about the reliability of the blood supply. Cadaveric studies and standardized nomenclature have advanced our collective understanding of the vascular anatomy. Successful harvest of trapezius muscle flaps with reliable blood supply is possible with knowledge of the complex vascular supply. Table 11.1 provides the various terms used in the literature to describe the flap modifications and vascular anatomy along with the nomenclature that will be used throughout this chapter.

In this chapter, we will review the history and development of the trapezius flap, discuss the relevant anatomy, and review the various modifications of the flap with case presentations. The flap types will be defined by their supplying arteries using the nomenclature proposed by Haas and Weiglein [14].

K. B. Wie · W. Wang (✉)
Department of Otolaryngology Head and Neck Surgery, University of Rochester, Rochester, NY, USA
e-mail: Kathryn_wie@urmc.rochester.edu; Weitao_wang@urmc.rochester.edu


F. Sokoya, A. G. Vincent (eds.), *Manual of Head and Neck Reconstruction*, https://doi.org/10.1007/978-3-031-65999-7_11

**Table 11.1** Flap nomenclature and anatomic description

| Muscle fibers, artery | Nomenclature in literature | Pedicle artery in literature | Authors |
|---|---|---|---|
| Middle/transverse superficial cervical artery (SCA) | Type 2: Trapezius flap based on SCA. Middle transverse fibers included | SCA | Haas [1] |
| | Upper musculocutaneous (myocutaneous) trapezius flap | *** | Nettervile [4] |
| | Trapezius myocutaneous flap | Superficial transverse cervical artery | Demergasso, [2] Panje [3] |
| | Lateral island trapezius musculocutaneous (myocutaneous) flap | Transverse cervical artery | Netterville [4] |
| | Extended trapezius musculocutaneous flap | Descending branch of TCA | Rosen [5] |
| | Vertical trapezius musculocutaneous flap | Descending branch of TCA | Papadopoulos [6] |
| Inferior/ascending DSA | Type 3: Trapezius flap based on DSA. Inferior (ascending) muscle fibers | DSA | Haas [1] |
| | Lower trapezius musculocutaneous (myocutaneous) flap | *** | Weiglein [7] |
| | | | Lynch [8] |
| | | | Ou [9] |
| | | | Haas [1] |
| | | | Yoon |
| | Extended lower trapezius myocutaneous flap | Descending branch of the transverse cervical artery | Zheng |
| | Extended lower trapezius island myocutaneous flap | DSA | Tan [10] |
| | Extended vertical lower trapezius island myocutaneous flap | Transverse cervical artery | Chen [11] |
| | | | Huang [12] |
| | Pear-shaped lower trapezius flap | DSA | Hamilton |
| | Vertical island myocutaneous trapezius flap | *** | Lee [13] |

***Dorsal scapular artery

## History

We will first review the development of the flap in clinical practice and then discuss the relevant anatomy, and how the terminology used to describe the trapezius flap has evolved over time.

In 1979, Demergasso and Piazza were the first to describe the trapezius musculocutaneous and osteomyocutaneous flaps. Their work demonstrated the versatility of the flap in head and neck reconstruction, using it to reconstruct large defects in the oral cavity, oropharynx, hypopharynx, and skin of the head and neck. Their flaps were pedicled on the superficial cervical artery, which they called the superficial transverse cervical vessels [2]. In 1980, Panje further described the anatomic basis of the same flap, referencing fluorescein perfusion studies performed by McGregor and Morgan which showed that the upper third of the trapezius muscle is supplied by transverse cervical artery. His work further promoted the trapezius flap as a safe and effective reconstructive option [3]. The vascular territories and physiologic basis of the flap were further elucidated by experimental studies [15, 16]. Baek et al. were the first to publish on a lower trapezius flap, which he described as the lower trapezius island flap with blood supply primarily from the transverse cervical artery. His work showed that the flap was a reliable reconstructive option for facial defects. In the following years, there were reports of flap complications specifically due to poor vascularity of the distal portion of the flap. Previous experimental studies identified the dorsal scapular artery (DSA) as a major portion of the blood supply to the lower part of the trapezius muscle and the overlying skin [17]. For that reason, in 1991, Netterville and Wood reinvestigated the blood supply to the lower trapezius muscle fibers by dissecting 15 cadavers. They found the dominant vessel to the lower trapezius muscle to be DSA in 50%, transverse cervical artery (TCA) in 30%, and co-dominance of DSA and TCA in 20%. The lack of clarity regarding the vascular anatomy led to further cadaveric studies that will be discussed below [1, 18].

Additional publications reporting various modifications and names of the flap led to further confusion about the anatomic basis of the flap and the vascular supply. Recent publications by Haas et al., Yang et al., and *many others* have clarified the vascular territories of the trapezius muscle and the nomenclature of the vascular supply [1, 18]. Successful utilization of the trapezius flap depends on a thorough understanding of the variations in the vascular anatomy that they have identified.

## Relevant Anatomy *[and Nomenclature]*

### The Trapezius Muscle

The trapezius muscle is a large, flat, triangular muscle that stabilizes and moves the scapula and elevates the shoulder. *There are three parts of the trapezius muscle, and each has distinct directional fibers*: upper/descending, middle/transverse, and lower/ascending. The trapezius muscle originates from the external occipital protuberance and the medial third of the superior nuchal line down the ligamentum nuchae and the spinous process of the seventh cervical and all thoracic vertebrae. The upper part of the muscle attaches to the lateral third of the clavicle and the middle part attaches to the acromion, while the fibers of the lower part of the muscle converge to form an aponeurosis that inserts on the medial tubercle of the scapular spine [4, 19, 20].

The muscle fibers of the upper/superior part of the muscle travel obliquely, downward, and laterally. As a result, this is frequently referred to as the descending part of the muscle. The upper part originates at the base of skull along the medial third of the superior nuchal line of the occipital bone, external occipital protuberance, ligamentum nuchae, and spinous process of the seventh cervical vertebra.

These fibers then descend to attach to the lateral third of the clavicle. The primary function of the upper muscle fibers is to elevate the scapula.

The fibers of the middle part of the trapezius muscle pass transversely, and as such this part of the muscle is frequently referred to as the transverse part. This part of the muscle originates from the spinous processes of the first through fifth thoracic vertebrae and attaches to the acromion. The function of the middle part is to adduct and retract the scapula.

Lastly, the fibers of the lower part of the trapezius muscle pass obliquely, upward and laterally from the spinous processes of the sixth through twelfth thoracic vertebrae and attach to the medial aspect of the spine of the scapula. This aspect of the muscle is frequently referred to as the ascending part. It functions to depress the scapula [4, 19, 20]. The middle (transverse) and lower (ascending) parts are the most frequently used in reconstruction [1]. Table 11.2 lists the trapezius muscle anatomy, attachments, function, and blood supply.

The spinal accessory nerve (cranial nerve 11) provides motor innervation to the trapezius muscle. *The nerve enters near the junction between the middle and lower fibers.* The blood supply to the trapezius muscle is via the occipital artery and direct or indirect branches of the subclavian artery. The vascular anatomy has been extensively investigated and is described in detail below [4].

**Table 11.2** Description of trapezius muscle

| Muscle "Portion" | Fiber direction | Origin | Attachment | Function | Blood supply |
|---|---|---|---|---|---|
| Upper/superior | Oblique, downward and laterally | Medial third of the superior nuchal line of the occipital bone | Lateral third of the clavicle | Elevate scapula | Occipital artery |
| | | External occipital protuberance | | | |
| | | Ligamentum nuchae | | | |
| | | Spinous process of C7 | | | |
| Middle | Transverse | Spinous processes of T1–T5 | Acromion | Adduct/retract scapula | Superficial branch of the transverse cervical artery (SCA)[a] |
| Lower/inferior | Oblique, upward and laterally | Spinous processes of T6–T12 | Medial tubercle of the spine of the scapula | Depress scapula | Dorsal scapular artery (DSA)[a] |
| | | | | | Minor intercostal perforators |

[a]Some publications refer to SCA as superficial branch of the transverse cervical artery and DSA as the deep branch of the transverse cervical artery in early publications

## Regional Anatomy

Muscles that lie deep to the trapezius muscle include the levator scapulae, the major and minor rhomboid muscles, and the latissimus dorsi.

## Blood Supply: Nomenclature

It is commonly taught that the thyrocervical trunk arises from the subclavian artery and gives risk to the inferior thyroid artery, the suprascapular artery, and the transverse cervical artery. *Nomina Anatomica* defines the transverse cervical artery as the common trunk that gives rise to a superficial and a deep branch. The superficial branch is also called the superficial cervical artery (SCA), and the deep branch is also called the dorsal scapular artery (DSA) [1]. However, cadaveric studies have shown that the origin of the SCA and DSA is variable [1, 7].

While there are many variations in the proximal vascular anatomy of the SCA and DSA, the distal course of these vessels is constant. Successful flap elevation with reliable blood supply is possible with the knowledge of the distal course of the SCA and DSA because their proximal components are not routinely explored during flap elevation.

The DSA is located deep to the levator scapulae and minor rhomboid muscles. In the vast majority of cases, it passes medial to the levator scapulae. The branch that supplies the trapezius muscle flap arises between the minor and major rhomboid muscles at the level of the spine of the scapula. It courses along the under surface of the trapezius muscles close to the medial border of the scapula in a more lateral course than the SCA. It is accompanied by the dorsal scalpular nerve.

## Flap Nomenclature

The middle part is referred to as the upper trapezius flap, and the lower part is referred to as the lower trapezius flap [20].

# Operative Technique

## Preoperative Evaluation

Proper counseling of the patient is essential in preparation for trapezius reconstruction. In cases of large defect reconstruction requiring a large amount of trapezius muscle and skin transfer, patients must be warned of associated shoulder morbidity and the likely need for postoperative physiotherapy and rehabilitation. History of prior neck dissection is in itself not a contraindication of this flap and does not necessarily preclude use of a trapezius flap even when the transverse cervical artery was previously sacrificed. The back and shoulder should be assessed for prior scars and trauma, which may compromise the vascular supply of anticipated flap designs.

## Positioning

Harvest techniques vary depending on the anticipated defect to be reconstructed. In many cases, if an upper trapezius flap is needed for a periauricular defect, a lazy lateral decubitus position is enough. In cases where a lower trapezius island myocutaneous flap is utilized, a lateral decubitus position may be necessary. Often a lateral decubitus position may be useful for both the ablative portion of malignancy involving periauricular areas, radical parotidectomy, and radical excision of the neck. In these scenarios, the advantage is no position change requirement prior to starting the reconstructive portion of the case.

## Harvest Technique

The lateral aspect of the designed skin paddle is typically incised first. When performing an upper trapezius flap, following incision, blunt dissection is carried out until the lateral border of the upper trapezius is identified. A simple way to consistently identify the lateral border of the trapezius is to first identify the upper border of the latissimus dorsi muscle with its muscle fibers in a horizontal orientation. This can then be traced medially until the more vertically oriented muscle fibers of the trapezius are encountered. Care is taken to avoid dissecting between the plane of the skin paddle and trapezius muscle owing to risk of injury of the musculocutaneous perforators. Once the lateral border is identified, blunt dissection is carried out under the trapezius muscle until it is dissected off of the underlying soft tissue. Care should be taken during this step as the transverse cervical artery contributions can be encountered deep to the trapezius muscle as it enters. In the event an island flap is utilized, this vessel must be preserved as it is the sole vascular supply for the skin paddle. In cases where a transposition flap is planned, the vessel can be ligated as the vascular supply is based off the superior trapezius and intercostal perforators. Once the trapezius muscle is well dissected off the underlying soft tissues, the inferior skin paddle or skin flap incision is then made as the skin is ensured to be positioned on the trapezius muscle. Rapid division of the trapezius muscle close to the spine of the scapula can then be performed to free the flap and allow adequate arc of rotation. The flap is then transposed to the defect and inset. The donor site is closed primarily with undermining of the surrounding skin and layered closure is performed with placement of a fenestrated drain via a separate incision.

Lower trapezius flap design should be that at least one-third of the skin paddle should be overlapping the inferior border of the trapezius muscle.

## Upper Trapezius Flap

The ideal defect for an upper trapezius flap is an infra-auricular, or posterior superior neck defect. Flaps can be designed along the upper back in both island and transposition fashion. The lateral border of the trapezius muscle is palpated above the spine of the scapula. The designed flap can be medially based off the intercostal perforators or laterally based off the transverse cervical artery, if the arch of rotation is enough.

Figure 11.1 demonstrates the upper trapezius flap. Flap is designed with a 90° arch of rotation to address a nonhealing periauricular wound secondary to prior radical resection and adjuvant radiation. The skin paddle should be elevated with the underlying trapezius muscle intact to keep as much of the musculocutaneous perforators intact. Width of the flap should be no narrower than 5 cm to minimize distal flap necrosis. The inferior aspect of the upper trapezius muscle is divided to allow arch of rotation and the flap is supplied by the superior and medial contributions of the occipital artery and intercostal perforators. The intervening skin bridge is divided. The flap is transposed and inset.

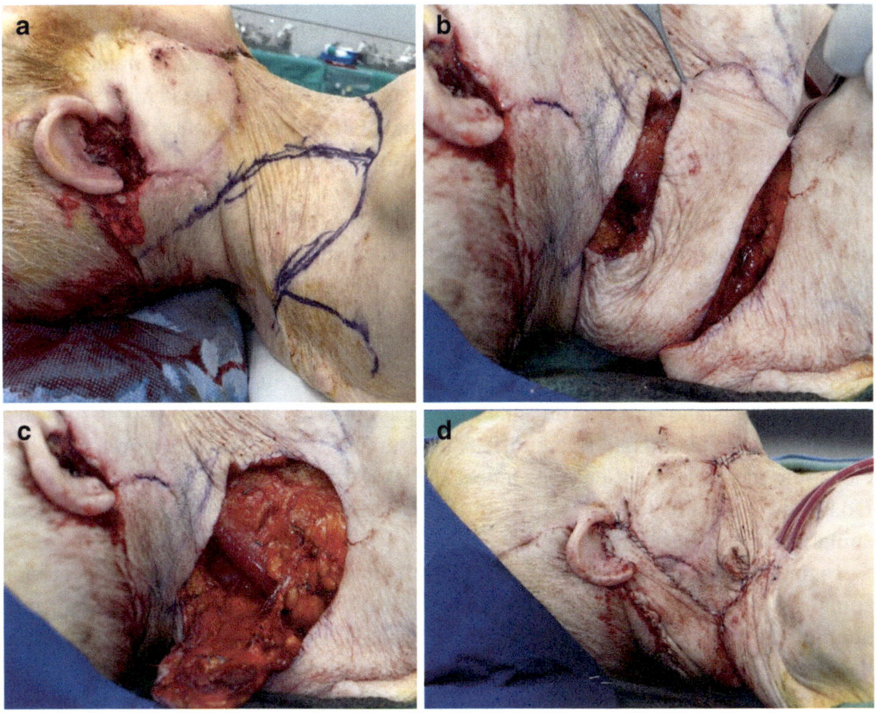


**Fig. 11.1** Upper trapezius flap reconstruction of preauricular defect. (**a**) Periauricular defect with upper trapezius flap designed. (**b**) Raised medially based upper trapezius flap. (**c**) Flap reflected to show the undersurface. (**d**) Inset into the defect

## Lower Trapezius Flap

The lower trapezius flap is more commonly utilized and described due to the increased arc of rotation to reach the midline neck, lateral cheek, and scalp. Typically, the flap has a dual vascular supply to include both the transverse cervical system as well as dorsal scapular artery, making it very robust. Even in cases where the transverse cervical artery was sacrificed from prior radical neck dissection, there is typically adequate supply from the dorsal scapular system for the flap to be reliable. No preoperative angiography is necessary for flap planning.

Intraoperatively, the vertebral process and medial and inferior border of the scapula are marked. The inferolateral border of the trapezius is approximated with a diagonal line along the inferior third of the medial border of the scapula to the lower thoracic vertebrae. The dorsal scapular artery lies just medial to the medial border of the scapula, and the transverse cervical artery supplies the flap above the scapular spine. This typically is on the undersurface of the trapezius muscle and can be doplered out intraoperatively if one encounters difficulty with visually identifying it. While the flap itself is versatile depending on the location of the defect, when designing the skin paddle, at least one-third of the paddle should be overlapping the trapezius muscle to ensure capture of an adequate number of musculocutaneous perforators. The inferior-most reliable skin paddle that can be harvested is generally 10 cm inferior to the lower border of the scapula. While the lower skin paddle is designed to provide increased arc of rotation and reach, this must be balanced with the understanding that the reliability of the distal most flap decreases. Myocutaneous flaps of the lower trapezius can be harvested with minimal donor-site morbidity particularly for central spinous defect coverage as the arc of rotation required is smaller.

Figure 11.2 shows a case of an elderly male who underwent prior radical neck dissection, composite oral resection, pectoralis flap reconstruction, and radiation several decades ago who developed a basal cell carcinoma on the right neck that was excised via Mohs surgery. Given his prior treatment, the neck did not heal, and he required vascularized tissue coverage of the carotid artery. Due to lack of recipient vessels as well as limited regional options, a lower trapezius myocutaneous flap was planned. The island flap was designed with the majority of the skin paddle overlapping the trapezius muscle to capture as many musculocutaneous perforators. After elevation, the flap was inset to the anterior neck defect with adequate arc of rotation. Donor-site morbidity was minimal in this case owing to the previously sacrificed spinal accessory nerve.

Figure 11.3 demonstrates a case of poor wound healing following a posterior spinal fusion approach, leading to chronic vertebral spine exposure after multiple attempts at primary closure. This case highlights the design of a skin paddle along the inferior trapezius requiring minimal arc of rotation once the trapezius muscle is fully mobilized and easily transferred to the defect for vascularized tissue coverage of the defect with minimal shoulder morbidity.

Figure 11.4 is a case of chronic occipital calvarial exposure following Mohs resection of nonmelanoma skin cancer in the setting of prior irradiation. A lower

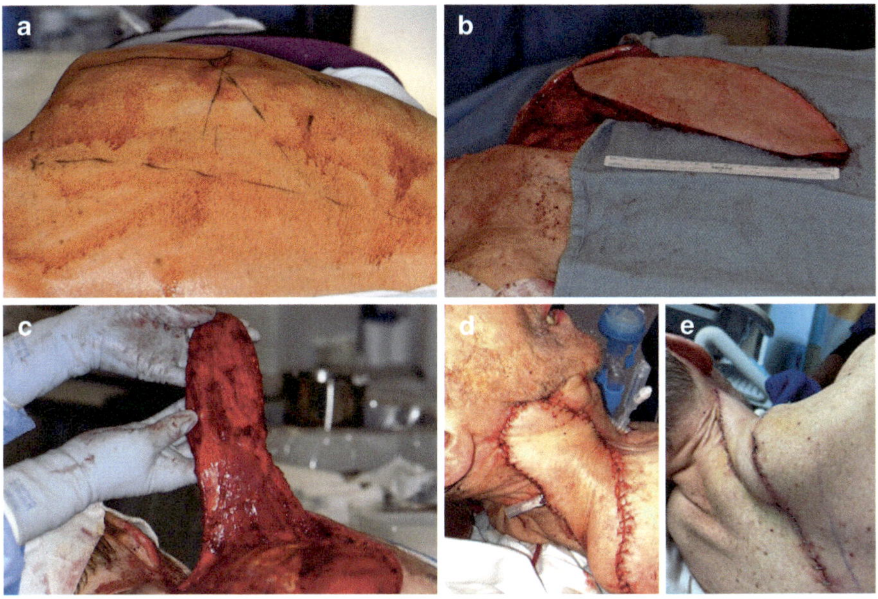

**Fig. 11.2** Lower trapezius flap reconstruction of carotid exposure neck wound in prior irradiated neck. (**a**) Inferior border of the trapezius demarcated. (**b**) Lower trapezius flap raised with distal skin paddle 5 cm inferior to the trapezius border. (**c**) Flap completely elevated with medial and lateral attachments released. (**d**) Inset along the right neck. (**e**) Donor site closure

trapezius myocutaneous flap was utilized to provide vascularized tissue coverage after debridement of non-viable bone. The trapezius flap can reach high along the occipital scalp, but typically defects along the vertex are more difficult to reach.

## Trapezius Free Flap

A lower trapezius myocutaneous flap can be designed with the benefit of a very long pedicle by tracing the dorsal scapular or transverse cervical vessels up to the origin point in the neck anteriorly. This can afford a flap pedicle of up to 25–30 cm in some cases. The trapezius free flap remains described in few case reports in the literature and has not achieved widespread use. Typically free tissue transfer use of the trapezius myocutaneous flap is limited in the head and neck owing to its wide reach as a pedicle flap. Alternative free flaps such as the latissimus dorsi provide the additional reach to areas such as the scalp with a similarly long pedicle length as well as superior muscle area coverage compared to the trapezius and are likely the reason why the trapezius flap remains largely a pedicled flap in most clinical scenarios.

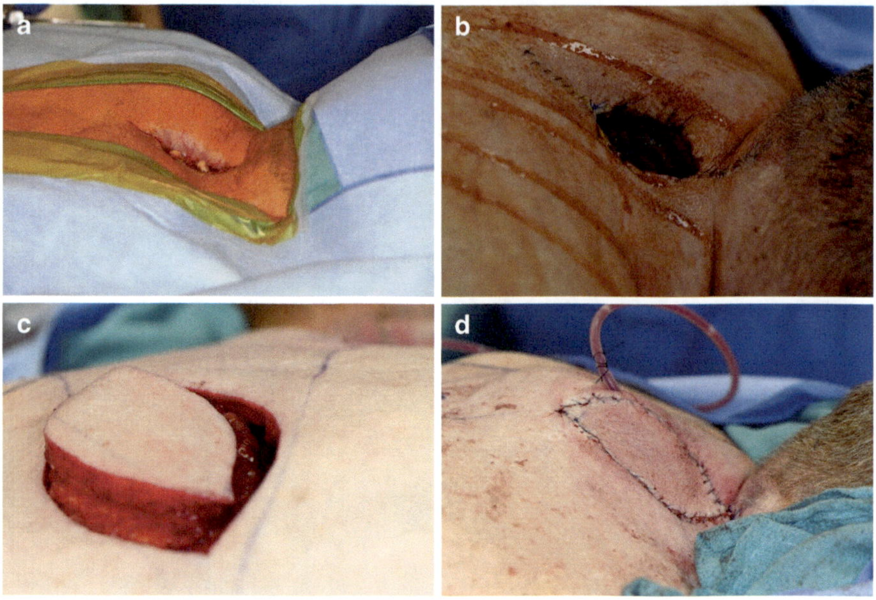


**Fig. 11.3** Posterior nape of neck wound from multiple failed complex closures following posterior spine approach. (**a**, **b**) Large wound with exposed vertebral processes. (**c**) Lower trapezius flap elevated. (**d**) Inset along the nape of neck/upper back defect

## Donor-Site Morbidity

Often the trapezius flap is not considered a first-line regional flap for head and neck reconstruction owing to the unfamiliarity of the anatomy by many head and neck surgeons despite its proven reliability and excellent reach. Donor-site morbidity in cases of salvage surgery is typically minimal in patients where the spinal accessory nerve is sacrificed. Considerations for the trapezius flap as the primary regional flap for reconstruction can be in cases that require sacrifice of the spinal accessory nerve. In such situations, use of the trapezius flap instead of the pectoralis myocutaneous flap prevents the added disability to the shoulder function that results from the loss of both muscles [21]. From a cosmetic standpoint, the trapezius flap is relatively less deforming for women when compared to the pectoralis major flap.

In situations where the spinal accessory nerve is intact, patients should be counseled on the possibility of shoulder weakness and need for physiotherapy to assist in ipsilateral shoulder abduction. To avoid functional impairments, a smaller cuff of trapezius muscle can be harvested with a skin paddle with perforator dissection. The small size of the perforators through the trapezius does make this technically challenging and risky.

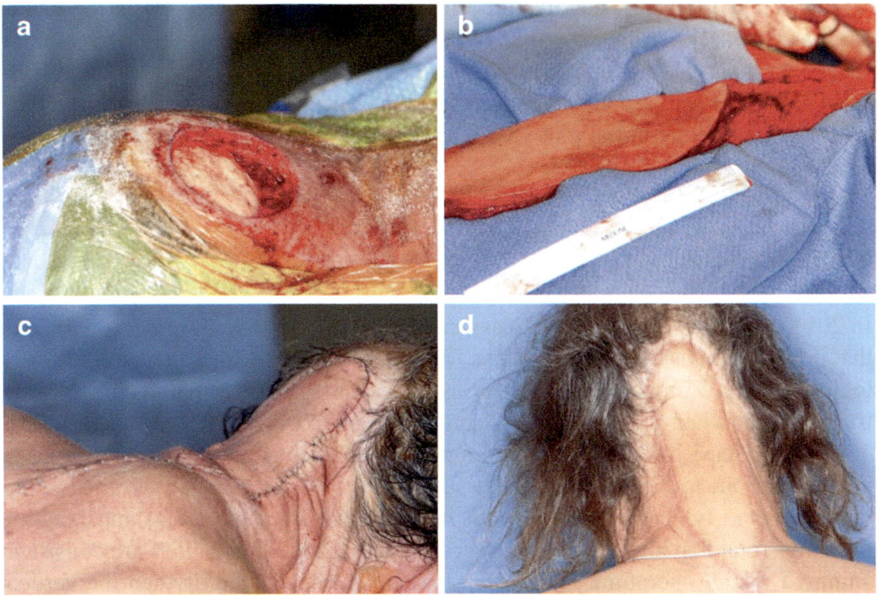


**Fig. 11.4** (**a**) Prior radiated occipital scalp nonhealing wound with bone exposure, s/p debridement. (**b**) Lower trapezius flap raised with long skin island to ensure distal perfusion. (**c**) Inset along occipital scalp defect. (**d**) 6 months postoperatively, well healed flap

## Limitations

The trapezius flap's major limitation is its arc of rotation. Its vertical reach is limited to the occipital scalp. Vertex, parietal, and anterior scalp defects would not be ideal for trapezius flap reconstruction; however, in these cases, rotational flaps can be borrowed from the remainder of the scalp, and the trapezius flap can be used to cover the donor site. Cheek and anterior facial defects are also limited by the reach of the flap, and additionally cosmesis of a bulky muscle pedicle is unfavorable. The flap can easily reach the anterior neck, periauricular region, and posterior neck regions and can be considered the optimal flap for reconstructing these areas.

## Indications

There are several advantages to using the trapezius flap as discussed above in terms of reach. The trapezius flap is viable in complex, salvage head and neck cases in that it does not require recipient vessels and is outside of the irradiated field. Additionally, a large skin island can be harvested; the muscle is thin and thus very pliable. While we discussed the limitations of reach of the trapezius flap, overall it has a very long pedicle length and wide arc of rotation making it a suitable reconstructive option for a wide range of defects [19, 22].

Can et al. suggested using the trapezius flap for the lateral face, posterior, lateral and anterior neck, scalp, temporal fossa, oral cavity involving floor of mouth or tongue, oropharynx, hypopharynx, cervical esophagus, and coverage of major vessels [23]. In the senior author's experience, the trapezius flap is not ideal for tubing to use as a circumferential pharynx defect, or bulky enough for hemiglossectomy reconstructions.

## Complications

In 2017, Sugrue et al. performed a systematic review of studies from 1985 to 2015 that involved the use of trapezius flaps for head and neck reconstruction after oncologic resection. Compared to other forms of head and neck free flap reconstruction, trapezius flaps had a similar complication rate to free flaps (15.9% trapezius vs. 15.1% free flap) [24]. The most common complication is donor-site seroma or hematoma. Due to the extent of soft tissue dissection, postoperative seroma is commonplace and typically resolves with incision and drainage (I&D) and pressure dressing. Total flap loss is rare, and success rates of greater than 95% are consistent among available literature. Partial flap loss can be encountered when the vertical skin paddle is extended beyond 10 cm inferior to the scapula border. When the skin paddle is too inferior, choke vessels are encountered, and the distal end of the skin paddle becomes essentially a random-pattern-based skin flap.

Figure 11.5 shows a lower trapezius flap used to reconstruct a lateral face defect following radical resection and parotidectomy with neck dissection. Small amount of flap of the distal most facial skin paddle developed over the course of a week postoperatively. This was managed with debridement of eschar and local wound care.

Delaying the flap in a staged fashion is a way to optimize the random pattern of the skin and improve distal flap survival. Intraoperatively, fluorescence imaging

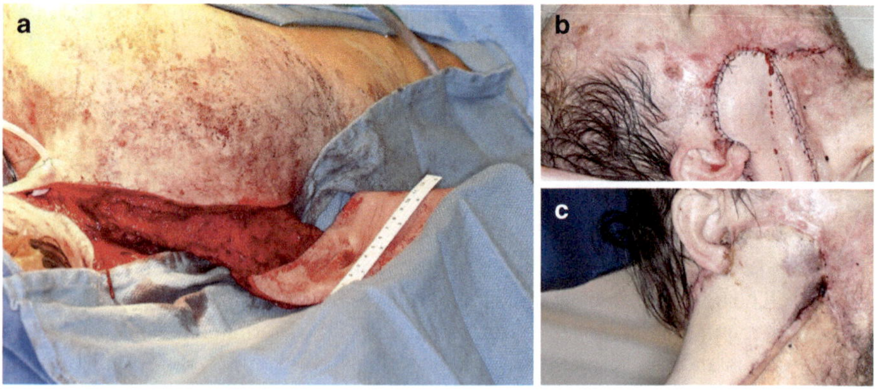


**Fig. 11.5** Large preauricular cutaneous defect follow-up ablation for squamous cell carcinoma. (**a**) Lower trapezius flap elevated with medial and lateral attachments freed. (**b**) Flap inset to face. (**c**) Post-operatively 1 week, with superficial sloughing of distal flap edge with limited perfusion

techniques can be utilized to assess the perfusion of the distal skin paddle after flap elevation, particularly when the distal portion covers vital structures such as the great vessels.

## Conclusions

The trapezius flap is a well-described myocutaneous flap that is versatile and reliable. Its arch of rotation makes it an obvious choice for lateral face, periauricular, lower scalp, and posterolateral neck defects. The dorsal scapular and transverse cervical artery supply the lower trapezius flap, while upper trapezius flaps can be based off the transverse cervical artery and occipital and intercostal perforators. Complication rates are comparable to other regional flaps, and donor-site cosmesis is improved in female patients when compared to other workhorse flaps such as the pectoralis major flap.

## References

1. Haas F, et al. The lower trapezius musculocutaneous flap from pedicled to free flap: anatomical basis and clinical applications based on the dorsal scapular artery. Plast Reconstr Surg. 2004;113(6):1580–90.
2. Demergasso F, Piazza MV. Trapezius myocutaneous flap in reconstructive surgery for head and neck cancer: an original technique. Am J Surg. 1979;138(4):533–6.
3. Panje WR. Myocutaneous trapezius flap. Head Neck Surg. 1980;2(3):206–12.
4. Netterville JL, Panje WR, Maves MD. The trapezius myocutaneous flap. Dependability and limitations. Arch Otolaryngol Head Neck Surg. 1987;113(3):271–81.
5. Rosen HM. The extended trapezius musculocutaneous flap for cranio-orbital facial reconstruction. Plast Reconstr Surg. 1985;75(3):318–27.
6. Papadopoulos ON, et al. Vertical trapezius musculocutaneous flap: a retrospective study. Scand J Plast Reconstr Surg Hand Surg. 2005;39(3):158–61.
7. Weiglein AH, Haas F, Pierer G. Anatomic basis of the lower trapezius musculocutaneous flap. Surg Radiol Anat. 1996;18(4):257–61.
8. Lynch JR, et al. The lower trapezius musculocutaneous flap revisited: versatile coverage for complicated wounds to the posterior cervical and occipital regions based on the deep branch of the transverse cervical artery. Plast Reconstr Surg. 2002;109(2):444–50.
9. Ou KL, et al. The lower trapezius musculocutaneous flap for head and neck reconstruction: two decades of clinical experience. Ann Plast Surg. 2013;71(Suppl 1):S48–54.
10. Tan KC, Tan BK. Extended lower trapezius Island myocutaneous flap: a fasciomyocutaneous flap based on the dorsal scapular artery. Plast Reconstr Surg. 2000;105(5):1758–63.
11. Chen WL, et al. Extended vertical lower trapezius Island myocutaneous flap for reconstruction of cranio-maxillofacial defects. Int J Oral Maxillofac Surg. 2007;36(2):165–70.
12. Huang ZQ, et al. Use of a folded extended vertical lower trapezius Island myocutaneous flap to repair large pharyngocutaneous fistulae developing after salvage total laryngectomy. Int J Oral Maxillofac Surg. 2018;47(10):1268–73.
13. Lee GK, Yamin F, Ho OH. Vertical island trapezius myocutaneous flap for cervical esophagoplasty: case report and review of the literature. Ann Plast Surg. 2012;68(4):362–5.
14. Wei F-C, Mardini S. Flaps and reconstructive surgery. 2nd ed. Edinburgh: Elsevier; 2017.
15. Mathes SJ, Nahai F. Classification of the vascular anatomy of muscles: experimental and clinical correlation. Plast Reconstr Surg. 1981;67(2):177–87.

16. Maruyama Y, et al. The definition of cutaneous vascular territories over the back using selective angiography and the intra-arterial injection of prostaglandin E1: some observations on the use of the lower trapezius myocutaneous flap. Br J Plast Surg. 1981;34(2):157–61.
17. Huelke DF. A study of the transverse cervical and dorsal scapular arteries. Anat Rec. 1958;132(3):233–45.
18. Yang D, Morris SF. Trapezius muscle: anatomic basis for flap design. Ann Plast Surg. 1998;41(1):52–7.
19. Achim V, Wenig BL. Understanding the vascular anatomy of the trapezius flap. Oper Tech Otolaryngol Head Neck Surg. 2019;30(2):156–60.
20. Krespi YP, Baek SM, Surek CL. Flap reconstruction of the upper face: free flaps vs. lower trapezius myocutaneous flap. Laryngoscope. 1983;93(4):485–8.
21. Singh A, et al. Utility and relevance of modified lateral trapezius myocutaneous flap as a locoregional reconstructive option for medium-sized ablative defects in head and neck cancer-our experience. Eur Arch Otorhinolaryngol. 2020;277(9):2539–49.
22. Gantz BJ, Panje WR. "How I do it"—plastic surgery. Practical suggestions on facial plastic surgery. Trapezius myocutaneous island flap. Laryngoscope. 1981;91(7):1196–9.
23. Can A, et al. The myocutaneous trapezius flap revisited: a treatment algorithm for optimal surgical outcomes based on 43 flap reconstructions. J Plast Reconstr Aesthet Surg. 2014;67(12):1669–79.
24. Sugrue CM, Rooney G, Sugrue RM. Trapezius flaps for reconstruction of head and neck defects following oncological resection—a systematic review. J Craniomaxillofac Surg. 2017;45(12):2115–9.

# Supraclavicular Flap

# 12

Arya Namin and Masoud Saman

## Introduction

The supraclavicular flap is a pedicled fasciocutaneous flap based off the supraclavicular artery that was originally described in the late 1970s. While various descriptions of shoulder flaps were present in the literature, Lamberty described the vascular anatomy of the supraclavicular flap in 1979 [1]. The cervicohumeral flap was described as a flap based off the transverse cervical artery and centered over the acromioclavicular joint with the option of extending the flap distally over the lateral arm [2]. The anatomic study by Lamberty included 30 cadaveric sides that described a superficial branch of the superficial transverse cervical artery that was present in 28 out of 30 cadaveric sides [1]. The course of the superficial branch of the superficial transverse cervical artery is described as originating from the superficial transverse cervical artery and then passing laterally toward the acromioclavicular joint and then sending branches laterally onto the lateral aspect of the upper arm [1]. Lamberty later went on to clarify that the cervicohumeral flap was a musculocutaneous flap with random extensions, explaining the higher failure rate in certain studies [3]. The use of the supraclavicular flap did not become widespread during the 1980s and 1990s likely because of the rise of free tissue transfer and lack of a clear understanding of the angiosome and therefore design of the supraclavicular artery flap.

The vascular anatomy, angiosome, flap design, and reliability were more robustly described by a series of studies in the late 1990s [4, 5]. In the 2000s, multiple studies were published supporting the utility of the supraclavicular flap in reconstructing a variety of cutaneous and aerodigestive tract defects [6–9]. Subsequently during

A. Namin
Otolaryngology and Facial Plastic Surgery Associates, Fort Worth, TX, USA

M. Saman (✉)
DallasFaceDoc, PLLC, Dallas, TX, USA
e-mail: drsaman@dallasfacedoc.com


F. Sokoya, A. G. Vincent (eds.), *Manual of Head and Neck Reconstruction*,
https://doi.org/10.1007/978-3-031-65999-7_12

the 2010s, the supraclavicular flap gained widespread use across many centers for the reconstruction of defects, including cutaneous defects of the head and neck, lateral skull base, parotidectomy, and aerodigestive tract [10–17]. Head and neck defects often have multiple reconstructive options that would result in acceptable form and function with minimal morbidity. The benefits of the supraclavicular flap include avoidance of distant donor site morbidity, microvascular anastomosis, rapidity of harvest, and thinness and pliability of the flap matching cutaneous defects of the head and neck.

## Anatomy

The supraclavicular flap is a pedicled fasciocutaneous flap based off the supraclavicular artery, which is most commonly a branch of the transverse cervical artery [4, 8]. The supraclavicular artery can be less commonly found as a branch of the suprascapular artery [8]. However, there is discrepancy in the published literature regarding the anatomy of the supraclavicular artery. In an anatomical study of 19 fresh cadavers, the supraclavicular artery arose 3–4 cm from the origin of the transverse cervical artery in 100% of the specimens [4]. Multiple anatomical studies have demonstrated the supraclavicular artery branching from the transverse cervical artery 3.0–3.6 cm above the clavicle, 8.2–8.6 cm from the sternoclavicular joint, and 2.1 cm dorsal to the sternocleidomastoid muscle with a mean diameter of 1.0–1.5 mm [4, 18]. Importantly, this study of 19 fresh cadavers defined the angiosome of the supraclavicular artery as the skin over the ventral surface of the deltoid extending from the supraclavicular region to the should cap, which was an important clarification of the early studies describing the cervicohumeral flap that centered the skin paddle over the acromioclavicular joint and extending distally over the lateral arm [2, 4]. Understanding this anatomy and typical course of the supraclavicular artery is important when designing the flap over the ventral surface of the deltoid muscle (Fig. 12.1). The area of the angiosome ranged from $10 \times 22\ cm^2$ to $16 \times 30\ cm^2$ [4]. More recently, Pallua et al. have described the anterior supraclavicular artery, which is also a branch of the transverse cervical artery, but branches more proximally above the clavicle directly lateral to the sternocleidomastoid muscle before passing through the platysma crossing the clavicle in the medial third and then running in the deltopectoral groove [19]. In the experience of Pallua et al., both the supraclavicular artery and the anterior supraclavicular artery are reliably present [19].

Multiple radiographic studies of cadaveric supraclavicular flaps have examined the angiosome of the supraclavicular artery [18, 20, 21]. A cadaveric study has been described where postcontrast CT scans were obtained after supraclavicular flaps were elevated, including the deltoid muscle in some of the flaps [21]. The course of the supraclavicular artery and the dimension of the vessel were in concordance with previously published studies [4, 21]. The supraclavicular artery was noted to cross the clavicle in the middle to lateral thirds in the suprafascial plane [21]. The skin superficial to the deltoid muscle was noted to have perfusion through musculocutaneous perforators originating from the anterior and posterior circumflex humeral

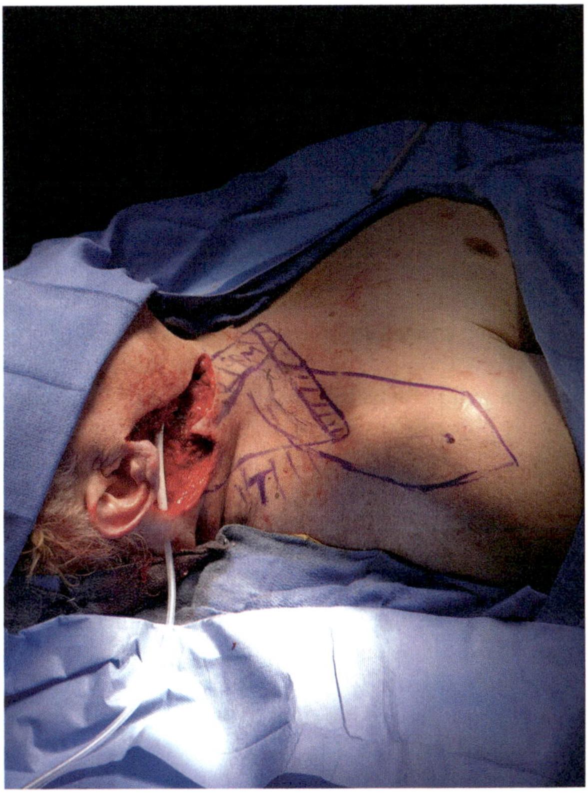

**Fig. 12.1** Supraclavicular flap design. The supraclavicular artery is identified with Doppler ultrasonography in the triangle formed by the posterior border of the sternocleidomastoid, the clavicle, and the external jugular vein. The skin paddle is designed over the ventral surface of the deltoid, not extending distal to the deltoid's insertion point into the humerus. (Courtesy of Masoud Saman, MD)

arteries [21]. The study concluded that it was anastomosis between the supraclavicular artery and the musculocutaneous perforators through the deltoid muscle that allow for a reliable flap design up to the insertion of the deltoid muscle, which is consistent with clinical findings [8, 12, 21]. A similar study of ten cadaveric supraclavicular flaps demonstrated concordant findings that the supraclavicular artery perfused the distal portions of the flap overlying the deltoid muscle through an interperforator flow from direct linking vessels and recurrent flow through the subdermal plexus [18]. Chan et al. found that one of the ten flaps was perfused only about 50% by the supraclavicular artery due to a smaller supraclavicular artery (0.7 mm) [18]. The venous drainage of the supraclavicular flap typically drains via the venae comitantes that subsequently drain into the transverse cervical veins and a second vein draining into the external jugular vein [4, 18, 21]. Prior to flap elevation, the skin overlying the distal aspect of the flap has venous drainage into the cephalic vein and circumflex humeral vein via the musculocutaneous branches through the deltoid muscle, which likely increases venous pressure within the distal portion of the flap after elevation [18, 21]. While the supraclavicular flap has been described as a free flap, the diameter of the veins requiring anastomosis and number of excellent low morbidity donor site alternatives has led to its infrequent use as a free flap [20].

## Indications

The indications for the supraclavicular flap have been widely expanded over the past two decades to include postburn neck scar contractures, noma orofacial defects, progressive hemifacial atrophy asymmetry, tracheal reconstruction, parotidectomy contour defects, cutaneous defects of the head and neck, lateral skull base defects, auriculectomy defects, and aerodigestive tract defects.

The supraclavicular flap initially gained more widespread use after its application in reconstructing postburn neck scar contractures [5, 22]. With pre-expansion of the supraclavicular flap, entire facial resurfacing of burn scars with the supraclavicular flap proved feasible [23]. Noma, a rapidly progressive, multifactorial, gangrenous condition of the mouth and face that is predominantly found in malnourished patients within the sub-Saharan region, is a challenging disease to treat with exceptionally high morbidity and mortality [24]. While management of the early stages of disease involves medical and nutritional support, late stage management involves reconstructing complex orofacial defects for which the supraclavicular flap has been utilized [24–26]. Progressive hemifacial atrophy is a rare disorder of unknown etiology that typically develops during the first or second decade of life that is characterized by slowly progressive unilateral atrophy of the skin, soft tissue, muscle, and bony skeleton [7, 27]. Soft tissue augmentation in the form of a scapular free tissue transfer has been found to correct the facial asymmetry and halt the progression of the disease [27]. The supraclavicular flap has also been described as an alternative to free tissue transfer in correcting the facial asymmetry in progressive hemifacial atrophy. [7]

The supraclavicular flap has been successfully applied to reconstruct auriculectomy and temporal bone defects [10, 28]. In order to obtain adequate pedicle length, a soft tissue back cut can be made superiorly over the posterior border of the sternocleidomastoid muscle, and the pedicle can also be elevated over the clavicle in a subperiosteal plane [10]. In cases where the lateral skull base defect is too large for free fat grafts or in cases where vascularized soft tissue coverage is needed, the supraclavicular flap is an option. The supraclavicular flap is not ideal in lateral skull base defects greater than 10–15 cm in width and deep defects that require substantial vascularized soft tissue bulk [10].

Contour irregularities and Frey's syndrome are common postoperative sequelae after parotidectomy. Fat grafts, superficial musculoaponeurotic system flaps, and buried free flaps have all been utilized to minimize the incidence of Frey's syndrome and contour abnormalities [29–31]. The supraclavicular flap has also been described as an excellent option for reconstructing parotidectomy contour defects [10, 13]. The supraclavicular flap provides an adequate volume of vascularized tissue for most parotidectomy contour defects while also avoiding the need for microvascular surgery and distant donor site morbidity. Typically, the supraclavicular flap is deepithelialized for contour defect reconstruction. However, if a cutaneous defect is present, the supraclavicular flap is an ideal regional reconstruction option (Figs. 12.2 and 12.3). The morbidity of a shoulder scar from the supraclavicular flap must be considered and discussed with the patient.

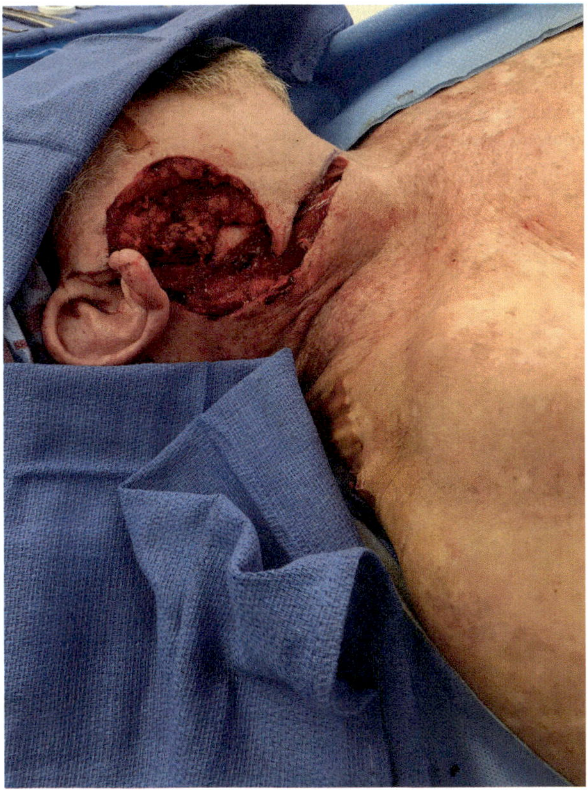

**Fig. 12.2** Preauricular defect amenable to supraclavicular flap reconstruction. (Courtesy of Masoud Saman, MD)

As experience has been gained with the supraclavicular flap in reconstructing cutaneous and soft defects, aerodigestive tract reconstruction with the supraclavicular flap has been demonstrated as a feasible option. A prefabricated supraclavicular flap with auricular cartilage has been described in reconstructing high-risk tracheal stenosis with eight out of eight patients being successfully decannulated [15]. In a series of ten patients who underwent patch graft reconstruction, a reconstruction of the anterior pharyngeal wall, of total laryngectomy defects with a supraclavicular flap two out of ten patients developed a pharyngocutaneous fistula with one of those patients having near total loss of the flap [11]. The circumferential pharyngoesophageal defect following salvage laryngectomy is a complex defect with high risk for complications [32]. While free tissue transfer is usually the preferred method of reconstructing circumferential pharyngoesophageal defects after salvage laryngectomy, the supraclavicular flap has been successfully utilized for this challenging problem [9]. Primary tracheoesophageal puncture with intraoperative prosthesis placement has been found to be safe and effective in patients undergoing reconstruction with the supraclavicular flap [33]. The supraclavicular flap provides a regional source of vascularized soft tissue that can be employed in reconstructing esophageal perforations after anterior cervical spine surgery [14].

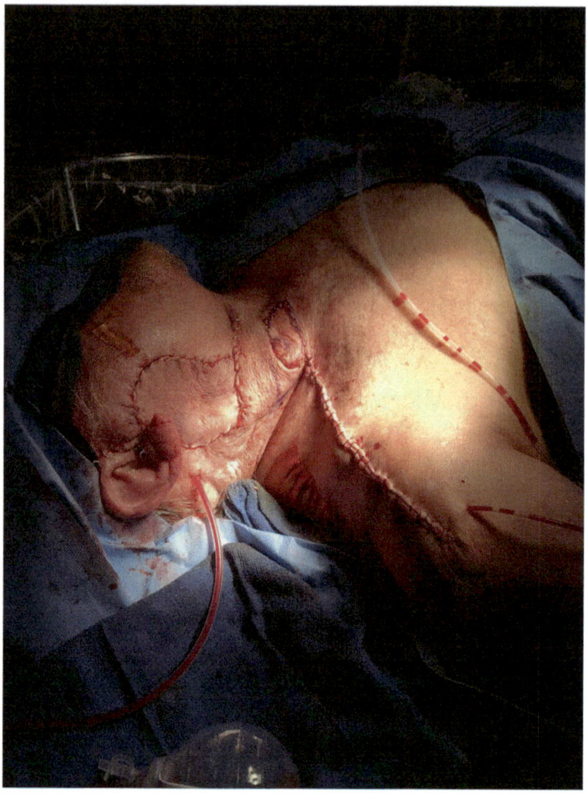

**Fig. 12.3** Supraclavicular flap inset into preauricular defect. Donor site successfully closed primarily. (Courtesy of Masoud Saman, MD)

As can be seen in the above discussion, the supraclavicular flap has been successfully applied to many reconstructive challenges. However, most defects often have many acceptable reconstructive options. As the supraclavicular flap has gained popularity, studies identifying limitations and comparing outcomes of the supraclavicular flap with free flaps have been published. In a retrospective series of 32 patients in whom all patients were candidates for either a free fasciocutaneous flap or a supraclavicular flap, the 16 patients who underwent supraclavicular flap reconstruction had significantly shorter operative times, significantly shorter ICU stays, and significantly less need for split thickness skin graft [17, 34, 35]. The rate of complications has been found to be significantly higher in patients undergoing mucosal reconstruction with the supraclavicular flap compared to patients undergoing cutaneous reconstruction with the supraclavicular flap [16, 36]. The supraclavicular flap can be utilized to reconstruct oral cavity defects in addition to pharyngeal defects (Fig. 12.4). While the supraclavicular flap has been successfully utilized in patients with prior radiation therapy to the neck and prior neck dissection, the presence and size of the supraclavicular artery should be more intensively scrutinized [9, 37]. The presence of an ipsilateral pacemaker or ports adds risk of contamination of these devices, particularly in clean contaminated surgery; however, the supraclavicular flap has been successfully utilized in patients with these devices [38].

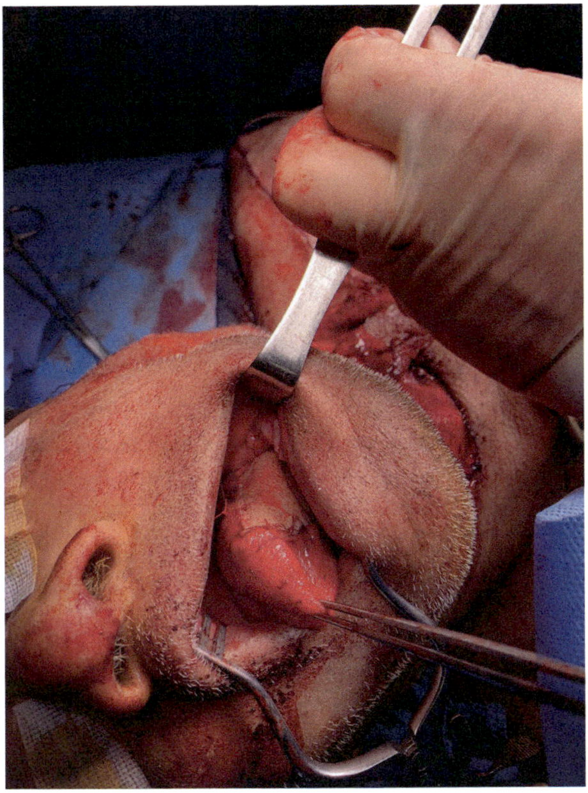

**Fig. 12.4** Supraclavicular flap inset into partial glossectomy defect. Many reconstructive options lend themselves to partial glossectomy reconstruction. Pedicle length of the supraclavicular flap does allow for utilization in oral cavity defects. (Courtesy of Masoud Saman, MD)

## Preoperative Planning

Preoperative confirmation of the presence of a supraclavicular artery should be performed either with a Doppler identifying the supraclavicular artery within the triangular fossa (sternocleidomastoid muscle, clavicle, and external jugular vein) or computed tomography angiography (CTA) [12, 39]. The neck should be examined for any prior scars. If the patient has had a prior neck dissection and/or radiation, the presence of a supraclavicular artery should be more thoroughly investigated. Preoperative discussion with the ablative surgeon should be had regarding plans for incorporating level 5b and 4, as the transverse cervical artery and supraclavicular artery will be at risk. The benefits of CTA allow the surgical team to have strong clinical data regarding the presence, location, diameter, and length of the pedicle [39]. If the surgical team has a donor side preference, the contrast bolus should be given contralaterally to minimize bolus artifacts, and the arms should be kept at the patients' side during the study [39].

## Instrumentation

- Bipolar electrocautery
- Monopolar electrocautery
- Skin hooks
- Suction drains
- Fine tip dissecting scissors
- Dissolvable and permanent sutures
- Doppler probe

## Surgical Technique

A Doppler probe is used to confirm the presence and location of the supraclavicular artery in the triangle bordered by the posterior border of the sternocleidomastoid muscle, the clavicle, and the external jugular vein. A fusiform skin paddle is then designed over the ventral aspect of the deltoid muscle. The neck and arm are then prepped and draped circumferentially down to the elbow. An incision is then made from the medial aspect of the skin paddle to triangle where the supraclavicular artery was identified. Subdermal flaps are then elevated to the lateral border of the sternocleidomastoid muscle and 3 cm lateral to the point where the supraclavicular artery crosses over the clavicle. Designing the soft tissue pedicle to include a wide base of soft tissue protects the pedicle, minimizes risk of kinking the pedicle, and also likely incorporates the anterior supraclavicular artery described by Pallua et al. in 2013 [12, 19].

The supraclavicular flap is then elevated in the subfascial plane from distal to proximal. As the clavicle is encountered, the pedicle is dissected over the clavicle in a subperiosteal plane. In the plane superficial to the pedicle, dissection is carried forth in the subdermal pane in order to protect the pedicle. Dissection continues in the subdermal plane superficially until a point over the sternocleidomastoid muscle is reached at which point the plane of dissection is transition to the subplatysmal plane and therefore allowing tunneling of the flap into the anterior neck, face, and aerodigestive tract [4, 11, 12].

## Postoperative Management

Standard postoperative care is undertaken. Suction drains are managed. The area is closely followed for signs of infection. Evidence of partial or complete flap loss are monitored for in cases where the flap is visible on examination. Signs of fistula are closely looked for in cases of mucosal reconstruction. The donor site is assessed for any evidence of dehiscence.

## References


1. Lamberty BG. The supra-clavicular axial patterned flap. Br J Plast Surg. 1979;32(3):207–12.
2. Mathes SJ, Vasconez LO. The cervicohumeral flap. Plast Reconstr Surg. 1978;61(1):7–12.
3. Lamberty BG, Cormack GC. Misconceptions regarding the cervico-humeral flap. Br J Plast Surg. 1983;36(1):60–3.
4. Pallua N, Magnus NE. The tunneled supraclavicular island flap: an optimized technique for head and neck reconstruction. Plast Reconstr Surg. 2000;105(3):842–51; discussion 852–4.
5. Pallua N, Machens HG, Rennekampff O, Becker M, Berger A. The fasciocutaneous supraclavicular artery island flap for releasing postburn mentosternal contractures. Plast Reconstr Surg. 1997;99(7):1878–84; discussion 1885–6.
6. Di Benedetto G, Aquinati A, Pierangeli M, Scalise A, Bertani A. From the "charretera" to the supraclavicular fascial island flap: revisitation and further evolution of a controversial flap. Plast Reconstr Surg. 2005;115(1):70–6.
7. Di Benedetto G, Aquinati A, Balercia P, Forlini W, Bertani A. Supraclavicular island fascial flap in the treatment of progressive hemifacial atrophy. Plast Reconstr Surg. 2008;121(5):247e–50e.
8. Chiu ES, Liu PH, Friedlander PL. Supraclavicular artery island flap for head and neck oncologic reconstruction: indications, complications, and outcomes. Plast Reconstr Surg. 2009;124(1):115–23.
9. Chiu ES, Liu PH, Baratelli R, Lee MY, Chaffin AE, Friedlander PL. Circumferential pharyngoesophageal reconstruction with a supraclavicular artery island flap. Plast Reconstr Surg. 2010;125(1):161–6.
10. Emerick KS, Herr MW, Lin DT, Santos F, Deschler DG. Supraclavicular artery island flap for reconstruction of complex parotidectomy, lateral skull base, and total auriculectomy defects. JAMA Otolaryngol Head Neck Surg. 2014;140(9):861–6.
11. Emerick KS, Herr MA, Deschler DG. Supraclavicular flap reconstruction following total laryngectomy. Laryngoscope. 2014;124(8):1777–82.
12. Herr MW, Emerick KS, Deschler DG. The supraclavicular artery flap for head and neck reconstruction. JAMA Facial Plast Surg. 2014;16(2):127–32.
13. Epps MT, Cannon CL, Wright MJ, Chaffin AE, Newsome RE, Friedlander PL, et al. Aesthetic restoration of parotidectomy contour deformity using the supraclavicular artery island flap. Plast Reconstr Surg. 2011;127(5):1925–31.
14. Gibson AW, Gobillot TA, Bass DI, Zakarevicius Z, Rizvi ZH, Ravanpay AC. Case of esophageal perforation and repair with a supraclavicular artery island fascial flap 15 years after anterior spine surgery. World Neurosurg. 2020;143:102–7.
15. Zender CA, Patel AV, Strohl M, Melki S, Maronian N. The prefabricated supraclavicular artery flap in high-risk tracheal stenosis patients. Laryngoscope. 2020;130(3):641–8.
16. Kokot N, Kim JH, West JD, Zhang P. Supraclavicular artery island flap: critical appraisal and comparison to alternate reconstruction. Laryngoscope. 2022;132 Suppl 3:1–14.
17. Kozin ED, Sethi RK, Herr M, Shrime MG, Rocco JW, Lin D, et al. Comparison of perioperative outcomes between the supraclavicular artery island flap and fasciocutaneous free flap. Otolaryngol Head Neck Surg. 2016;154(1):66–72.
18. Chan JWH, Wong C, Ward K, Saint-Cyr M, Chiu ES. Three- and four-dimensional computed tomographic angiography studies of the supraclavicular artery island flap. Plast Reconstr Surg. 2010;125(2):525–31.
19. Pallua N, Wolter TP. Moving forwards: the anterior supraclavicular artery perforator (a-SAP) flap: a new pedicled or free perforator flap based on the anterior supraclavicular vessels. J Plast Reconstr Aesthetic Surg. 2013;66(4):489–96.
20. Cordova A, Pirrello R, D'Arpa S, Jeschke J, Brenner E, Moschella F. Vascular anatomy of the supraclavicular area revisited: feasibility of the free supraclavicular perforator flap. Plast Reconstr Surg. 2008;122(5):1399–409.
21. Ross RJ, Baillieu CE, Shayan R, Leung M, Ashton MW. The anatomical basis for improving the reliability of the supraclavicular flap. J Plast Reconstr Aesthetic Surg. 2014;67(2):198–204.

22. Vinh VQ, Van Anh T, Ogawa R, Hyakusoku H. Anatomical and clinical studies of the supraclavicular flap: analysis of 103 flaps used to reconstruct neck scar contractures. Plast Reconstr Surg. 2009;123(5):1471–80.
23. Pallua N, von Heimburg D. Pre-expanded ultra-thin supraclavicular flaps for (full-) face reconstruction with reduced donor-site morbidity and without the need for microsurgery. Plast Reconstr Surg. 2005;115(7):1837–44; discussion 1845–7.
24. Srour ML, Marck K, Baratti-Mayer D. Noma: overview of a neglected disease and human rights violation. Am J Trop Med Hyg. 2017;96(2):268–74.
25. Heitland AS, Pallua N. The single and double-folded supraclavicular island flap as a new therapy option in the treatment of large facial defects in noma patients. Plast Reconstr Surg. 2005;115(6):1591–6.
26. Hartman EHM, Van Damme PA, Suominen SHH. The use of the pedicled supraclavicular flap in noma reconstructive surgery. Plast Reconstr Surg. 2006;118(1):270–1.
27. Chen JT, Schmid DB, Israel JS, Siebert JW. A 26-year experience with microsurgical reconstruction of hemifacial atrophy and linear scleroderma. Plast Reconstr Surg. 2018;142(5):1275–83.
28. Levy JM, Eko FN, Hilaire HS, Friedlander PL, Melgar MA, Chiu ES. Posterolateral skull base reconstruction using the supraclavicular artery Island flap. J Craniofac Surg. 2011;22(5):1751–4.
29. Curry JM, Fisher KW, Heffelfinger RN, Rosen MR, Keane WM, Pribitkin EA. Superficial musculoaponeurotic system elevation and fat graft reconstruction after superficial parotidectomy. Laryngoscope. 2008;118(2):210–5.
30. Cannady SB, Seth R, Fritz MA, Alam DS, Wax MK. Total parotidectomy defect reconstruction using the buried free flap. Otolaryngol Head Neck Surg. 2010;143(5):637–43.
31. Loyo M, Gourin CG. Free abdominal fat transfer for partial and total parotidectomy defect reconstruction. Laryngoscope. 2016;126(12):2694–8.
32. Microvascular Committee of the American Academy of Otolaryngology-Head & Neck Surgery. Salvage laryngectomy and laryngopharyngectomy: multicenter review of outcomes associated with a reconstructive approach. Head Neck. 2019;41(1):16–29.
33. Sethi RKV, Kozin ED, Lam AC, Emerick KS, Deschler DG. Primary tracheoesophageal puncture with supraclavicular artery island flap after total laryngectomy or laryngopharyngectomy. Otolaryngol Head Neck Surg. 2014;151(3):421–3.
34. Sukato DC, Timashpolsky A, Ferzli G, Rosenfeld RM, Gordin EA. Systematic review of supraclavicular artery island flap vs free flap in head and neck reconstruction. Otolaryngol Head Neck Surg. 2019;160(2):215–22.
35. Granzow JW, Suliman A, Roostaeian J, Perry A, Boyd JB. Supraclavicular artery island flap (SCAIF) vs free fasciocutaneous flaps for head and neck reconstruction. Otolaryngol Head Neck Surg. 2013;148(6):941–8.
36. Kadakia S, Agarwal J, Mourad M, Ashai S, Lee T, Ducic Y. Supraclavicular flap reconstruction of cutaneous defects has lower complication rate than mucosal defects. J Reconstr Microsurg. 2017;33(4):275–80.
37. Razdan SN, Albornoz CR, Ro T, Cordeiro PG, Disa JJ, McCarthy CM, et al. Safety of the supraclavicular artery island flap in the setting of neck dissection and radiation therapy. J Reconstr Microsurg. 2015;31(5):378–83.
38. Zenga J, Chen J, Deschler DG. Supraclavicular artery island flap in patients with ports or pacemakers. JAMA Facial Plast Surg. 2018;20(3):256–7.
39. Adams AS, Wright MJ, Johnston S, Tandon R, Gupta N, Ward K, et al. The use of multislice CT angiography preoperative study for supraclavicular artery island flap harvesting. Ann Plast Surg. 2012;69(3):312–5.

# Part IV

# Osseous and Osteocutaneous Flaps and Grafts

# The Free Fibula Flap

# 13

Jason Cohn and Fiyin Sokoya

## Introduction/History

First described by Hidalgo in 1989, the free fibular flap (FFF) is the workhorse for reconstructing soft tissue and bony defects of the head and neck [1]. FFF is a diverse flap that may be harvested as an osseous, osteocutaneous or osteofascial flap and may be precisely tailored to the defect by using multiple osteotomies, double perforator-based skin flaps, muscle component, and "double-barreling", amongst others [2–7].

The fibula is a long, bicortical bone that can be harvested up to 25 cm in length [8]. This allows for complete angle-to-angle mandibular reconstruction [9]. Using a two-team approach, simultaneous ablation and free tissue harvest are attainable. Multiple osteotomies can be performed and precise shaping of the flap can be achieved, with up to five bony segments generally used [8].

Due to its rich periosteal blood supply, the FFF permits the placement of osseointegrated implants [9]. Not only does this allow the patient to masticate, but implants have been shown to improve aesthetics and lip support aiding in oral competence [10].

J. Cohn
Sunrise ENT and Facial Plastics, Lindenhurst, NY, USA

F. Sokoya (✉)
Wellstar Health Systems, Atlanta, GA, USA


F. Sokoya, A. G. Vincent (eds.), *Manual of Head and Neck Reconstruction*,
https://doi.org/10.1007/978-3-031-65999-7_13

## Anatomy

The main blood supply to the osteocutaneous fibular flap is the peroneal artery via perforators, which are divided into septocutaneous, musculocutaneous, and septo-musculocutaneous [11, 12]. One study defined the peroneal skin branches into three patterns:

Type A located in the proximal third of the leg, pass through the peroneus longus or the soleus muscles;
Type B located throughout the leg, pass between the soleus and peroneal muscles and branch to adjacent muscles;
Type C located in the middle and distal thirds of the leg, same as Type B but do not branch to adjacent muscles [12].

Yoshimura et al. determined the average number of cutaneous branches to be 4.8 per leg. Cutaneous branches from the peroneal artery were located 6–30 cm distal from the fibular head, with the greatest confluence of vessels 24 cm distal from the fibular head [12].

## Indication/Contraindications

Maxillary and mandibular reconstruction are performed after resection due to malignant tumors, nonmalignant tumors, congenital conditions, trauma, osteoradio-necrosis, infection, and previous flap failure [7–9]. FFF is often the flap of choice for mandibular reconstruction including bone-only defects, anterior reconstruction requiring external replacement of the skin and internal floor of mouth, as well as hemi-mandible defects with adjacent lateral floor of mouth and buccal mucosa loss [13] (Fig. 13.1).

One main disadvantage of the FFF is that the skin island is not reliable in every patient. Retromolar trigone defects have large mucosal requirements with a short bone gap. In these situations, a unicortical radial forearm flap would be more appropriate. Lateral defects with large internal and external tissue loss would also exclude FFF reconstruction. For this scenario, the scapular free flap would provide enough reliable soft tissue coverage [13]. Anatomical variants and peripheral arterial disease of the lower extremity can also preclude the use of this flap [11].

## Preoperative Planning

Preoperative models with or without prefabricated reconstruction plates and cutting guides may be used and have shown to decrease ischemia time, operative time, and length of stay and in some reports also improve operative outcome [4, 7, 14–16]. In addition, virtual planning allows the surgical team to customize the operation to the patient needs within 2–4 mm of accuracy [16].

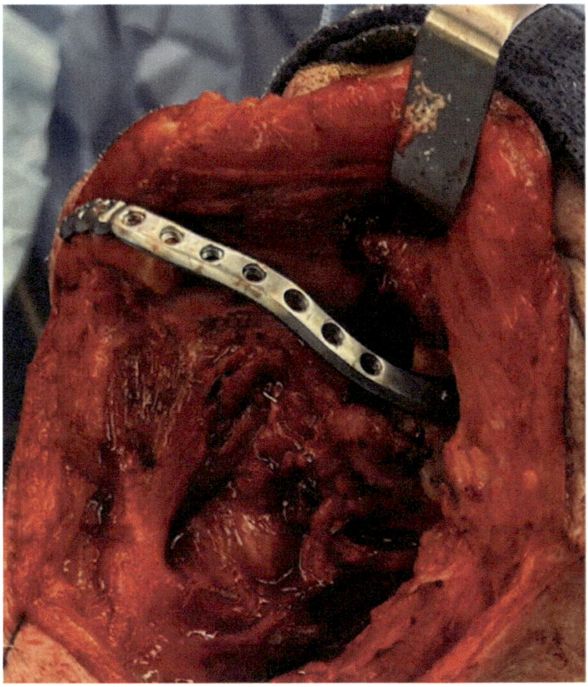

**Fig. 13.1** Segmental mandible defect from symphysis to angle after plate reconstruction

Computer planning sessions typically occur with vendors via virtual meetings. Each session can take up to 1 h; however, with each successive session, meetings can be streamlined. During the session, data is extracted from the patient's CT scan and it is used to plan the resection and reconstruction. Following this, a surgical plan is created and reviewed by the surgical team, allowing for changes prior to the surgery. The ablative and reconstructive teams then coordinate how many osteotomies and bone segments will be required. Surgical models including cutout templates of the various angles of the dentoalveolar arch are then prepared with cutting guides. Finally, plate bending is planned, further saving of operative time [7, 16].

The need for preoperative angiography remains controversial. One study indicated that there is low-quality evidence to suggest the need for lower limb angiography with flap. However, physical examination alone is insufficient in detecting poor limb perfusion [9]. Specifically, the ankle–brachial index was found to be insufficient in detecting vascular anomalies or subclinical peripheral arterial disease [17, 18]. A more recent study demonstrated that computed tomographic angiography accurately predicted the course and location of the peroneal artery and perforators. However, perforator size was less accurately estimated [19].

Intraoperative indocyanin green (ICG) videoangiography can be used to assess perfusion to the fibula flap to ensure flap viability especially in individuals at risk for flap loss [20, 21]. However, ICG imaging cannot visualize the macrovascular (tibioperoneal) and fibula bony anatomy and is only available intraoperatively, not allowing for preoperative planning [19].

## Instrumentation

Standard operative instrumentation and microsurgical instrumentation are required. These include major plastic surgery/otolaryngology trays and biceps forceps trays. Specifically, necessary instruments include dissecting scissors, such as Stevens and Metzenbaum, hemoclip appliers, and nylon sutures. Additionally, Browns, Addison-browns, and jeweler forceps are also helpful during dissection. Iris and double skin hooks, Army-Navy, and Senn retractors all have a role in exposure. Finally, bovie cautery and various blade sizes are necessary for dissection dependent on surgeon preference and experience. The specific details of tool vary by surgeon preference and institutional tray setup. In most cases, a dermatome will be required for skin graft harvest, and a pneumatic tourniquet cuff will be utilized during flap dissection.

## Flap Design and Surgical Technique

### Flap Design and Preparation

Hidalgo, the first to describe fibula free flap for mandibular reconstruction, proposed that the skin island should span the entire length of the fibula. It should taper proximally and distally relative to the main skin island and should be centered over the midpoint of the fibula [1]. Based upon further anatomical studies, osteocutaneous free fibular flaps should be designed 10–20 cm from the fibular head and should include the soleus and flexor hallicus longus muscle cuff to incorporate potential septocutaneous perforators [22]. The long axis of the skin island is centered over the posterior border of the fibula in order to capture the septal blood supply [13].

During hemimandibular reconstruction, the ipsilateral leg is typically selected (Fig. 13.2). The rationale is that the flexor hallucis longus muscle lies directly underneath the fibula. In addition, the skin island can easily be rotated up and over the fibula to reach the oral cavity for mucosal reconstruction. Reconstruction is

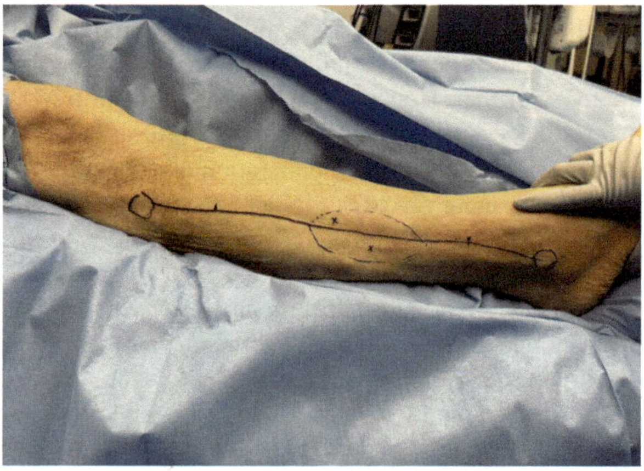

**Fig. 13.2** Skin paddle and perforators identified. Note depiction of lateral malleolus and ankle mortise and distance from the joints marked

planned so that the pedicle enters the bone at the angle of the mandibular flap. This maximizes the pedicle length. For more anterior defects, the flap design is shifted more distally. The proximal bone is removed in the subperiosteal plane, adding more pedicle length [13].

A helpful rule in determining the laterality of leg selection is the rule of the surgeon's fist. The surgeon's fist with the thumb up can be used to replicate the fibula and the peroneal vessels. The skin and the lateral surface of the fibula bone are represented by the back of the hand and fingers, and the pedicle is represented by the thumb. This method is helpful in vessel selection, skin paddle selection, and orientation and complication avoidance.

## Dissection and Elevation

The tunneling technique popularized by Dr. Ducic makes for expedited harvest of the fibular free flap. First, the flap is designed by centering it along a vertical line slightly anterior to the posterior intermuscular septum. The skin paddle, if needed, is oriented lengthwise and is centered over this line. Under tourniquet control of 350 mmHg, the skin paddle is incised and relaxing incisions carried inferiorly to within 5–6 cm of the ankle mortise and superiorly to within 6 cm of the head of the fibula (Fig. 13.3). Care is taken to avoid the peroneal nerve in this region. The incision is carried right down to the peroneal muscles. The peroneus longus and brevis are retracted anteriorly. Dissection is then carried anteriorly past the lateral surface of the fibula. The anterior septum is traversed at this point. Dissection is then carried past the extensor digitorium longus and the extensor hallucis longus. Next a small perforation is made in the central portion of the interosseous membrane. Finger dissection is then performed superiorly and inferiorly along the anticipated portion of fibula harvest (Fig. 13.4).

Next, the periosteum in the area of proposed osteotomy is then elevated using a periosteal elevator. The elevator is then placed medial to the bone in the area of elevated periosteum to help protect the pedicle. An oscillating saw is then used to perform an osteotomy distally then proximally. The hallucis longus muscle is then sectioned and the distal pedicle controlled with hemoclips. Finger dissection is performed in the tunnel of dissection deep to the tibialis posterior and medial to the vessels. This is a loose areolar, avascular plane that runs superiorly to the takeoff of the peroneal artery in all cases. The tibialis posterior muscle superficial to the index finger which rests within the dissection tunnel can be divided with Metzenbaum scissors. Now, the fibula osteomyocutaneous flap should be pedicled just on the peroneal artery and its paired venae comitantes. The pedicle is then divided at the takeoff (Fig. 13.5). The tourniquet is removed and the pedicle is tied off once vascularity is verified [23]. Typical microvascular anastomosis is performed with 9.0 nylon sutures and venous couplers. One or both veins may be utilized, depending on flow (Fig. 13.6).

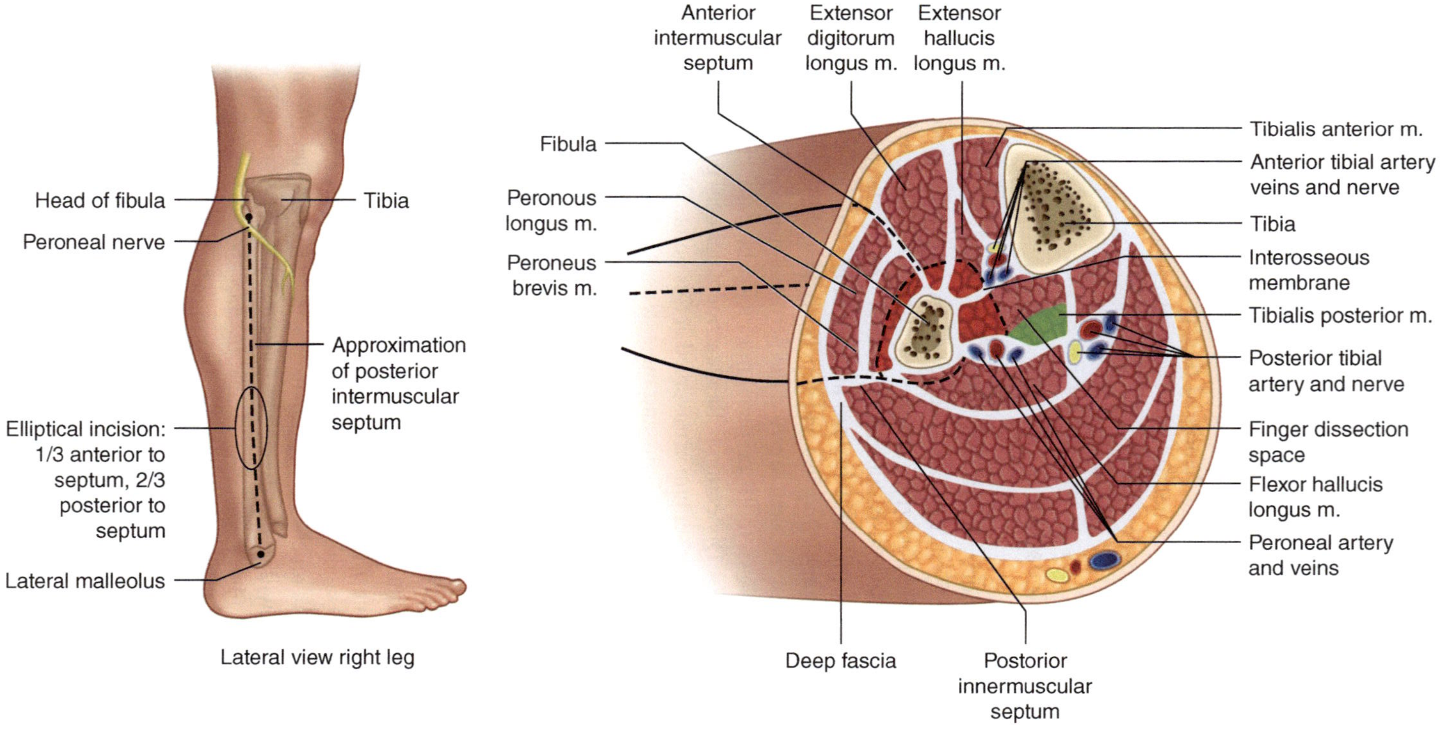


**Fig. 13.3** Compartments of the leg. Fibula anatomy

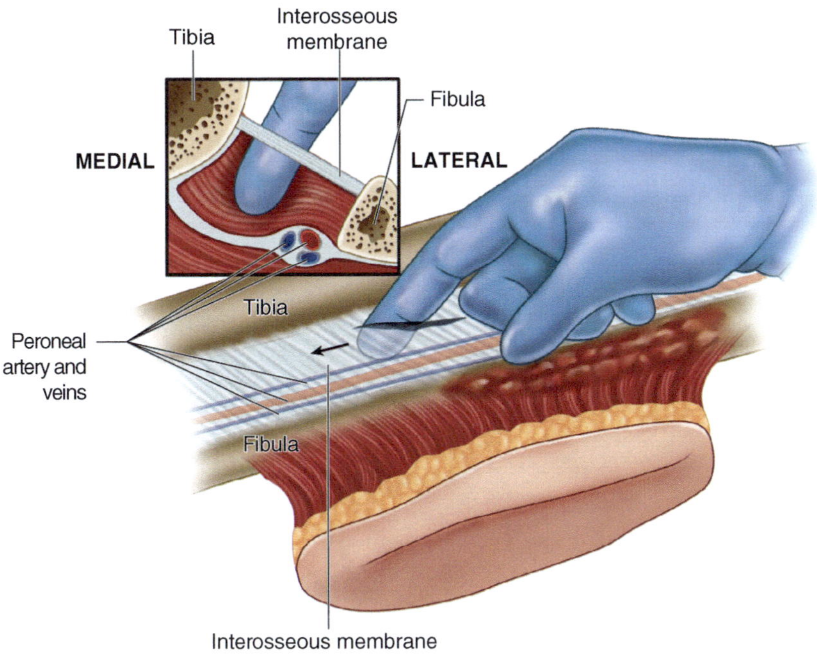


**Fig. 13.4** Traversing the interosseous membrane

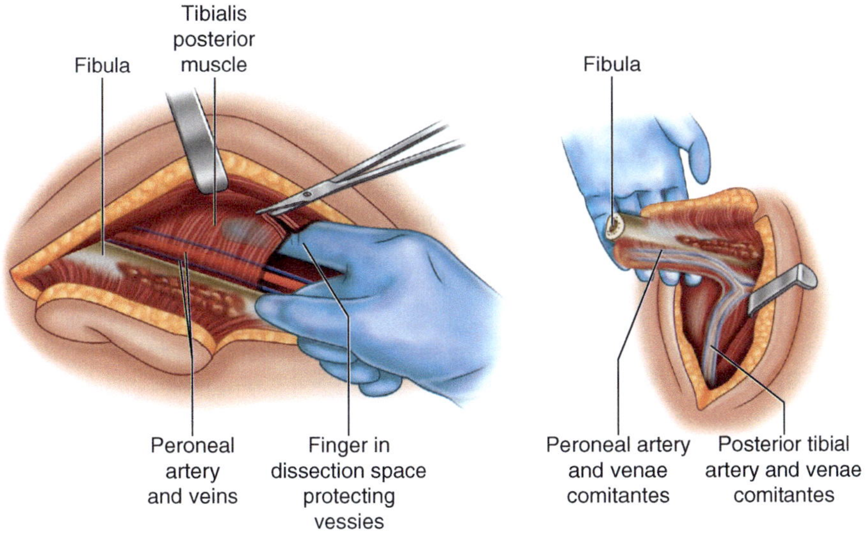


**Fig. 13.5** Tunneling method

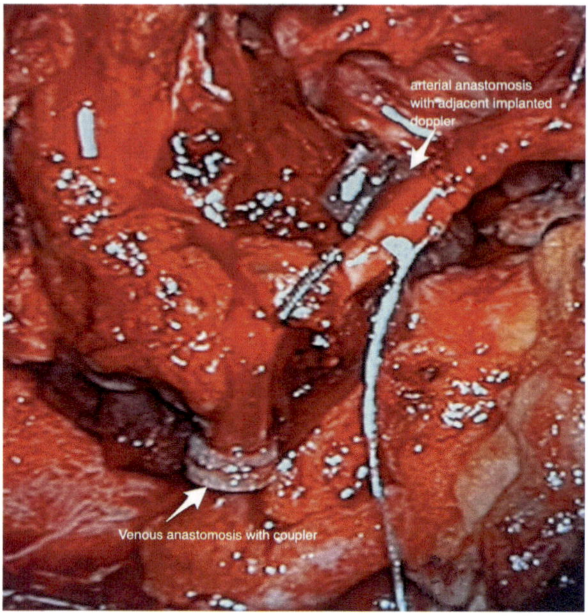


**Fig. 13.6** Venous anastomosis with coupler and arterial anastomosis with adjacent implantable Doppler

## Donor Site Closure

The donor site was initially thought to be closed primarily the majority of the time [12]. However, primarily closure is sometimes associated with excess tension which can lead to wound breakdown, necrosis, infection, and compartment syndrome. It is now recommended to use a skin graft to close most defects, regardless of the width of the skin paddle. Some studies advocate for the placement of a bolster dressing or negative-pressure wound therapy, while others state that it has no impact on donor site healing [24]. One systematic review and meta-analysis concluded that flap reconstruction of the donor site resulted in less short-term complications compared to skin grafting [25]. However, most studies have shown overall complication rates to be the same regardless of closure technique [26].

## Postoperative Management

One of the main drawbacks of the FFF is monitoring its blood supply because the flap is often buried within the mandible. This can be mitigated by externalizing a small skin island, monitoring an intraoral skin island, selective angiography, and technetium-99m bone scanning [12, 13]. An implanted Doppler can also be used to monitor arterial and/or venous flow.

Flap checks of the peroneal artery with a pencil Doppler are recommended every 1–2 h for the first 48 h postoperatively. In one study, the use of an implantable Doppler device reduced flap failure from 56% to 21% [8]. Panoramic X-ray studies or CT scans are utilized to monitor bone stock healing. Patient free of disease can receive osseointegrated implants 6–12 months following reconstruction [13]. Although radiation exposure can show a trend toward implant failure, this has not been shown to be significant. Some advocate waiting 6 months following radiation for implantation [10]. As in most scenarios, edentulous bone experiences significantly higher rates of bone resorption and atrophy when compared to the dentulous mandible [27].

Ambulation is encouraged as soon as 2 days postsurgery, but this can be negatively impacted by skin grafting and donor site morbidity for up to 3 weeks. Some advocate the use of a splints, and boots for 6 weeks with weight-bearing [12, 26]. In the initial 60 patient series by Hidalgo, all patients were eventually able to ambulate normally. Two patients experienced running limitations. In this same series, most individuals were able to maintain an oral diet. Specifically, 51% had no restrictions, 42% tolerated a soft diet and only 7% required tube feedings. Furthermore, speech was documented as normal in 39%, mildly impaired in 32%, hard to understanding in 19%, and unintelligible in 10% of patients [28].

## Pearls/Pitfalls

- The mainstay option for mandibular reconstruction is the fibula free flap. Other options include rib, metatarsal, ilium, radius, and scapula [28].
- When elevating the flap proximally, care should be taken to not transect the pedicle near its origin as it crosses the tibialis posterior muscle raphae from medial to lateral [13].
- Flap failure can occur in up to 13% of cases due to arteriovenous complications and difficulties of monitoring buried flaps [8, 12].
- The more common recipient site complications include wound dehiscence, hardware extrusion, inadequate fixation, fistula formation, bone loss, osteoradionecrosis, and surgical-site infections [8, 28].
- Donor site morbidity can affect up to 30% of patients [8].
  - Long-term effects can include persistent pain, edema, numbness, cold intolerance, compartment syndrome, and decreased strength and range of motion of the ankle [9, 13, 24, 29].
  - Planar flexion and foot eversion can be preserved provided foot flexors and peroneus brevis muscle remains intact [12].
  - Early ambulation, less bedrest, and physical therapy before and after surgery play an important role in minimizing these issues [9, 24].
- One should consider an alternate reconstructive option in high-performance athletes, as they will not tolerate any degree of functional impairment due to the need for lateral mobility offered by the fibula bone [9].
- Computer-assisted virtual planning has been shown to achieve high rates of dental rehabilitation [7].

## References


1. Hidalgo DA. Fibula free flap: a new method of mandible reconstruction. Plast Reconstr Surg. 1989;84(1):71–9.
2. Hidalgo DA. Aesthetic improvements in free-flap mandible reconstruction. Plast Reconstr Surg. 1991;88(4):574–85; discussion 586–7.
3. Smith ML, Clarke-Pearson E, Dayan JH. Fibula osteo-adipofascial flap for mandibular and maxillary reconstruction. Head Neck. 2012;34(10):1389–94.
4. Chang EI, Jenkins MP, Patel SA, Topham NS. Long-term operative outcomes of preoperative computed tomography-guided virtual surgical planning for osteocutaneous free flap mandible reconstruction. Plast Reconstr Surg. 2016;137(02):619–23.
5. Shpitzer T, Neligan PC, Gullane PJ, et al. Oromandibular reconstruction with the fibular free flap. Analysis of 50 consecutive flaps. Arch Otolaryngol Head Neck Surg. 1997;123(9):939–44.
6. Inbal A, Gur E, Zaretski A, Barnea Y, Khafif A, Amir A. The "origami" composite free fibula flap for complex defects of the mandible, floor of the mouth, and tongue. J Oral Maxillofac Surg. 2015;73(08):1617–26.
7. Avraham T, Franco P, Brecht LE, Ceradini DJ, Saadeh PB, Hirsch DL, Levine JP. Functional outcomes of virtually planned free fibula flap reconstruction of the mandible. Plast Reconstr Surg. 2014;134(4):628e–34e.
8. Fliss E, Yanko R, Bracha G, Teman R, Amir A, Horowitz G, Muhanna N, Fliss DM, Gur E, Zaretski A. The evolution of the free fibula flap for head and neck reconstruction: 21 years of experience with 128 flaps. J Reconstr Microsurg. 2021;37(4):372–9.
9. Anthony JP, Rawnsley JD, Benhaim P, Ritter EF, Sadowsky SH, Singer MI. Donor leg morbidity and function after fibula free flap mandible reconstruction. Plast Reconstr Surg. 1995 Jul;96(1):146–52.
10. Jackson RS, Price DL, Arce K, Moore EJ. Evaluation of clinical outcomes of osseointegrated dental implantation of fibula free flaps for mandibular reconstruction. JAMA Facial Plast Surg. 2016;18(3):201–6.
11. Alolabi N, Dickson L, Coroneos CJ, Farrokhyar F, Levis C. Preoperative angiography for free fibula flap harvest: a meta-analysis. J Reconstr Microsurg. 2019;35(05):362–71.
12. Cho BC, Kim SY, Park JW, Baik BS. Blood supply to osteocutaneous free fibula flap and peroneus longus muscle: prospective anatomic study and clinical applications. Plast Reconstr Surg. 2001;108(7):1963–71.
13. Hidalgo DA. Fibula free flap mandible reconstruction. Microsurgery. 1994;15(4):238–44.
14. Barr ML, Haveles CS, Rezzadeh KS, et al. Virtual surgical planning for mandibular reconstruction with the fibula free flap: a systematic review and meta-analysis. Ann Plast Surg. 2020;84(01):117–22.
15. Powcharoen W, Yang WF, Yan Li K, Zhu W, Su YX. Computerassisted versus conventional freehandmandibular reconstruction with fibula free flap: a systematic review andmeta-analysis. Plast Reconstr Surg. 2019;144(06):1417–28.
16. Cannady SB, Rosenthal EL, Knott PD, Fritz M, Wax MK. Free tissue transfer for head and neck reconstruction: a contemporary review. JAMA Facial Plast Surg. 2014;16(5):367–73.
17. Klein S, Hage JJ, van der Horst CM, Lagerweij M. Ankle-arm index versus angiography for the preassessment of the fibula free flap. Plast Reconstr Surg. 2003;111(02):735–43.
18. Futran ND, Stack BC Jr, Zachariah AP. Ankle-arm index as a screening examination for fibula free tissue transfer. Ann Otol Rhinol Laryngol. 1999;108(08):777–80.
19. Garvey PB, Chang EI, Selber JC, Skoracki RJ, Madewell JE, Liu J, Yu P, Hanasono MM. A prospective study of preoperative computed tomographic angiographic mapping of free fibula osteocutaneous flaps for head and neck reconstruction. Plast Reconstr Surg. 2012;130(4):541e–9e.
20. Beckler AD, Ezzat WH, Seth R, Nabili V, Blackwell KE. Assessment of fibula flap skin perfusion in patients undergoing oromandibular reconstruction: comparison of clinical findings, fluorescein, and indocyanine green angiography. JAMA Facial Plast Surg. 2015;17(6):422–6.

21. Fichter AM, Ritschl LM, Georg R, et al. Effect of segment length and number of osteotomy sites on cancellous bone perfusion in free fibula flaps. J Reconstr Microsurg. 2019;35(02):108–16.
22. Schusterman MA, Reece GP, Miller MJ, Harris S. The osteocutaneous free fibula flap: is the skin paddle reliable? Plast Reconstr Surg. 1992;90(5):787–93; discussion 794–8.
23. Ducic Y, Defatta R, Wolfswinkel EM, Weathers WM, Hollier LH Jr. Tunneling technique for expedited fibula free tissue harvest. Craniomaxillofac Trauma Reconstr. 2013;6(4):233–6. https://doi.org/10.1055/s-0033-1349208.
24. Harris BN, Bewley AF. Minimizing free flap donor-site morbidity. Curr Opin Otolaryngol Head Neck Surg. 2016;24(5):447–52.
25. Shimbo K, Okuhara Y, Yokota K. Closure of a free osteofasciocutaneous fibula flap donor site using local skin grafts or flaps: a systematic review and meta-analysis. Microsurgery. 2022;42(2):192–8.
26. Momoh AO, Yu P, Skoracki RJ, Liu S, Feng L, Hanasono MM. A prospective cohort study of fibula free flap donor-site morbidity in 157 consecutive patients. Plast Reconstr Surg. 2011;128(3):714–20.
27. Shokri T, Stahl LE, Kanekar SG, Goyal N. Osseous changes over time in free fibular flap reconstruction. Laryngoscope. 2019;129(5):1113–6.
28. Hidalgo DA, Rekow A. A review of 60 consecutive fibula free flap mandible reconstructions. Plast Reconstr Surg. 1995;96(3):585–96; discussion 597–602.
29. Ling XF, Peng X. What is the price to pay for a free fibula flap? A systematic review of donor-site morbidity following free fibula flap surgery. Plast Reconstr Surg. 2012;129(3):657–74.

# Scapular Free Tissue Transfer for Head and Neck Reconstruction

# 14

Wesley Mcilwain and Weitao Wang

## History

In 1978, Saijo et al. [1] used dye injection cadaveric dissections to study the suitability of the dorsal thoracic anatomy suitable for flap harvesting. He predicted that the fasciocutaneous flap based on the circumflex scapular artery (CSA) could supply up to $15 \times 20$ cm$^2$ of thin, pliable skin supplied by a pedicle sufficient for microvascular reconstruction. The scapular flap was reportedly first described by dos Santos in 1980 [2, 3]. In 1982, Gilbert and Teot [4] successfully used the scapular flap in four lower extremity reconstructions. In 1981, Teot et al. [5] described the use of the lateral scapular border as a pedicled osteocutaneous flap. In 1982, Nassif et al. [6] described the parascapular flap via designing the skin paddle along the lateral border of the scapula using the descending branch of the CSA. In 1986, Koshima and Soeda [7] described the ability for use of a chimeric flap, combining both the scapular and parascapular skin paddles to cover a large leg defect. In 1986, Swartz et al. [8] described their experience with osteocutaneous scapular flap for mandibular and maxillary reconstruction in 26 patients. This group reported that the lateral border of the scapula can be harvested with up to 14 cm of thick, straight, corticocancellous bone.

The angular artery was subsequently described as a major blood supply to the scapular tip, facilitating a longer vascular pedicle [9]. Coleman and Sultan [10] described a bipedicled osteocutaneous flap for mandibular and midface reconstruction, using the angular artery to harvest the scapular tip and the CSA to harvest a fasciocutaneous paddle. This study demonstrated the longer arc of rotation between

W. Mcilwain
Otolaryngology and Facial Plastic Surgery Associates, Fort Worth, TX, USA

W. Wang (✉)
Department of Otolaryngology Head and Neck Surgery, University of Rochester, Rochester, NY, USA



F. Sokoya, A. G. Vincent (eds.), *Manual of Head and Neck Reconstruction*,
https://doi.org/10.1007/978-3-031-65999-7_14

the skin supplied by the CSA the bone supplied by the angular branch of the thoracodorsal artery. Baker and Sullivan [11] reported the advantage of the separate pedicles for simultaneously reconstructing soft tissue defects up to 12 × 10 $cm^2$ and segmental bone gaps of up to 14.5 cm. Moscoso et al. [12] reported that the thickest portion of the scapula is distal to the glenohumeral joint and that 78% of cadaveric specimens were suitable for dental implants. With newer positioning technique described to facilitate a two-team approach [13], this flap has gained significant popularity to reconstruct complex head and neck defects [14–16].

## Anatomy of the Scapular Flap

### Vascular System

The versatility of the scapular system is due to its robust vascularity. Roswell et al. [17] performed 100 cadaveric dissections to study the subscapular-thoracodorsal arterial system. The subscapular artery originates from the axillary artery in 97% of cases and absent in 3% of cases. The subscapular artery divides into the CSA and the thoracodorsal artery. The CSA may originate directly from the axillary artery in 3% of cases [17].

The CSA proceeds to give off the superficial circumflex scapular artery, a descending branch to the lateral scapular border, and branches to the subscapularis, teres major, teres minor, and infraspinatus muscles. The superficial CSA travels toward the subcutaneous tissue through areolar tissue through a triangular space bounded by the long head of triceps brachii muscle laterally, teres minor muscle superiorly, and the teres major muscle inferiorly. The artery pierces through the deep fascia and subsequently divides into the horizontal (transverse), vertical (descending), ascending, and lateral branches. The horizontal and vertical arteries supply the scapular and parascapular fasciocutaneous flaps, respectively [18]. Paired venae comitantes, with one frequently larger than the other, are associated with the circumflex scapular and subscapular arteries that drain into the axillary vein.

The thoracodorsal artery is a branch of the subscapular artery in 94% of cases but can be a direct branch of the axillary artery in 5% of cases and direct branch of the lateral thoracic artery in 1% of cases [17]. The thoracodorsal artery, with an average length of 8.4 cm and diameter of 3 mm, gives at least one branch to the serratus anterior muscle [17]. The angular artery supplying the scapular tip is a branch of the thoracodorsal artery in 59% of cases and travels deep to the latissimus dorsi muscle within a fat pad lateral to the scapular bone. The branch terminates at the dorsal surface of the angle of the scapula. In 41% of the cases, the angular artery may originate from the serratus anterior pedicle, as a trifurcation with the latissimus dorsi and serratus anterior pedicles, or proximal to the latissimus dorsi and serratus anterior pedicles [10]. If a combined latissimus-scapula flap is planned, one should remember that up to 6% of cases that the subscapular artery will not be available as a single pedicle for both components [17].

The length of the pedicle available depends on the flap type harvested. The distance of the combined subscapular and circumflex scapular pedicle from the axillary artery to the lateral scapular border varies from 4 to 9 cm, and the pedicle from bone to the overlying horizontal skin paddle is approximately 2–3 cm [10, 17, 18]. The descending parascapular flap is 11–14 cm [6]. If the angular artery is used, an additional length can be obtained between the bone harvested and the skin paddle, with up to 15 cm of vascular pedicle from the bone to the axillary artery [10].

## Muscle

The muscles encountered during flap elevation include the infraspinatus, teres minor, teres major, and the latissimus dorsi muscles. The infraspinatus muscle originates medially at the infraspinous fossa and the teres minor originates from the lateral border of the scapula. Both muscles insert at the greater tubercle of the humerus and primarily function to externally rotate and adduct the arm. The teres major muscle originates from the inferior angle and lateral border of the scapula and inserts into the lesser tubercle of the humerus. This muscle acts to extend, adduction, and internally rotate the humerus.

The latissimus dorsi muscle is a large superficial posterior trunk muscle originating from the lower thoracic spine, posterior iliac crest, and the thoracolumbar fascia. The muscle inserts in the intertubercular groove of the humerus. The muscle's primary function is to adduct the arm and internally rotate the shoulder. The latissimus dorsi is innervated by the thoracodorsal nerve (C6–C8) [19]. The nerve is usually located 3 cm medial to the origin of the subscapular artery in the axilla. The nerve runs in proximity to the thoracodorsal artery to innervate the deep surface of the latissimus dorsi muscle. The nerve divides into lateral and medial branches with its vascular counterparts. This nerve can be harvested with the latissimus dorsi muscle with minimal donor morbidity. The latissimus dorsi can be harvested as a component of the subscapular system flap with or without an overlying skin paddle and has the potential to cover a large surface area ($25 \times 40$ cm$^2$) [20]. Simultaneous harvest of the latissimus dorsi allows for significant versatility given its own vascular source of the thoracodorsal artery.

The serratus anterior muscle originates from the first through eighth ribs on the lateral chest and inserts along the entire medial border of the scapula. The muscle is deep to the subscapularis muscle. The muscle functions to pull the scapula anteriorly toward the thorax. The muscle is innervated by the long thoracic nerve. The long thoracic nerve originates from the C5, C6, and C7 cervical spinal nerves, pierces through the scalene muscles, travels deep to the clavicle, and lies along the superficial surface of the serratus anterior muscle [19]. Injury to this nerve can lead to scapula alata (i.e., winged scapula). Scapula alata can limit a person's ability to lift their arm and push against resistance. Therefore, harvest of this nerve is not recommended.

### Bone

The scapula bone is primarily cancellous with a thin cortical rim, contrary to the more robust cortex associated with the fibula or iliac crest. The thickest bone available is approximately midway between the inferior angle and the glenoid. The entire lateral scapula and angle may be available to harvest, with a straight segment of bone up to 14 cm in males and 10 cm in females [8]. An additional 3–4 cm of bone at the inferior angle can be harvested based on the angular artery.

### Fasciocutaneous Flaps

The horizontal fasciocutaneous flap is most used. The limits of dissection typically include the scapular spine, the inferior scapular angle, the posterior axillary line, and the midline. The maximum width that allows primary closure is approximately 12 cm. The parascapular fasciocutaneous flap is based on the descending branch and can extend 25–30 cm from the scapular spine. However, distal blood supply to this flap beyond the scapular angle may be questionable [18]. The approximate width harvested to allow primary closure is approximately 14 cm [6]. The ascending oriented flap can also be used based on the ascending branch [21]. The lateral margin of the ascending flap is the axilla, and the superior margin is the root of the neck. The width can be approximately 10 cm, and the distal portion of this flap may receive a large component of its blood supply through communication with the perforating branches of the transverse cervical and suprascapular arteries.

## Operative Technique

### Preoperative Evaluation

The primary objectives for defect reconstruction should be analyzed to determine the most appropriate type of flap. Moreover, each patient's soft tissue should be assessed, as body habitus and skin elasticity can vary from patient to patient. The fasciocutaneous paddle thickness can vary significantly between patients. Moreover, the pedicle length must be considered. For instance, the flap should be designed on the angular branch for longer pedicle length to reach from the midface defect to the neck. If a scapular system flap is determined to be appropriate for reconstructing the defect, the preoperative workup is minimal compared to other flaps. There are no age restrictions for this flap, but the patient should be medically fit for prolonged general endotracheal anesthesia. The medium-sized vessels of this flap system are typically not compromised by diabetes and arteriosclerosis. No preoperative imaging is thus required to investigate vascular integrity. Relative contraindications to flap harvest include prior history of axillary dissection or extensive trauma involving the scapula or humeral joint as this can potentially result in compromise of the pedicle. If possible, the nondominant arm is preferred. Moderate to severe obesity can make the thickness of the skin paddle difficult to use for intraoral contouring and inset. Most of donor skin defects can be closed primarily. There is minimal donor site morbidity [18]. Sullivan et al. [22] reported that flexion, abduction, and external rotation were most affected initially postoperatively, but all patients subjectively felt that their function was adequate. Nonetheless, a structured physical therapy program focused on shoulder range of motion is typically provided for 1–2 weeks postoperatively.

## Positioning and Marking

The patient is placed in the lateral decubitus position supported by a vacuum bean bag and the contralateral arm protected with an axillary roll, while the ipsilateral arm is completely prepped into the field. This allows manipulation intraoperatively to facilitate deep axillary dissection. The supine position has been described as well, which may facilitate two-team harvest [13]. Once positioned, the CSA is found within the triangular space on the lateral border of the scapula approximately two-fifth of the distance from the scapular spine to the inferior angle. [4] The Doppler probe can locate the arterial pulse passing through this triangle. In obese patients, these landmarks are distorted, and a Doppler probe should be used to mark out the main cutaneous perforator. For a scapular fasciocutaneous flap, a line is drawn at this point medially parallel approximately 5–6 cm superior to the superior border of the latissimus dorsi muscle. The proximal end of the flap is located at the posterior axillary line. The distal endpoint may be extended to reach the medial border of the contralateral scapular bone. The parascapular fasciocutaneous flap travels in line with the lateral border of the scapula when the arm is adducted. The proximal end of this flap can originate at the axillary crease, and the distal flap has been shown to end at the 12th rib. In general, the subcutaneous tissue is thicker in the scapular flap compared to the parascapular flap. When harvesting a chimeric flap including the latissimus muscle, the anterior border of the latissimus is marked as a line between the mid-axillary and posterior superior iliac spine and the skin paddle designed just posterior to this line. The angular artery does not require Doppler and will be identified during flap harvest. The ipsilateral arm is abducted 90° and medially rotated to expose the lateral border. A third assist may be necessary to support the arm during flap harvest, or alternatively a spider-arm rest/mayo stand can be used to support the arm. For scapula tip and latissimus chimeric flaps, a lazy (30° rotation of the upper torso) lateral decubitus position can be used to afford rapid two team harvest. The senior author prefers full lateral decubitus positioning when harvesting the lateral border for ease of making osteotomies.

## Flap Harvest

The fasciocutaneous paddle is elevated from distal to proximal in the direction of the pedicle. The depth of dissection is superficial to the deep muscular fascia overlying the muscle. The dissection proceeds proximally by bluntly separating the fasciocutaneous flap from the infraspinatus and teres minor muscles. The cutaneous branch of the CSA will be identified superior to the teres major muscle attachment to the lateral scapular border. Once the cutaneous branch is identified laterally, the lateral portion of the fasciocutaneous paddle is dissected circumferentially to mobilize the flap.

Next, the CSA is traced proximally between the fascia of the teres minor and teres major. As the teres minor is retracted medially, the perforators to the bone are identified and protected. The lateral border of the scapula is then accessed via incising the infraspinatus and teres minor muscles parallel to the scapular border inferiorly and then transected perpendicularly superior to the perforator artery to prepare for the osteotomy. The teres major muscle is then undermined and retracted to visualize the angular artery. If not planning on using the thoracodorsal artery system, then this artery can be divided. The teres major muscle is then divided to fully expose the inferior lateral border of the scapula. The deep surface of the scapular border is bluntly dissected, and the osteotomies are planned by harvesting approximately 3 cm in width and 12 cm in length. Cutting guides can be placed at this time if planned. Otherwise, the osteotomies are created inferiorly, medially, and superiorly usually using an oscillating or reciprocating saw. Once the osteotomies are completed, the bone flap is rotated laterally, and the subscapularis muscle is divided on its deep surface. The remaining soft tissue attachments are divided as the pedicle is traced proximally. Complete mobilization of the vascular pedicle requires division of several muscular branches to the teres major, subscapularis, and infraspinatus muscles. If the latissimus dorsi muscle is not harvested, you can divide the thoracodorsal artery at its origin, and the pedicle can be dissected to the axillary artery to include the subscapular artery. However, the extra length obtained with the subscapular artery is nominal, so you may want to preserve vascularity to the latissimus dorsi for future flap harvest by dividing the CSA at its origin.

Every patient has different skin elasticity and subcutaneous tissue components. However, flaps less than 10 cm wide are typically closed directly. For osteocutaneous flaps, the teres minor and major muscles are reattached to the scapular remnant. Suction drains are placed. Shoulder range of motion exercises are begun as soon as the patient is capable clinically.

## Scapular Tip Flap

The scapular tip is similar in size and shape to the anterior wall of the maxilla and the hard palate and has been extensively used for midface reconstruction. The vascular supply via the angular branch facilitates harvesting a longer vascular pedicle to reach the neck for anastomosis. The dissection is similarly performed as described in detail above, but with careful attention to preserving the angular branch from the thoracodorsal artery. This angular branch is parallel to the lateral border of the scapula within the areolar tissue deep to the latissimus dorsi muscle. As described previously, the teres major, teres minor, and the infraspinatus muscles are divided with a small cuff of muscle to visualize the scapular tip. Occasionally, rhomboid major muscle is partially released from the medial border of the scapula. The planned osteotomies are marked and performed. The vascular pedicle based on the angular branch is then traced out, and the subsequent branches to the latissimus dorsi and serratus anterior are divided. Yet, each of these muscles can be harvested as described, which may be useful for dead space obliteration for midface reconstruction. Case example demonstrates the use of a chimeric scapula tip and latissimus dorsi flap for reconstruction of a composite oral resection defect of the floor of mouth, mandibular symphysis, mentum and neck skin for recurrent oral cavity squamous cell carcinoma (See Figs. 14.1, 14.2 and 14.3).

## Chimeric Flaps

The subscapular system provides significant flexibility with bringing in multiple types of flaps depending on the defect needed to be reconstructed. The large skin paddle options can be manipulated completely separately from the bone flap making it an excellent option in otherwise challenging composite defects for fibula osteocutaneous free flaps where the skin paddle and bone are relatively fixed in configuration. The flap can be designed to include multiple skin paddles with or without muscle, scapular bone, and rib. Knowledge of the anatomy of this system can facilitate complex three-dimensional reconstruction with multiple tissue types based on a single vascular pedicle. See Fig. 14.4 for the anatomic considerations regarding chimeric flap design. Chimeric flaps are useful for a combination of intraoral and extraoral defect reconstruction.

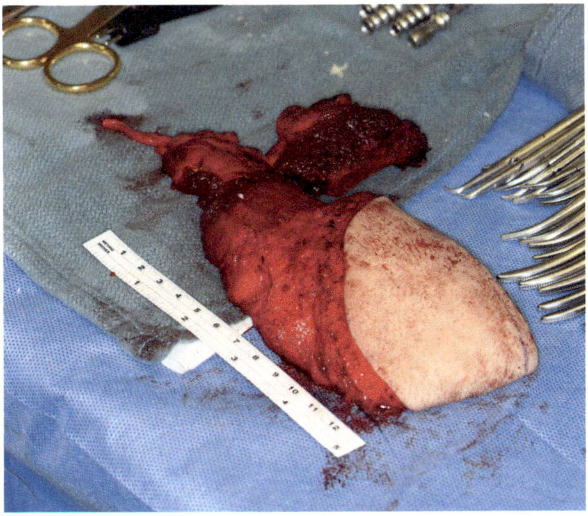

**Fig. 14.1** Latissimus myocutaneous with scapula tip free flap for floor of mouth and external skin reconstruction

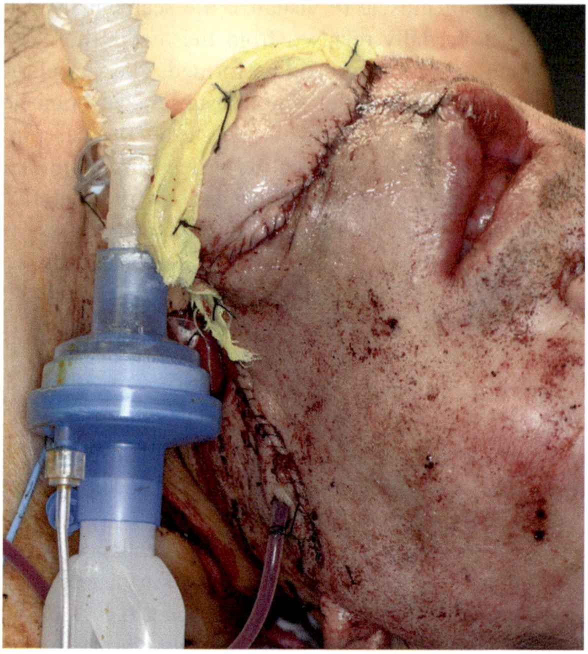

**Fig. 14.2** Scapula tip secured along anterior body with pre-milled reconstruction plate. Latissimus skin paddle is de-epithelialized for intraoral and extraoral reconstruction

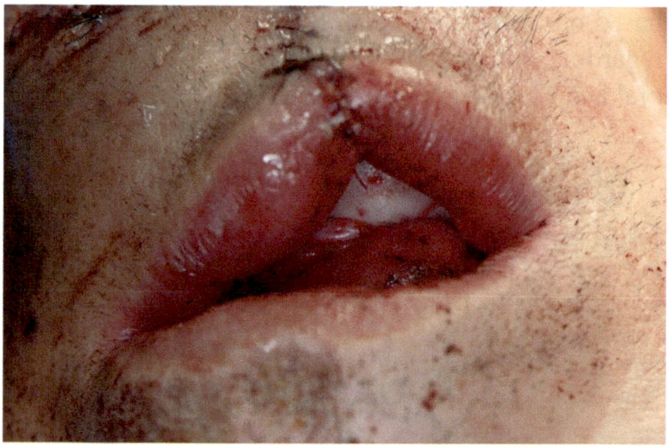

**Fig. 14.3** Intraoral skin paddle inset

## Fascial Flaps

Any of the previously mentioned fasciocutaneous flaps can be harvested without the overlying epidermis and dermis. This allows for greater harvest of tissue for the flap without concerns for primary closure of the donor defect. The fascia of the scapular and parascapular flaps are supplied by vasculature originating from the CSA that courses superficial to the fascia. These flaps must be carefully elevated in a subcutaneous plane, leaving enough tissue overlying the fascia to preserve its blood supply.

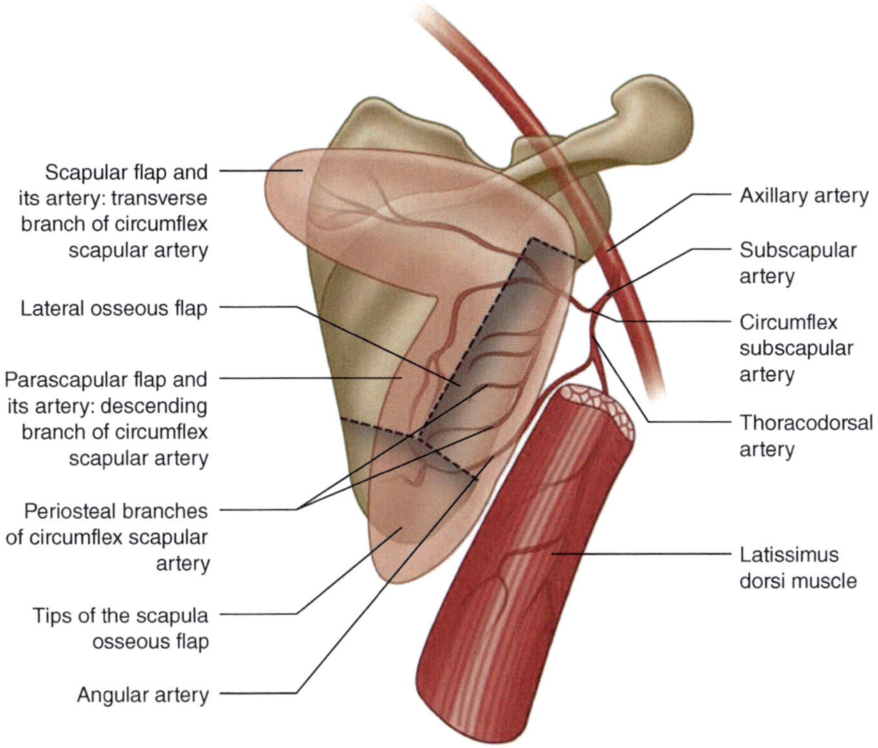


**Fig. 14.4** Scapular system flap schematic, respective osseous flap options, and relative blood supply for chimeric flap designs

## Virtual Surgical Planning

Stereolithography generates a highly accurate three-dimensional (3D) model from data of a computed tomography (CT) scan to assist with preoperative planning of complex craniofacial defects. The technology has enhanced, and its expense has been proven cost-effective by reducing operative times [23]. Virtual surgical planning ranges from printing of a stereolithographic model alone to allow for analysis of the case preoperatively, to custom 3D models with cutting guides and patient-specific implants [24]. Free-hand osteotomies or two-dimensional (2D) cutting guides require significant experience and often require intraoperative adjustments, prolonging operative times. With virtual surgical planning (VSP), surgeons can virtually plan osteotomies and subsequently generate preoperative models and intraoperative cutting guides. Moreover, patient-specific implants can be designed to support complex reconstructions. Reconstructive surgeons meet in a virtual session to mark out resection margins and decide on how many segments of bony reconstruction are required. Once this is determined, the software outlines the harvest margins of the free bone flap and determines the trajectory of the osteotomies, and an overlay of the resection and reconstruction is finalized. Kass et al. [25] recommended from their initial experience with VSP and scapular flaps to use a cup-shaped guide that can accommodate the various fibrous tip and muscle at the scapular tip to facilitate stabilizing the guide to the scapula. Surgical guides and models are created and sterilized for use intraoperatively. The major advantage of using VSP with the scapula is that it can determine the highest quality bone stock preoperatively [25]. VSP also minimizes excess osseous and soft tissue bulk of the flap, facilitating easier inset and maximizing bony contact to increase the chances of bony union [24]. Once the lateral border of the scapula is exposed as described previously, the clearly labeled cutting guides are placed in the precise position, and osteotomies are rapidly performed. Patient-specific reconstruction plates and/or implants are used to facilitate rapid and more accurate inset of the flap into the maxillary or mandibular reconstruction. Midface reconstruction is particularly challenging, and VSP has been shown to improve the anatomical accuracy of defect reconstruction and the bony apposition of the scapular bone segments to native bone [26].

## Midface Reconstruction

The scapula tip can be used in a vertical dimension to reconstruct the anterior maxilla and alveolar ridge, and the soft tissue of the flap can be used to obliterate the maxillary sinus and close an oroantral fistula. The vertical orientation improves the ability to use dental implants, although often additional bone grafting and soft tissue surgery is required [24, 27]. Infrastructure maxillary defects can be reconstructed with the scapular tip in the horizontal dimension, but the bone must be secured with plates on the premaxilla and posteriorly intraorally to prevent inferior displacement of the bone with time [26].

## Mandible Reconstruction

The lateral border of the scapula and the scapula tip have had success with reconstructing mandibular defects and have been shown to achieve dental implantation [22]. Large angle to angle composite oral defects including floor of mouth and cutaneous chin and neck defects are ideal for chimeric flaps. The lateral border of the scapula is of adequate length to reconstruct the mandible from angle to angle via two or three segment osteotomies. The lateral border is relatively forgiving in regard to need for wedge osteotomies commonly necessary for fibula free flaps given the thin nature of the bone and thus the entire lateral border is often usable. The limitation of the scapula for extensive mandible reconstruction lies in the short pedicle length, which typically limits the donor recipient vessels to be a facial artery and vein or an external jugular vein branch. In salvage cases, vein grafts or transpositions may be necessary. As discussed previously, pedicle length can be improved with the scapular tip flap but large segment mandibular defects typically require more bone than this can offer. Preservation of the angular and circumflex scapular artery contributions are ideal when making osteotomies to ensure each segment maintains their separate blood supply. In the event there is inadequate bone for complete mandibular reconstruction, priority should be focused on reconstructing the symphysis and body as bony gaps along the angle and ramus are generally better tolerated with less risk of plate extrusion as long as technically sound plate reconstruction is completed.

## Dental Implants

In 1994, Moscoso et al. [12] found that implants were only suitable in men and limited to the proximal and distal portion of the lateral border of the scapula. However, shorter and narrower implants have been used successfully in smaller bone volumes, negating these previous claims. Patients have decreased mastication forces after mandibular reconstruction, thus decreasing the stress on dental implants compared to normal population. Lanzer et al. [28] demonstrated that bone density increased after implants, favoring use for both males and females. Therefore, the scapula is suitable for osseointegrated implants [27–30]. The scapular tip flap has also been shown to be suitable for dental implants but may require additional bone grafting and soft tissue surgery prior to implant placement and restoration [27].

### Limitations

This flap has few limitations, as its versatility and robust vascular supply have been described. However, positioning can still be a challenge during two-team approach. Larger skin paddles cannot be closed primarily and may require skin grafting. Obese patients have thicker, less pliable skin, so a fascial-only flap may be considered in these patients. This flap is not a sensate flap.

## Conclusions

The subscapular flap system has many options for flap components and can be used to reconstruct simple to very complex head and neck defects. The scapula should be considered for midface reconstruction and considered for mandibular reconstruction when a fibula or iliac crest may not be suitable. Familiarity with this flap is imperative for head and neck reconstruction in cases where fibula harvest is contraindicated due to one or two vessel runoffs to the extremity. Donor site morbidity is minimal, and the vascularity is consistent. Newer position techniques allow for simultaneous harvest of the flap.

## References


1. Saijo M. The vascular territories of the dorsal trunk: a reappraisal for potential flap donor sites. Br J Plast Surg. 1978;31(3):200–4. https://doi.org/10.1016/s0007-1226(78)90082-6.
2. Dos Santos LF. Retalho escapular um novo retalho livre microcirurgio. Rev Brasil Cirurgia. 1980;70:133–44.
3. dos Santos LF. The vascular anatomy and dissection of the free scapular flap. Plast Reconstr Surg. 1984;73(4):599–604. https://doi.org/10.1097/00006534-198404000-00014.
4. Gilbert A, Teot L. The free scapular flap. Plast Reconstr Surg. 1982;69(4):601–4. https://doi.org/10.1097/00006534-198204000-00002.
5. Teot L. The scapular crest pedicled bone graft. J Microsurg. 1981;3:257–62.
6. Nassif TM, Vidal L, Bovet JL, Baudet J. The parascapular flap: a new cutaneous microsurgical free flap. Plast Reconstr Surg. 1982;69(4):591–600. https://doi.org/10.1097/00006534-198204000-00001.
7. Koshima I, Soeda S. Repair of a wide defect of the lower leg with the combined scapular and parascapular flap. Br J Plast Surg. 1985;38(4):518–21. https://doi.org/10.1016/0007-1226(85)90013-x.
8. Swartz WM, Banis JC, Newton ED, Ramasastry SS, Jones NF, Acland R. The osteocutaneous scapular flap for mandibular and maxillary reconstruction. Plast Reconstr Surg. 1986;77(4):530–45. https://doi.org/10.1097/00006534-198604000-00003.
9. Deraemaecker R, Thienen C, Lejour M, Dor P. The serratus anterior-scapular free flap: a new osteomuscular unit for reconstruction after radical head and neck surgery. New York: Springer; 1988.
10. Coleman JJ 3rd, Sultan MR. The bipedicled osteocutaneous scapula flap: a new subscapular system free flap. Plast Reconstr Surg. 1991;87(4):682–92. https://doi.org/10.1097/00006534-199104000-00013.
11. Baker SR, Sullivan MJ. Osteocutaneous free scapular flap for one-stage mandibular reconstruction. Arch Otolaryngol Head Neck Surg. 1988;114(3):267–77. https://doi.org/10.1001/archotol.1988.01860150049015.
12. Moscoso JF, Keller J, Genden E, et al. Vascularized bone flaps in oromandibular reconstruction. A comparative anatomic study of bone stock from various donor sites to assess suitability for enosseous dental implants. Arch Otolaryngol Head Neck Surg. 1994;120(1):36–43. https://doi.org/10.1001/archotol.1994.01880250032004.
13. Eskander A, Kang SY, Ozer E, et al. Supine positioning for the subscapular system of flaps: a pictorial essay. Head Neck. 2018;40(5):1068–72. https://doi.org/10.1002/hed.25051.
14. Gibber MJ, Clain JB, Jacobson AS, et al. Subscapular system of flaps: an 8-year experience with 105 patients. Head Neck. 2015;37(8):1200–6. https://doi.org/10.1002/hed.23738.
15. Brown J, Bekiroglu F, Shaw R. Indications for the scapular flap in reconstructions of the head and neck. Br J Oral Maxillofac Surg. 2010;48(5):331–7. https://doi.org/10.1016/j.bjoms.2009.09.013.
16. Urken ML, Bridger AG, Zur KB, Genden EM. The scapular osteofasciocutaneous flap: a 12-year experience. Arch Otolaryngol Head Neck Surg. 2001;127(7):862–9.
17. Rowsell AR, Davies DM, Eisenberg N, Taylor GI. The anatomy of the subscapular-thoracodorsal arterial system: study of 100 cadaver dissections. Br J Plast Surg. 1984;37(4):574–6. https://doi.org/10.1016/0007-1226(84)90152-8.
18. Funk GF. Scapular and parascapular free flaps. Facial Plast Surg. 1996;12(1):57–63. https://doi.org/10.1055/s-2008-1064494.
19. Netter F. Atlas of human anatomy. 5, Saunders/Elsevier; 2011.
20. Friedrich W, Herberhold C, Lierse W. Vascularization of the myocutaneous latissimus dorsi flap. Injection study on the thoracodorsal artery. Acta Anat (Basel). 1988;131(2):97–102. https://doi.org/10.1159/000146494.

21. Ohsaki M, Maruyama Y. Anatomical investigations of the cutaneous branches of the circumflex scapular artery and their communications. Br J Plast Surg. 1993;46(2):160–3. https://doi.org/10.1016/0007-1226(93)90152-2.
22. Blumberg JM, Walker P, Johnson S, et al. Mandibular reconstruction with the scapula tip free flap. Head Neck. 2019;41(7):2353–8. https://doi.org/10.1002/hed.25702.
23. Toto JM, Chang EI, Agag R, Devarajan K, Patel SA, Topham NS. Improved operative efficiency of free fibula flap mandible reconstruction with patient-specific, computer-guided preoperative planning. Head Neck. 2015;37(11):1660–4. https://doi.org/10.1002/hed.23815.
24. Breik O, Idle M, Martin T, Praveen P, Parmar S. Three-dimensional computer-assisted surgical planning and manufacturing in complex maxillary reconstruction. Atlas Oral Maxillofac Surg Clin North Am. 2020;28(2):151–64. https://doi.org/10.1016/j.cxom.2020.05.008.
25. Kass JI, Prisman E, Miles BA. Guide design in virtual planning for scapular tip free flap reconstruction. Laryngoscope Investig Otolaryngol. 2018;3(3):162–8. https://doi.org/10.1002/lio2.162.
26. Swendseid BP, Roden DF, Vimawala S, et al. Virtual surgical planning in subscapular system free flap reconstruction of midface defects. Oral Oncol. 2020;101:104508. https://doi.org/10.1016/j.oraloncology.2019.104508.
27. Mertens C, Freudlsperger C, Bodem J, Engel M, Hoffmann J, Freier K. Reconstruction of the maxilla following hemimaxillectomy defects with scapular tip grafts and dental implants. J Cranio Maxillofac Surg. 2016;44(11):1806–11. https://doi.org/10.1016/j.jcms.2016.08.010.
28. Lanzer M, Gander T, Gratz K, Rostetter C, Zweifel D, Bredell M. Scapular free vascularised bone flaps for mandibular reconstruction: are dental implants possible? J Oral Maxillofac Res. 2015;6(3):e4. https://doi.org/10.5037/jomr.2015.6304.
29. Frodel JL Jr, Funk GF, Capper DT, et al. Osseointegrated implants: a comparative study of bone thickness in four vascularized bone flaps. Plast Reconstr Surg. 1993;92(3):449–55; discussion 456–8.
30. Burgess M, Leung M, Chellapah A, Clark JR, Batstone MD. Osseointegrated implants into a variety of composite free flaps: a comparative analysis. Head Neck. 2017;39(3):443–7. https://doi.org/10.1002/hed.24609.

# The Osteocutaneous Radial Forearm Free Flap

# 15

Fatemeh Mirzamohammadi, Spenceer R. Anderson, Kaitlynne Pak, Sunishka M. Wimalawansa, and Sameep P. Kadakia

## Introduction

Head and neck microvascular reconstructive procedures are often challenging because of the extent of resection and anatomical structures involved. When dealing with complex segmental resections, composite tissue flaps can reconstruct such soft tissue and bony deficits in a single-stage procedure. Flap options must provide adequate and reliable soft tissue coverage, appropriately match tissue thickness, and, in some cases, donate adequate bone stock. To optimize the final results, these recipient site reconstructive needs must be balanced against the risks of donor site morbidity.

The radial forearm free flap (RFFF) is a well-known and well-described flap commonly utilized in head and neck reconstruction [1–5]. The RFFF offers thin, pliable soft tissue ideal for both intra- and extra-oral reconstruction [2, 5]. With a long vascular pedicle, the RFFF can be quite versatile for coverage and allows the ability to perform vascular anastomoses outside a zone of radiation, even reaching the contralateral neck when needed. The RFFF's forearm donor site is often reconstructed using split-thickness skin grafts and/or local soft tissue advancement flaps.

F. Mirzamohammadi · S. R. Anderson · S. M. Wimalawansa
Department of Orthopedic and Plastic Surgery, Boonshoft School of Medicine at Wright State University, Dayton, OH, USA

K. Pak
Boonshoft School of Medicine at Wright State University, Dayton, OH, USA
e-mail: pak.5@wright.edu

S. P. Kadakia (✉)
Department of Orthopedic and Plastic Surgery, Boonshoft School of Medicine at Wright State University, Dayton, OH, USA

Premier Comprehensive Head and Neck Oncology and Reconstructive Surgery Program, Miami Valley Hospital, Dayton, OH, USA



F. Sokoya, A. G. Vincent (eds.), *Manual of Head and Neck Reconstruction*,
https://doi.org/10.1007/978-3-031-65999-7_15

While the donor site reconstruction may appear unsightly, its functional deficits and morbidity are generally minimal.

The osteocutaneous radial forearm free flap (OCRFFF) offers all of the benefits of the RFFF while including vascularized bone. It is indicated in head and neck reconstruction when thick bone stock is not required or available, such as in the case of midfacial reconstruction, reconstruction of the edentulous mandible, or in scenarios when there are contraindications to utilizing the fibula-free flap, such as poor vasculature of the lower extremity (Figs. 15.1 and 15.2) [6–9].

Previously, the OCRFFF fell out of favor secondary to donor site pathologic fracture of the radius. However, the advent of prophylactic plating of the radius harvest site to prevent pathologic fracture complications has renewed surgeon interest in this flap option [4, 7, 8]. In this chapter, we describe important considerations when applying the OCRFFF in the reconstruction of head and neck defects, including key local anatomy and anatomical variations, preoperative planning, operative technique, postoperative management, and complication management.

## Historical

The RFFF, otherwise known as the "Chinese Forearm Flap," was first described in 1978 when Guofan, Baoqui, and Yuzhi utilized this flap for the correction of severe neck burn contractures at the Shenyang Military Hospital [2, 10]. The introduction of the RFFF became a mainstay for head and neck defect reconstruction, especially those defects out of reach of local pedicle flap options. In 1982, Biermer extended the RFFF technique to include a vascularized segment of the radius as an osteocutaneous forearm flap for reconstruction of the thumb [10]. With similarities to the RFFF, the OCRFFF offered familiarity amongst reconstructive surgeons and was adopted as a reconstructive modality.

However, in the late 1990s, the OCRFFF faced a temporary decline in popularity when several publications reported high rates of donor site morbidity secondary to radius fracture at the osteotomy donor site [2, 5, 8]. Thereafter, alternative

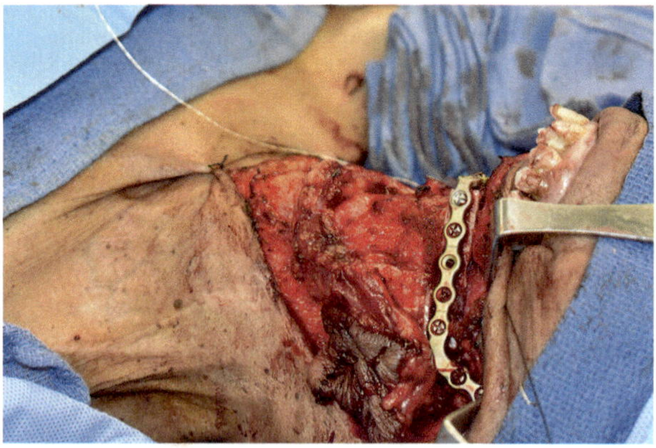

**Fig. 15.1** Intraoperative photograph of the OCRFF being used to reconstruct an edentulous mandible in conjunction with a preplanned titanium mandible plate

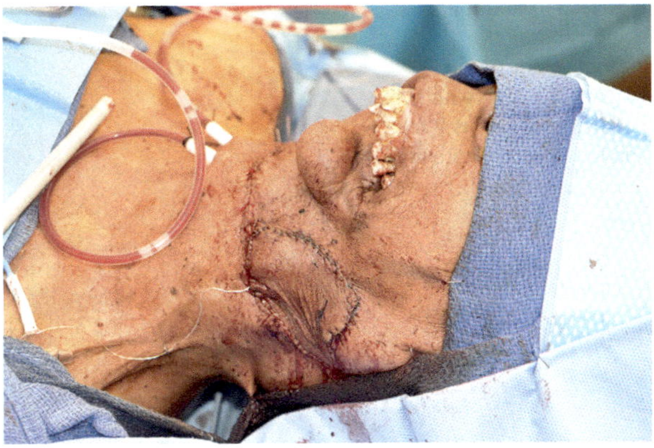

**Fig. 15.2** Intraoperative photograph from the same patient from Fig. 15.1 following inset of the external skin paddle utilized to augment the external skin closure and serve as a monitoring paddle with Doppler stitch in place

bone-based flaps from the fibula, scapula, and iliac crest increased in popularity, seemingly replacing the need to perform the OCRFFF.

Subsequently, orthopedic surgeons and otolaryngologists at the University of Kansas Medical Center described how immediate prophylactic plating of the donor radius harvest defect significantly reduced the incidence of donor site radius fracture. This modification essentially reintroduced the OCRFFF as a versatile and reliable option for modern head and neck reconstruction [1, 6–8, 11].

## Anatomy

The OCRFFF is an excellent and versatile flap for complex head and neck reconstructive cases because of its consistent donor site anatomy, low-profile bony donor site, long reliable vascular pedicle, and potential for complex flap design with multiple skin islands [2, 9]. The standard approach to this flap involves harvesting radial forearm skin and subcutaneous tissues overlying the radial artery, which can be extended ulnarly and proximally as needed, to include a section of volar radius and a cuff of flexor pollicis longus muscle (Fig. 15.3). The palmaris longus can also be included if a tendon graft is needed for the reconstruction. Concomitant prophylactic donor site plating facilitates safe harvest of up to 50% of the radial bone circumference [8, 12].

The OCRFFF is supplied by the radial artery. Here, fasciocutaneous perforators pierce the antebrachial fascia superficially to supply the skin paddle while deep perforating branches traverse the radial septum to feed the radius bone (Fig. 15.4). The distal radial artery is easily identifiable via palpation in the distal forearm and averages about 3 mm in diameter and 14–22 cm in length for an average adult [13]. At the antecubital fossa, the radial and ulnar arteries arise from the bifurcation of the brachial artery. Physiologic variants of the radial artery have been documented in the literature. The most commonly reported adjacent arterial variation is the persistence of the median artery, which is found parallel to the median nerve in the carpal tunnel in approximately 8–10% of the population [14].

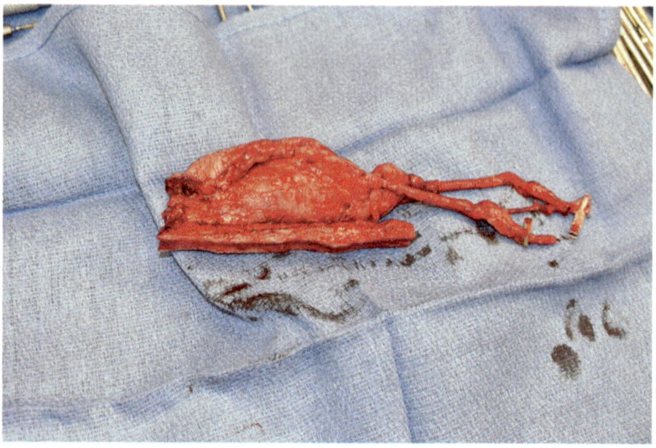

**Fig. 15.3** Photograph demonstrating the osteocutaneous radial forearm free flap with skin paddle, volar radius bone, and long pedicle with dual drainage system

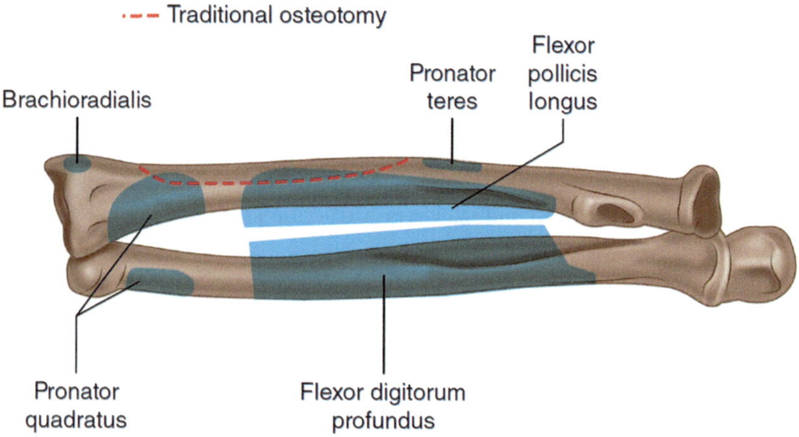


**Fig. 15.4** Illustration of traditional radius osteotomy planning. (This figure was modified from Matthews et al. by Springer Nature. Matthews J, Ng W, Archibald S, Levis C. The use of the radial styloid in the extended osteocutaneous radial forearm free flap. Plast Surg (Oakv). 2016;24(2):89–95)

Most radial artery vascular variations occur proximally in the forearm. Therefore, tracing the radial artery from distal to proximal can be beneficial to identifying its true anatomy. Most commonly, the brachial artery bifurcates into the radial and ulnar arteries approximately 1 cm distal to the antecubital fossa; however, this occurs in only 70% of patients. The radial artery then runs between the brachioradialis and pronator teres muscles in the proximal third of the forearm and follows the lateral (radial) intermuscular septum between the brachioradialis and flexor carpi radialis at the distal forearm. A high bifurcation off the axillary or brachial artery was reported in 9.2% of 120 cadavers, with 18.1% originating in the axilla and 81.8% in the bicipital groove [15, 16]. Distally, the radial artery becomes more superficial. At this level, it is covered by the deep fascia, superficial fascia, and the skin. Other variations reported in the reconstructive literature include duplication of the radial artery (most commonly lateral to the dominant radial artery), congenital absence of radial artery, or unique anatomical pathways, including under the pronator teres muscle [17, 18].

Several anatomical variations of the superficial and deep palmar arches have been described and may be complete or incomplete. Complete superficial palmar arches are reported to be as common as 84.4%, with the most common subtype involving communication of the radial artery superficial volar branch with the ulnar artery [19]. Incomplete arch variations may result in either part or the entire hand being solely dependent upon either the radial or ulnar artery alone.

OCRFFF flap harvest candidates have ulnar arteries that sufficiently supply the entire hand, including the thumb, via the palmar arch vessels. Clinically, this may be evaluated by the Allen test. Dr. Edgar V Allen first described the "Allen's test" in 1929 while studying three thromboangiitis obliterans patients [20]. Here, the patient is directed to make a fist with the radial artery simultaneously occluded by the examiner for 1 min, followed by release of the artery and observing for return of rubor in the hand while the patient performs active extension and flexion of the digits. The original technique has been since adjusted and is now termed the "modified Allen's test" [21]. Now, the patient is directed to make a fist for 30 s while occlusive pressure is applied over both the radial and ulnar arteries. The patient is then instructed to open the fist, and the ulnar artery is selectively released. If sufficient collateral circulation is present, there should be a normal return of color to the hand within about 3–12 s. If skin rubor does not occur, this raises concern for incomplete palmar arch connections and is deemed a positive modified Allen's test. As the modified Allen's test is subjective in nature, it can be prone to false positive or negative results because of observer biases or anatomical variations. Therefore, various objective noninvasive tests have since been added to the modified Allen's test to improve its reliability, including plethysmography, Doppler ultrasound, duplex ultrasonography, and pulse oximetry. There is no general consensus on the single best test for assessing collateral circulation of the hand, and the selection of a specific noninvasive test versus clinical diagnosis alone depends upon the preference of the investigating surgeon.

The addition of Doppler ultrasound to a modified Allen's test may significantly improve the objectivity of this evaluation. Here, an 8-MHz pen Doppler probe confirms intact pulses at the radial and ulnar arteries at the wrist. The probe is then placed over the palmar arch on the palmar border of the thenar eminence for arch flow confirmation. Then, direct occlusive pressure is applied over the radial and ulnar arteries simultaneously, attenuating the Doppler signal and confirming the absence of distal blood flow. At this time, the ulnar artery is released to resume palmar blood flow, confirmed with a Doppler signal. Loss of Doppler signal with radial artery compression suggests the absence of ulnar artery supply to the radial side of the hand and is considered a positive test finding [22–24].

Forearm venous drainage is primarily through the paired venae comitantes alongside the radial artery. Deep venae comitantes drain into the median cubital vein at the level of the elbow, where the superficial veins communicate to the deep system via the profunda cubital vein. Superficial venous drainage is through the cephalic vein, which can be included with flap elevation alone or as an additional outflow system option. The radial venae comitantes lumen diameter is generally 1.5 mm, while the cephalic vein diameter is often 3 mm or larger. The cephalic vein is simple to harvest and is most commonly employed as a single venous drainage system. The downside of single cephalic venous drainage is the risk of vessel thrombosis and possible OCRFFF failure [25, 26]. Venae comitantes join into a single larger caliber vein just before draining into the medial cubital vein at the bifurcation point of the brachial artery. The length of the coalesced vein is about 0.25–1.5 cm. Employing a large diameter coalesced vein gives effective venous drainage from the hemodynamically superior deep venous system as well as an appropriate lumen width for microanastomosis [27].

In general, there are multiple options for flap venous outflow designs, including the deep or superficial system alone or dual combination configurations. Prior studies have reported similar outcomes using superficial venous drainage systems compared to the deep alone or dual combination systems and ultimately may be selected per reconstructive surgeon preference and/or prior experience [28, 29].

## Preoperative Planning

Preoperative planning for the OCRFFF is both integral and critical for achieving a successful reconstructive outcome. This investigation includes thorough patient history and comprehensive clinical exam, complemented with diagnostic imaging as needed.

### Medical and Social History

The patient history establishes hand dominance and occupation, if applicable, as this will contribute to selecting the appropriate donor site arm. It is important to determine if the patient has had any prior surgery on the upper extremity that could jeopardize the vascularity of the flap.

### Clinical Exam

Following identification of the patient's preferred or dominant hand, the contralateral limb is evaluated for quality of skin, tissue bulk and consistency, as well as the presence of any prior scars or surgical interventions. The continuity of the palmar arch is assessed by employing Allen's test. A modified version of Allen's test can also be performed, utilizing either Doppler evaluation of the radial palmar arch or a pulse-oxygen monitor for evaluation of saturation throughout the study. This evaluation can identify if the ulnar artery is robust enough to perfuse the hand through the palmar arch after flap harvest radial artery sacrifice.

In our experience, we have found a combined approach of using an in-office Allen's test with an ultrasound duplex exam improves our accuracy of arterial flow dominance, thereby eliminating the need for intraoperative treatment of hand ischemia related to ulnar artery insufficiency. Furthermore, this more thorough preoperative workup minimizes the need for intraoperative preflap harvest tourniquet deflation (i.e., to assess radial hand perfusion prior to definitive donor radial artery ligation), thereby minimizing operative field bleeding and shortening our subsequent surgical times.

## Imaging

Image-based investigation is not a mandatory portion of the preoperative workup with a stable clinical evaluation, but it can certainly augment the clinical exam findings and provide clarification when clinical findings are equivocal. For example, if Allen's test lacks brisk hand reperfusion, an arterial duplex scan can objectively elucidate functional extremity vasculature and confirm whether radial artery harvest is safe.

## Instrumentation/Requirements

Positioning/Prep

- Split or universal draping system
- Betadine or ChloraPrep
- Supine positioning with arm accessible via arm table

Pharmacy

- Preoperative antibiotic per surgeon preference
- "Tsai solution" (vessel lumen irrigation) in 10 cc aliquots
  - 250 cc lactated ringers with 30 cc 1% lidocaine *without* epinephrine and 3000 units of heparin
- 0.5% marcaine or Ropivicaine for postoperative pain control
- Consider analgesic catheter placement in the forearm (i.e., *On-Q* pain pump; Avanos Medical, Inc., Alpharetta, Georgia)
- Heparin available
- Bone wax available

Instruments

- Microinstrument tray
  - Two sets available: one opened and one emergency backup tray.
- Head and neck/plastics tray
- Hand set
- Osteotomes
- Sagittal and reciprocating saw
- Dermatome
- Wound vacuum-assisted closure device

Suture

- Monocryl 4-0

- Vicryl 3-0 and 4-0
- Ethilon 8-0 BV (2815G)
- 2-0 Silk sutures for drains

Drains

- 10 flat JP, fully fluted or Blake round drain

Requests

- High-definition microscope, 250 lenses, preferably with monitor screen for the staff to follow along
- Maintain 70–75 F degree room temperature
- Two operative scrub teams—donor and recipient site assistance
- Bilateral lower extremity sequential compression devices (SCDs)
- Pressure point padding
- Foley catheter placement
- Arterial line placement per anesthesia assessment

## Design/Technique

### Patient Positioning

The patient is placed in a supine position with the head slightly over the upper edge of the bed. Belt and extremity straps are employed to secure the patient to the OR table. Sequential compression devices are placed on the bilateral lower extremities for DVT prophylaxis. The patient's neck is extended with a shoulder roll and a gel or polyfoam cushion under the head. The upper extremity from which the OCRFFF will be harvested is placed on a hand surgery side table or extended arm board, with attention paid to shoulder positioning to avoid excessive shoulder abduction/extension that could potentially cause a traction injury to the brachial plexus. An Allen test can be repeated prior to initiating harvest in a modified fashion with a pulse oximeter, or alternatively, an intraoperative Allen test can be performed when the radial artery has been isolated prior to ligation.

### Prepping and Draping

The entire donor limb is prepped from the axilla to the fingertips. An extremity drape, or two split drapes, is placed up to the axilla, and then a well-padded sterile tourniquet is placed to the root of the extremity/upper arm, leaving the antecubital fossa well exposed.

### Flap Design and Harvest

A template of the recipient site head and neck defect is created using a spare sterile surgical glove, sterile glove paper, or a piece of the sterile Esmarch elastic bandage.

The template is then transposed over the donor radial artery while ensuring the capture of the cephalic vein radially. Prior to making the incision, donor site closure is preplanned, whether by a skin graft or adjacent perforator flap, to guide the proximal forearm incision toward the antecubital fossa. Local flap reconstruction techniques often include the proximal flap harvest incision in the flap design, usually requiring a more radially positioned forearm access incision to allow recruitment of more ulnar artery-based tissues for donor site reconstruction. If a skin graft is selected to reconstruct the donor defect, a curvilinear incision is marked from the proximal marking of the template to the antecubital fossa.

The limb is partially exsanguinated with manual occlusion of the brachial artery at the elbow and elevation of the limb for approximately 60 s. This allows gravity to partially exsanguinate the limb while leaving enough blood in the vessels to aid in visual identifications of all key structures during the subsequent dissection. Alternatively, the tourniquet can be inflated to 250 mmHg for exsanguination as well.

The skin paddle incision is then carried down through the skin and the subcutaneous tissue where fascia of the muscles of the forearm is identified, taking extreme care to avoid injuring the cephalic vein and radial sensory nerve, both of which run subcutaneously above the antebrachial forearm fascia in the distal forearm. The radial artery is identified at the wrist and isolated with delicate dissection and vessel loops. The distal venae comitantes and other small veins are clipped and divided. The cephalic vein is dissected for an additional 1–2 cm distally and then clipped and divided. Axially oriented fascial incisions made over the brachioradialis (radially) and the flexor carpi radialis (ulnarly) tendons will allow safe *en bloc* elevation of the radial septum connecting the skin flap with the radial artery and its venae comitantes—the fascial incisions should not violate the radial septum. Care must be taken to preserve deep periosteal branches of the radial artery to the radius bone—these are the perforating vessels that will nourish the vascularized bone graft of the OCRFFF. The cephalic vein is also raised *en bloc* with the flap to provide a secondary drainage system for the flap as a backup or dual combination.

Identification of the superficial branch of the radial sensory nerve (RSN) as it courses close to the cephalic vein at the wrist is paramount. Meticulous preservation of the RSN branches prevents debilitating future painful neuromata and chronic pain syndromes; of note, the RSN runs in the deeper layer of subcutaneous fat, in a plane just deep to the cephalic vein. In contrast, the lateral antebrachial cutaneous (LABC) nerve runs in the same plane as the cephalic vein, closely following the path of this vein.

The proximal incision is then made through the skin and subcutaneous tissue taking care to identify and preserve the superficial venous system as well as the sensory nerves. The LABC nerve is located adjacent to the cephalic vein, and the medial antebrachial cutaneous nerve is adjacent to the basilic vein. The superficial drainage system generally runs superficial to the brachioradialis. It is isolated and followed proximally, where it is commonly seen converging with the deep venous system near the antecubital fossa. The radial artery and its venae commitantes run proximally under the brachioradialis muscle belly and are exposed by retracting the plane between the brachioradialis and flexor carpi radialis muscles.

Next, the skin island of the flap can be elevated off of the muscles of the forearm. If desired, the tourniquet can now be released to evaluate hand perfusion. Meticulous hemostasis is achieved. Microvascular clamps are applied to the distal radial artery, and hand perfusion can be observed to confirm intact ulnar circulation of the hand. The distal radial artery and cephalic vein should be divided no less than 1 cm beyond the skin paddle. With the vascular pedicle included with the skin paddle, the radial and ulnar aspects of the distal skin island are elevated off the tendons of the brachioradialis and flexor carpi radialis, taking care to maintain the integrity of the overlying paratenon in an effort to prevent them from adhering to the skin graft postoperatively. Alternatively, a suprafascial skin paddle harvest may provide an additional vascularized fascial soft tissue gliding barrier between the tendons and the overlying soft tissue coverage or skin graft.

## Radius Osteotomy

The brachioradialis muscle is retracted with careful preservation of the deep tissue of the muscle belly containing fascio-osseous perforator branches of the radial artery. Care must also be taken to preserve the deep course of the superficial branch of the radial nerve. The flexor digitorum superficialis is then released along the ulnar aspect of the radius and retracted to visualize the flexor pollicis longus. The pronator quadratus is transected at its insertion to the radius. The periosteum and the flexor pollicis longus are longitudinally dissected down over the radius.

Following exposure of the radius, the next step is planning the osteotomy. The length of the bone to be harvested is delineated following close evaluation and measurement of the defect to be reconstructed. The radius bone is generally harvested in the middle and distal one third of the forearm, between the pronator teres and brachioradialis tendon insertions (Fig. 15.5). The distal osteotomy must be made at least 2.5 cm proximal to the radius styloid process to allow a minimum of two

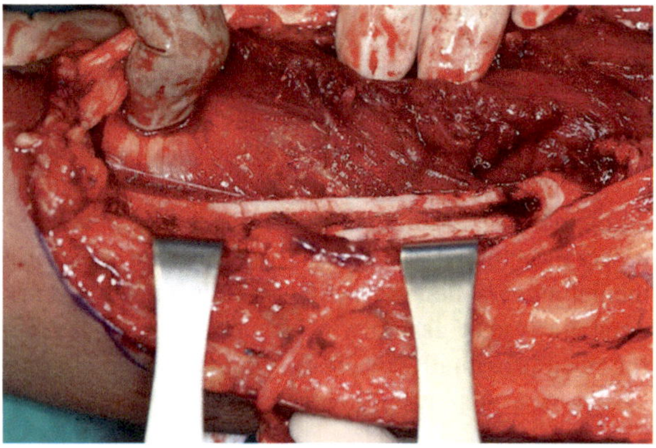

**Fig. 15.5** Intraoperative photograph showing radius bone following harvest of osteocutaneous free flap. Note the thickness of bone remaining and the beveled cut at the proximal osteotomy site, which is a commonly utilized osteotomy angle

screws to be inserted during prophylactic plating. Proximally, the bone can be harvested even beyond the pronator teres (PT) muscle insertion. In this case, the PT tendon would require reattachment to the remaining radius or suture directly to the plate. Figure 15.6 demonstrates the radius bone following the harvest of the free flap.

A reciprocating saw is used to first make the proximal and distal transverse osteotomy cuts, which are subsequently connected longitudinally with a sagittal saw. Up to 50% of the radius' thickness can be successfully and safely harvested. It is best to initiate the cut beginning proximally on the radius, followed by advancing distally. Extreme care must be taken to avoid injuring adjacent neurovascular and musculotendinous structures. This proximal-to-distal technique approach can minimize the risk of an overly thickened bone harvest where the radius diameter is anatomically smaller. Irrigating the saw blade prevents thermal necrosis of the peripheral margins of the bone flap and is essential to maintaining osteocyte viability within the flap. The periosteum is preserved over the bone graft and incised dorsally, completing the vascularized bone graft harvest. Extreme care must be taken to avoid separating the bone graft from the vascular pedicle.

## Proximal Donor Vessel Preparation

Once the osteotomies are complete, the flap is then elevated distal to proximal. The proximal venous and arterial anatomy is carefully evaluated and defined prior to ligation. The deep and superficial venous systems often come together to create a single large-caliber vein ideal for anastomosis. If this large caliber vein is traced proximal to the antecubital fossa, it may branch into two large outflows if a dual drainage flap is desired. The radial artery is followed distal to proximal. The most distal bifurcation observed is most likely found at the location of the radial artery and the recurrent radial artery. Labeling the pedicle's artery and veins in situ prior to flap harvest (we recommend using microvascular clamps of differing sizes for artery vs. vein) simplifies subsequent vessel identification and preparation for anastomosis (Fig. 15.7). Once the flap is ready to be transferred, the donor vein and

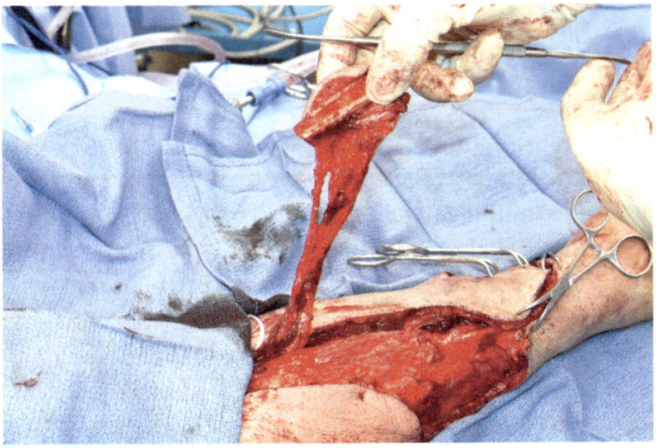

**Fig. 15.6** Intraoperative photograph showing completed proximal pedicle dissection following harvest of radius bone. Note dual drainage system utilizing deep and superficial venous outflow

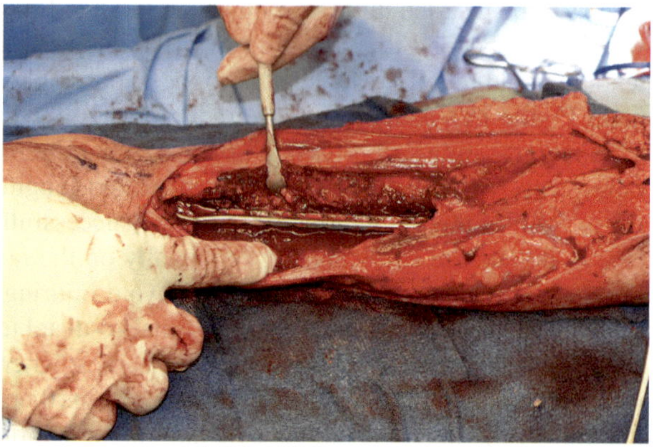

**Fig. 15.7** Intraoperative photograph showing prophylactic radius plating following harvest of osteocutaneous radial forearm free flap

artery are ligated, the flap is transferred to the recipient site and inset, bony fixation is performed (thereby defining pedicle orientation and length), and microvascular anastomosis is performed.

## Prophylactic Plating of the Radius

Forearm fracture following bone-harvesting radius osteotomy carries significant morbidity [30]. The incidence of pathologic fracture of the radius after radial osteotomy in older series reporting conventional approaches without radius reinforcement is reported between 20% and 67% [12, 30–33]. Biomechanical studies on cadaveric radii have demonstrated even small osteotomies, up to one-third of the radius diameter, may result in up to 24% loss of cortical integrity and radius strength [34]. In an animal bone-based biomechanical study, removal of 25%, 33%, and 50% of the cross-section area of the bone resulted in a 70%, 80%, and 85% decrease in bone tensile strength, respectively [35].

The use of prophylactic internal fixation of the radius after OCRFFF harvest to strengthen the donor site was first described in 1999; it has been shown to restore 75% of the bone strength of an intact radius and decrease the overall fracture rate to 0.5–2.6% [6, 12, 36–38]. With prophylactic plating, the amount of bone that can safely be harvested may increase to as much as 50% of the radial circumference [8, 12, 37].

Various plates have been used for radius prophylactic internal fixation. A straight 3.5 mm stainless steel dynamic compression plate (DCP), applied in neutral mode as a neutralizing tension band, is the most commonly used plate that has been described. This specific plate design is bridged over the osteotomized radius surface with bicortical screw fixation to redistribute tensile and torsion forces and avoid their stress concentration on the fulcrum otherwise created by the bone harvest osteotomy. Recently, low profile and anatomically contoured titanium or stainless steel plates have been introduced and secured by unicortical locking screw systems; these can be T-shaped or straight and vary in thickness from 2.4 or 3.5 mm [39, 40]. A biomechanical study of various prophylactic plates applied in sheep tibia found the straight 3.5 mm stainless DCP plate with bicortical screw fixation demonstrated the highest defined strain criteria, as compared to unicortical locking systems [38].

In our experience, we routinely use 3.5 mm stainless DCP plates for internal fixation of the radius following osteocutaneous harvest via anterior approach (Fig. 15.8). The plate is placed on the anterior surface of the radius over the bony defect and adapted in place with bicortical screw fixation with a minimum of two screws at each end of the osteotomy defect. Usually, an 8- to 14-hole plate is required depending on the length of the osteotomy defect. The plate's screws are applied in neutral mode (i.e., non-compressive) and act as neutralizing tension bands to provide bridging reinforcement and prevent tensile forces from stress concentrating on the intact radius cortex (i.e., prevent hinging on the intact cortex of the radius that would otherwise produce a pathologic fracture). This technique also increases our safe bone harvest limit up to 50% of the radial circumference [8, 12]. Distally, extreme care must be taken to ensure that the tips of the screws engaging the dorsal radius cortex do not impinge upon the extensor tendons, as this can risk tendon ruptures. The anterior approach is simple and effective [41].

Posterior plate positioning can also be employed by retracting the extensor tendons to allow dorsal radius plating opposite the donor site defect. Distally, the radial wrist extensors are retracted, and two to three standard bicortical screws are placed. Proximally, the supinator muscle is subperiosteally elevated, and the plate is placed beneath it. Care must be taken in this step to protect the posterior interosseous nerve (PIN), which pierces the supinator muscle; injury to the PIN can cause finger and thumb extensor paralysis. No screws are placed in the defect cavity because it is shown to increase the rate of fracture at the screw site. The soft tissue coverage over a posterior plate is relatively thin, and there is a higher chance of extensor tendon rupture.

Both anterior and posterior approaches have been successfully used in a number of clinical series with an overall fracture rate decrease to 2.6% [11, 38, 42, 43]. However, posterior plate fixation can be more demanding compared to the anterior

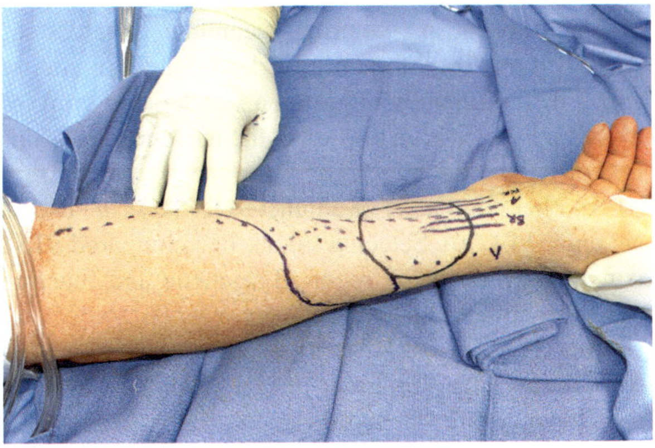

**Fig. 15.8** Intraoperative photograph showing preoperative forearm markings planning for local ulnar flap closure of flap donor site

approach and increase risks of extensor tendon-related complications. Because of this, we prefer the anterior method of fixation in our practice.

## Closure of the Donor Site

In order to optimize closure of the forearm donor site, vascularized soft tissue, including underlying muscle, should be reapproximated over the fixation plate to prevent plate extrusion. The flexor pollicis longus is sutured over the plate, and the flexor digitorum superficialis is brought over the flexor carpi radialis tendon to the radial skin edge. This provides a second muscular layer over the plate and bony donor site and facilitates skin graft take should one be used. The pronator quadratus can also be repaired to the radial edge of the brachioradialis tendon to provide an interposed vascularized muscle layer to separate the plate from the flexor tendons to decrease the risk of tendon rupture.

Multiple different techniques for the closure of the OCRFFF donor site have been described. Direct closure may be possible in certain scenarios, but generally not performed as the size of skin paddles typically harvested precludes this [44, 45]. Preexpansion of the OCRFFF donor site is another technique that can facilitate the primary closure of the donor site [46]. However, preexpansion requires an additional surgical procedure and delays the treatment of oncologic patients requiring immediate surgery and reconstruction. Furthermore, tissue expanders are not without the risk of implant infection or extrusion.

Secondary OCRFFF donor site closure techniques can be divided into two major categories: nonvascularized versus vascularized soft tissue based closure.

## Nonvascularized Donor Site Reconstruction Techniques

Split-thickness skin grafts (STSG) have conventionally been used to close OCRFFF donor sites. They are technically simple to apply, but associated complications reported include partial loss of the skin graft, tendon exposure with poor skin graft bed preparation, and suboptimal aesthetic results.

The purse-string suturing technique or cross-suturing technique have been described and used to partially close the donor site, reducing the size of the donor site defect, ultimately requiring a smaller skin graft [47, 48]. Care must be taken to avoid applying undue tension to the wrist crease, as this can risk causing subsequent loss of wrist motion.

Another alternative or adjunct to STSG is the use of dermal substitutes for donor coverage [49, 50]. Selected studies that compared STSG-alone versus dermal matrix combined with STSG reported aesthetic and functionally favorable results in the dermal matrix augmentation group.

Full-thickness skin graft (FTSG) reconstruction is another alternative to STSG. The FTSG provides thicker wound coverage compared to STSG, reducing the rate of wound breakdown in addition to providing a superior aesthetic result

[51]. FTSGs can be harvested from multiple locations, including the abdomen, groin, inner arm, or neck [52–55]. Harvest of an FTSG adjacent to the OCRFFF donor has also been described in an attempt to improve secondary donor-related outcomes and better skin color match [51, 56–58]. However, the size of donor site defects that can be covered with this technique is limited. FTSG techniques also depend on a robust and well-vascularized recipient site wound bed capable of supporting the skin graft.

Few studies have described the innovative use of local tissue rearrangement and skin grafting to be able to close a larger donor defect in the forearm. In a series of 100 patients with OCRFFF donor reconstruction using local FTSG, Morino Sanchez et al. describe a graft technique using between two and four local FTSG triangles in a geometric model for the reconstruction of large donor site defects up to 70 $cm^2$ [59].

## Vascularized Soft Tissue Donor Site Reconstruction Techniques

OCRFFF donor site reconstruction by local flaps may achieve primary closure of the donor site without an additional limb donor site (as seen with skin grafts), provide the optimally matched soft tissue for forearm donor site closure (often with superior aesthetics), and provide the optimal soft tissue gliding barrier over exposed tendons and the underlying reconstruction plate. These local flap techniques can be performed in a single stage but are limited by the amount of tissue required and available for defect closure and can be complicated by issues such as dehiscence/partial tip flap loss.

Since 1988, when Elliot et al. used the ulnar artery perforator flap to close a radial forearm donor defect, multiple modifications have been introduced to optimize the RFFF tissue coverage based on this technique [60, 61]. The ulnar artery is radial to the flexor carpi ulnaris muscle. Dominant perforators of the ulnar artery emerge approximately at the distal one-third of the forearm. One or two perforators of the ulnar artery are consistently observed 8–10 cm proximal to the pisiform [62]. By preserving these perforating vessels of the ulnar artery, the remaining forearm fasciocutaneous tissue can be lifted off the underlying musculature and advanced forward to close the radial forearm free flap donor defect.

If a V-to-Y advancement flap is selected for donor site reconstruction, the radial forearm flap is better to be elevated with its long axis parallel to the wrist crease rather than the anatomical design along the radial artery to facilitate closure using proximal forearm local tissues. However, this approach may decrease radial forearm flap viability. The ulnar perforator flap closure is not without risk. It has been associated with the risk of sensory deficit or marginal necrosis because of extensive undermining required for advancement closure.

A variety of different local tissue rearrangements based on the fasciocutaneous perforators of the ulnar artery have been described, facilitating anatomical long-axis harvest of the radial forearm flap and the ability to cover a larger donor defect size. These techniques include using a bilobed flap, a double-opposing rhomboid transposition flap, and z-plasty [63–66]. The Keystone flap is also a feasible alternative technique for RFFF donor site closure that offers a smaller size donor wound closure with the advantage of no secondary donor site associated morbidity associated with a skin graft [67].

However, the elimination of a second donor site alone should not entirely dictate decision-making on selecting a donor site closure modality. In a systematic review of 24 studies describing different types of RFFF donor site closures, Shimbo et al. reported that the FTSG method based on V-to-Y closure was an effective technique that could be adapted to a large and variable RFFF donor defect size with reasonably low short-term complications. Their data suggested that perforator flaps may be associated with higher complication rates [68].

In our experience, we may select either STSG or a local perforator-based flap to close the radial forearm donor site, depending on the size of the defect and the sufficiency of local tissue (Fig. 15.9). If a skin graft is used, we routinely dress the graft with antibiotic ointment and nonadherent gauze and overlay a negative pressure dressing as a bolster for approximately 5 days. If the closure is obtained with a local perforator flap, our wound care regimen is minimal, with non-adherent gauze dressings around the perimeter of the flap, leaving a window open over the flap for bedside assessments.

## Postop Management

Please review the radial forearm free flap postoperative management chapter for details.

## Complications

Prior to the incorporation of prophylactic plating, the most common complication secondary to OCRFFF was a radial bone fracture at the donor site, which has been reported to be as high as 40% by Satteson et al. [4]. With this presentation, operative

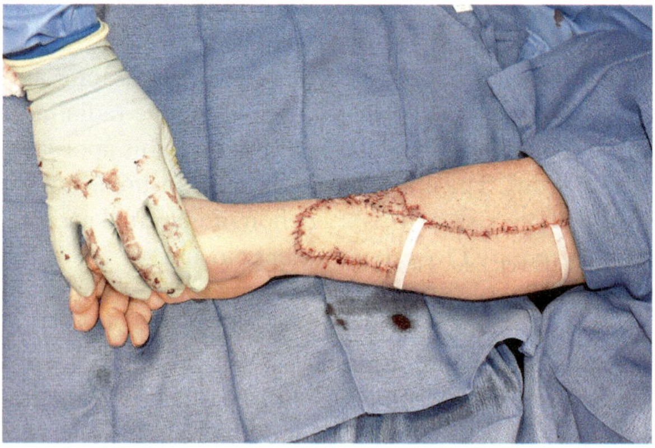

**Fig. 15.9** Intraoperative photograph from the same patient from Fig. 15.8 following ulnar flap reconstruction of the donor site augmented by a small adjacent split-thickness skin graft

intervention for open reduction and internal fixation with plating is required to reduce and stabilize the fracture. Fracture of the radial bone despite prophylactic plating has been reported in 0.5–1% of cases [4–6]. In this setting, management includes open reduction and revision of the operative fixation plate with the possibility of a different plate style or in conjunction with iliac crest bone grafting [5]. Periprosthetic fractures can be technically challenging to treat, given the surgically altered and scarred anatomy, the presence of adjacent hardware (which may sometimes require removal), and the more limited and less forgiving bone stock in which to anchor the new hardware.

Skin graft breakdown or failure over the donor site may also be encountered postoperatively. In mild cases, simple local wound care may facilitate adequate healing and closure. However, in more severe cases, the loss of soft tissue coverage can potentially risk severe complications of tendon and/or hardware exposure. Reports have shown major skin graft breakdown, described as greater than 50% of the graft, to manifest in approximately 4–5% of performed cases [4, 5]. Following skin graft coverage, as many as 16% of patients report restricted function of the donor's forearm, and up to 28% of patients, particularly females, complain of poor aesthetic results [34, 69].

Hardware extrusion can occur at the donor site and manifest either in the short- or long-term setting. Because of the nature of the procedure (i.e., flap elevation of the overlying native soft tissues with underlying bone harvest), the plate can be quite vulnerable to exposure despite attempts to cover it with underlying local muscle prior to donor site skin grafting. If sufficient adjacent muscle tissue is not adequate for durable hardware coverage, consideration should be placed on performing a local fasciocutaneous advancement flap in an effort to ensure viable hardware coverage with additional soft tissue security to prevent the possibility of hardware exposure. However, despite best efforts, tissue may break down, leading to hardware exposure. Unlike tendon exposure, if hardware becomes exposed, biological acellular matrices are not viable treatment options, as direct placement over the exposed hardware will not facilitate matrix incorporation. Acellular matrices require vascularized wound beds and will not "take" over exposed metal implants. Therefore, the provision of vascularized tissue coverage is required. The level to which the hardware is exposed, as well as the available surrounding soft tissue, will direct the plan of care for coverage. For small- to medium-sized wounds, there are a variety of fasciocutaneous local skin flap options available for wound reconstruction. However, if local soft tissue is not available or inadequate, a two-stage groin flap can be performed based on the superficial circumflex iliac arterial system. In the first stage, the flap is elevated and inset over the exposed hardware defect; the second stage requires division of the flap and closure of both donor and recipient sites, generally 2–3 weeks later. Alternatively, if all local or pedicle options are exhausted or unavailable, a second free flap can be considered for coverage of the exposed hardware.

Tendon exposure is reported to occur in as high as 28% of cases [4, 6]. Efforts to prevent tendon exposure require focus both during flap elevation as well as donor site closure. The goal during flap elevation is to ensure paratenon is not violated and preserved over the underlying tendons. This adds benefits both for tendon nourishment, protection, and prevention of restrictive tendon adhesions, as well as ease of donor site management with a skin graft adherence and take. However, despite good intentions, tendons may be exposed at the donor site secondary to paratenon compromise, poor skin graft secondary to graft adherence or patient-specific healing deficits, or a secondary trauma involving the donor site [70]. In these cases, an intervention must be performed to ensure no resultant loss of tendon. Similarly described for hardware extrusion, reconstructive options include local soft tissue advancement, fasciocutaneous, or pedicle-based flaps. In more severe cases where local soft tissue may not be immediately available or sufficient (and assuming the absence of hardware exposure), multistage management with acellular biologic matrix application followed by definitive skin grafting coverage is an option. Two-stage groin flaps remain a backup option for recalcitrant cases.

Donor site tendon rupture is a severe postoperative complication that may manifest in some patients. Tendon ruptures in this setting occur either secondary to postoperative tendon exposure with desiccation and/or infection; or secondary to hardware impingement upon the affected tendon (i.e., attritional tendon ruptures caused by direct contact with the sharp tip of a screw or the plate and/or head of a screw). Tendons at risk for rupture are those located on the radial aspect of the forearm, including brachioradialis (BR), flexor pollicis longus (FPL), flexor digitorum profundus (FDP), abductor pollicis longus (APL), flexor carpi radialis (FCR), and extensor pollicis longus (EPL). The most common ruptured flexor tendons are the FPL and the index finger FDP, as they are the deepest flexor tendons at the level of the wrist and, therefore, most likely to rub on the hardware. Dorsally, the most commonly injured tendon is the EPL.

In these cases, the patient would likely present complaining of persistent precursory pain followed by a sudden loss of a previous hand function (i.e., acute loss of the ruptured tendon's specific function). Ideally, if a patient presents with early precursor signs of focal persistent radial wrist pain and crepitation (a "crunching" sensation in the wrist) in conjunction with a specific tendon gliding motion causing concern for impending tendon rupture, then X-ray and/or CT studies should be performed to evaluate hardware placement/migration. If these studies indicate mechanical tendon impingement, urgent revision of the hardware and tenolysis may be able to prevent subsequent tendon rupture.

However, if the patient presents with an obvious and established tendon rupture, reconstruction becomes much more complicated. Diagnosis in these cases is generally clinical; however, it can be augmented with ultrasound and/or MRI studies if needed. Additionally, ruptured tendons are rarely, if ever, amenable to a simple primary tendon repair. Because of the nature of hardware induced tendinopathy/ruptures, the tendon injury site is often frayed and scarred with nonviable stumps that require excisional debridement that will produce a significant tendon gap. If the proximal muscle remains viable with an adequate tendon stump, interpositional tendon grafting can restore native length and function to the tendon. Primary donor tendons for free grafting include the palmaris tendon when present or the plantaris tendon; other options exist as well.

If the proximal muscle is scarred, contracted, or otherwise not viable, transfer of a redundant tendon for de novo reconstruction of the missing tendon function is another option. Excellent tendon transfer donor options to reconstruct the FPL include BR, ring finger FDS, and EIP. The primary tendon transfer donor option to reconstruct the index and/or long finger FDPs is a side-to-side FDP tendon transfer of the distal ruptured FDP tendon into the intact functional ring and small finger FDP tendons. The specific anatomy of the FDP makes this modality possible, as the four FDP tendons share a common muscle belly; thereby, all four FDP tendons act in a concerted fashion for handgrip function.

Sensory neuropathy or weakness may present following reconstruction and may manifest as either a short-term or long-term complication pending the index injury. During flap harvest and dissection, the median nerve and superficial radial nerve may be at risk for injury. Studies report neuropathy or weakness/numbness anywhere from 0% to 9% of cases [4–6]. Prevention of nerve injury is directed upon a thorough knowledge of local anatomy and meticulous dissection technique. Nerve injuries sustained during flap harvest should be immediately reconstructed. Sharp nerve lacerations are amenable to direct repair; however, segmental or other complex injuries that generate nerve gaps require either nerve grafting or nerve transfer. If the RSN or median nerves are injured, the LABC nerve serves as an obvious autologous nerve donor. Alternatively, cadaveric nerve allograft is emerging as another alternative graft source with evolving indications.

Hand ischemia is the most devastating potential complication. Multiple barriers throughout the initial patient clinical evaluation, and the intraoperative flap dissection and elevation should be in place to prevent this complication. However, if this complication arises, immediate steps must be taken. If the patient is systemically hypoperfused, all four limbs may show end-organ vasoconstriction; in this case, the patient should be adequately resuscitated and carefully observed for response. Also, it is essential to confirm the absence of any upstream vascular occlusions (i.e., persistently inflated or tightly applied tourniquet), warm the hand, and continue to observe for any acute changes in flow or presentation of the hand. If hand ischemia persists, the ulnar artery and palmar arch should be evaluated for patency and flow. Doppler exams may identify a site of focal occlusion or insufficiency; however, any uncertainty warrants operative exploration. If the ulnar artery is unable to sustain perfusion to the entire hand, it must be revascularized. Options include repairing the radial artery donor site defect with an autologous vein graft bypass graft (options include a reversed saphenous vein graft or an in situ dorsal forearm vein-based bypass following an in situ valvulotomy), autologous end-to-side vein graft anastomosis of the distal radial artery stump to the ulnar artery distally, or an autologous vein graft bypass within the palmar arch.

## Outcomes

In comparison to the fibula, iliac crest, or scapula-based flap alternatives, the OCRFFF has comparable functional outcomes with high rates of success [1, 71, 72]. One such study demonstrated 218 cases of OCRFFF with successful flap viability, minimal donor site morbidity, and flap success [5]. Another retrospective study highlighted the utility of OCRFFF for nonmandibular head and neck cases, where 25 of 142 patients received OCRFFF as their flap choice due to its versatility and malleability, reporting the osseous components of other bone-based flaps may be too bulky for the complex recipient site [2]. As supported extensively by literature, the utility of the OCRFFF has greatly evolved in its versatility from the originally intended oromandibular reconstruction to include functionality and success for orbital, nasomaxillary, maxillofacial, naso-sinus, palatomaxillary, laryngeal, cricotracheal, and clavicular complex reconstructions [1, 2, 6, 13].

## Conclusion

The osteocutaneous radial forearm free flap is a highly advantageous flap that can be successfully used in the reconstruction of numerous head and neck defects requiring skin and bone. Prophylactic plating of the radius has proven to be a significant improvement in donor site outcome as well as renewing physician interest and preference in this flap option. The modern OCRFFF has shown low donor site morbidity and high versatility secondary to both its thin pliable soft tissue and osseous bulk [2, 5]. However, the OCRFFF does have limited osseous bulk compared to the free fibula flap. Specific indications for the OCRFFF flap are beneficial in certain populations where a limited amount of bone is sufficient for successful reconstruction, such as midface or an edentulous mandible, or in situations where the fibula is not available. No single flap is superior to the other as each has its own benefits and drawbacks, and associated comorbidities, which must be evaluated prior to initiation. The OCRFFF is a proven viable and reliable flap option and should be included in the reconstructive surgeon's armamentarium.

## References

1. Kim J, Rosenthal E, Ellis T, Wax M. Radial forearm osteocutaneous free flap in maxillofacial and oromandibular reconstructions. Laryngoscope. 2005;115:1697–701. https://doi.org/10.1097/01.MLG.0000174952.98927.9F.
2. Ahmad F, Means C, Labby A, Troob S, Gonzalez J, Kim M, et al. Osteocutaneous radial forearm free flap in nonmandible head and neck reconstruction. Head Neck. 2017;39:1888–93. https://doi.org/10.1002/HED.24863.
3. Yajima H, Tamai S, Yamauchi T, Mizumoto S. Osteocutaneous radial forearm flap for hand reconstruction. J Hand Surg Am. 1999;24:594–603. https://doi.org/10.1053/JHSU.1999.0594.

4. Satteson E, Satteson A, Waltonen J, Li Z, Wiesler E, Apel P, et al. Donor-site outcomes for the osteocutaneous radial forearm free flap. J Reconstr Microsurg. 2017;33:544–8. https://doi.org/10.1055/S-0037-1602740.
5. Sinclair C, Gleysteen J, Zimmermann T, Wax M, Givi B, Schneider D, et al. Assessment of donor site morbidity for free radial forearm osteocutaneous flaps. Microsurgery. 2012;32:255–60. https://doi.org/10.1002/MICR.21950.
6. Arganbright JM, Tsue TT, Girod DA, Militsakh ON, Sykes KJ, Markey J, et al. Outcomes of the osteocutaneous radial forearm free flap for mandibular reconstruction. JAMA Otolaryngol Neck Surg. 2013;139:168–72. https://doi.org/10.1001/JAMAOTO.2013.1615.
7. Silverman D, Przylecki W, Shnayder Y, Tsue T, Girod D, Andrews B. Expanding the utilization of the osteocutaneous radial forearm free flap beyond mandibular reconstruction. J Reconstr Microsurg. 2016;32:361–5. https://doi.org/10.1055/S-0035-1571251.
8. Werle AH, Tsue TT, Toby EB, Girod DA. Osteocutaneous radial forearm free flap: its use without significant donor site morbidity. Otolaryngol Head Neck Surg. 2000;123:711–7. https://doi.org/10.1067/MHN.2000.110865.
9. Burget G, Walton R. Optimal use of microvascular free flaps, cartilage grafts, and a paramedian forehead flap for aesthetic reconstruction of the nose and adjacent facial units. Plast Reconstr Surg. 2007;120:1171–207. https://doi.org/10.1097/01.PRS.0000254362.53706.91.
10. Kruavit A, Visuthikosol V, Punyahotra N, Srimuninnimit V. Radial forearm free flap. Thai J Surg. 2004;25:7–22.
11. Militsakh O, Wallace D, Kriet J, Tsue T, Girod D. The role of the osteocutaneous radial forearm free flap in the treatment of mandibular osteoradionecrosis. Otolaryngol Head Neck Surg. 2005;133:80–3. https://doi.org/10.1016/J.OTOHNS.2005.03.018.
12. Bowers KW, Edmonds JL, Girod DA, Jayaraman G, Chua CP, Toby EB. Osteocutaneous radial forearm free flaps. The necessity of internal fixation of the donor-site defect to prevent pathological fracture. J Bone Joint Surg Am. 2000;82:694–704.
13. Bigcas J-LM, Bond J. Osteocutaneous radial forearm flap. StatPearls; 2021.
14. Acarturk T, Tuncer U, Aydogan L, Dalay A. Median artery arising from the radial artery: its significance during harvest of a radial forearm free flap. J Plast Reconstr Aesthet Surg. 2008;61:e5–8. https://doi.org/10.1016/J.BJPS.2007.10.026.
15. Rodríguez-Niedenführ M, Vázquez T, Nearn L, Ferreira B, Parkin I, Sañudo J. Variations of the arterial pattern in the upper limb revisited: a morphological and statistical study, with a review of the literature. J Anat. 2001;199:547–66. https://doi.org/10.1046/J.1469-7580.2001.19950547.X.
16. Haładaj R, Wysiadecki G, Dudkiewicz Z, Polguj M, Topol M. The high origin of the radial artery (brachioradial artery): its anatomical variations, clinical significance, and contribution to the blood supply of the hand. Biomed Res Int. 2018;2018:1520929. https://doi.org/10.1155/2018/1520929.
17. Marchese RM, Geiger Z. Anatomy, shoulder and upper limb, forearm radial artery. StatPearls; 2020.
18. Breik O, Selbong U, Laugharne D, Jones K. Dealing with vascular anomalies during radial forearm free flap harvest: report of two cases and review of the literature. Int J Oral Maxillofac Surg. 2019;48:1509–15. https://doi.org/10.1016/J.IJOM.2019.06.003.
19. Gellman H, Botte M, Shankwiler J, Gelberman R. Arterial patterns of the deep and superficial palmar arches. Clin Orthop Relat Res. 2001;383:41–6. https://doi.org/10.1097/00003086-200102000-00007.
20. Allen E. Thromboangiitis obliterans: methods of diagnosis of chronic occlusive arterial lesions distal to the wrist with illustrative cases. Am J Med Sci. 1929;178:237–44.
21. Fuhrman T, Pippin W, Talmage L, Reilley T. Evaluation of collateral circulation of the hand. J Clin Monit. 1992;8:28–32. https://doi.org/10.1007/BF01618084.
22. Kamienski R, Barnes R. Critique of the Allen test for continuity of the palmar arch assessed by Doppler ultrasound. Surg Gynecol Obs. 1976;142:861–4.

23. Mozersky D, Buckley C, Hagood C, Capps W, Dannemiller F. Ultrasonic evaluation of the palmar circulation. A useful adjunct to radial artery cannulation. Am J Surg. 1973;126:810–2. https://doi.org/10.1016/S0002-9610(73)80077-7.
24. Cooke R, Lawson I. Use of Doppler in the diagnosis of hypothenar hammer syndrome. Occup Med (Chic Ill). 2009;59:185–90. https://doi.org/10.1093/OCCMED/KQP040.
25. Vaughan E. The radial forearm free flap in orofacial reconstruction. Personal experience in 120 consecutive cases. J Craniomaxillofac Surg. 1990;18:2–7. https://doi.org/10.1016/S1010-5182(05)80596-7.
26. Beckingham IJ, Wilson GR, McLean NR, Soames JV. Free flap failure due to venous occlusion secondary to previous intravenous cannulation: a case report. Microsurgery. 1992;13:348–9. https://doi.org/10.1002/MICR.1920130613.
27. Cha Y, Nam W, Cha I, Kim H. Revisiting radial forearm free flap for successful venous drainage. Maxillofac Plast Reconstr Surg. 2017;39:14. https://doi.org/10.1186/S40902-017-0110-8.
28. Liu Y, Jiang X, Huang J, Wu Y, Wang G, Jiang L, et al. Reliability of the superficial venous drainage of the radial forearm free flaps in oral and maxillofacial reconstruction. Microsurgery. 2008;28:243–7. https://doi.org/10.1002/MICR.20489.
29. Futran N, Stack B. Single versus dual venous drainage of the radial forearm free flap. Am J Otolaryngol. 1996;17:112–7. https://doi.org/10.1016/S0196-0709(96)90006-X.
30. Clark S, Greenwood M, Banks R, Parker R. Fracture of the radial donor site after composite free flap harvest: a ten-year review. Surgeon. 2004;2:281–6. https://doi.org/10.1016/S1479-666X(04)80098-2.
31. Soutar D, McGregor I. The radial forearm flap in intraoral reconstruction: the experience of 60 consecutive cases. Plast Reconstr Surg. 1986;78:1–8. https://doi.org/10.1097/00006534-198607000-00001.
32. Boorman J, Brown J, Sykes P. Morbidity in the forearm flap donor arm. Br J Plast Surg. 1987;40:207–12. https://doi.org/10.1016/0007-1226(87)90197-4.
33. Thoma A, Khadaroo R, Grigenas O, Archibald S, Jackson S, Young J, et al. Oromandibular reconstruction with the radial-forearm osteocutaneous flap: experience with 60 consecutive cases. Plast Reconstr Surg. 1999;104:368–78. https://doi.org/10.1097/00006534-199908000-00007.
34. Swanson E, Boyd J, Manktelow R. The radial forearm flap: reconstructive applications and donor-site defects in 35 consecutive patients. Plast Reconstr Surg. 1990;85:258–66.
35. Meland N, Maki S, Chao E, Rademaker B. The radial forearm flap: a biomechanical study of donor-site morbidity utilizing sheep tibia. Plast Reconstr Surg. 1992;90:763–73.
36. Nuñez V, Pike J, Avery C, Rosson J, Johnson P. Prophylactic plating of the donor site of osteocutaneous radial forearm flaps. Br J Oral Maxillofac Surg. 1999;37:210–2. https://doi.org/10.1054/BJOM.1999.0021.
37. Edmonds JL, Bowers KW, Toby EB, Jayaraman G, Girod DA. Torsional strength of the radius after osteofasciocutaneous free flap harvest with and without primary bone plating. Otolaryngol Head Neck Surg. 2016;123:400–8. https://doi.org/10.1067/MHN.2000.109474.
38. Avery C, Danford M, Johnson P. Prophylactic internal fixation of the radial osteocutaneous donor site. Br J Oral Maxillofac Surg. 2007;45:576–8. https://doi.org/10.1016/J.BJOMS.2006.08.025.
39. Downing N, Karantana A. A revolution in the management of fractures of the distal radius? J Bone Joint Surg Br. 2008;90:1271–5. https://doi.org/10.1302/0301-620X.90B10.21293.
40. Jupiter J, Marent-Huber M. Operative management of distal radial fractures with 2.4-millimeter locking plates: a multicenter prospective case series. Surgical technique. J Bone Joint Surg Am. 2010;92 Suppl 1 Pt 1:96–106. https://doi.org/10.2106/JBJS.I.01340.
41. Waits C, Toby E, Girod D, Tsue T. Osteocutaneous radial forearm free flap: long-term radiographic evaluation of donor site morbidity after prophylactic plating of radius. J Reconstr Microsurg. 2007;23:367–72. https://doi.org/10.1055/S-2007-992342.
42. Shnayder Y, Tsue TT, Toby EB, Werle AH, Girod DA. Safe osteocutaneous radial forearm flap harvest with prophylactic internal fixation. Craniomaxillofac Trauma Reconstr. 2011;4:129. https://doi.org/10.1055/S-0031-1279675.

43. Avery C. Review of the radial free flap: still evolving or facing extinction? Part two: osteocutaneous radial free flap. Br J Oral Maxillofac Surg. 2010;48:253–60. https://doi.org/10.1016/J.BJOMS.2009.09.017.
44. Elliot D, Bardsley A, Batchelor A, Soutar D. Direct closure of the radial forearm flap donor defect. Br J Plast Surg. 1988;41:358–60. https://doi.org/10.1016/0007-1226(88)90073-2.
45. Li H, Xu W, Wang Y, Liu Z, Cao Y, Han W. A novel design of V-shaped radial forearm free flap facilitates the direct closure of donor site wound. J Craniofac Surg. 2020;32:1136–9. https://doi.org/10.1097/SCS.0000000000007211.
46. Bergé S, Wiese K, von Lindern J, Niederhagen B, Appel T, Reich R. Tissue expansion using osmotically active hydrogel systems for direct closure of the donor defect of the radial forearm flap. Plast Reconstr Surg. 2001;108:1–5. https://doi.org/10.1097/00006534-200107000-00001.
47. Winslow C, Hansen J, Mackenzie D, Cohen J, Wax M. Pursestring closure of radial forearm fasciocutaneous donor sites. Laryngoscope. 2000;110:1815–8. https://doi.org/10.1097/00005537-200011000-00009.
48. Moazzam A, Gordon D. Cross-suturing as an aid to wound closure: a prospective randomised trial using the forearm flap donor site as a model. Br J Plast Surg. 2003;56:695–700. https://doi.org/10.1016/S0007-1226(03)00213-3.
49. Abbate V, Laconetta G, Sani L, Bonavolontà P, Di Lauro AE, Masone S, et al. The use of dermal substitutes for donor site closure after radial forearm free flap harvesting. J Craniofac Surg. 2021;32:e205–8. https://doi.org/10.1097/SCS.0000000000006808.
50. Pilkington R, Bhatia S. Acellular dermal regenerative matrix material "Integra™" as an adjunct for radial forearm free flap donor site closure. Br J Oral Maxillofac Surg. 2020;58:726–7. https://doi.org/10.1016/J.BJOMS.2020.01.034.
51. Karimi A, Mahy P, Reychler H. Closure of radial forearm free flap donor site defect with a local meshed full-thickness skin graft: a retrospective study of an original technique. J Craniomaxillofac Surg. 2007;35:369–73. https://doi.org/10.1016/J.JCMS.2007.07.004.
52. Sleeman D, Carton A, Stassen L. Closure of radial forearm free flap defect using full-thickness skin from the anterior abdominal wall. Br J Oral Maxillofac Surg. 1994;32:54–5. https://doi.org/10.1016/0266-4356(94)90176-7.
53. Jang HW, Kim N-K, Lee W-S, Kim HJ, Cha I-H, Nam W. Mandibular condyle and infratemporal fossa reconstruction using vascularized costochondral and calvarial bone grafts. J Korean Assoc Oral Maxillofac Surg. 2014;40(2):83–6. https://doi.org/10.5125/jkaoms.2014.40.2.83.
54. Kaltman J, McClure S, Lopez E, Pedrolett F. Closure of the radial forearm free flap donor site defect with a full-thickness skin graft from the inner arm: a preferred technique. J Oral Maxillofac Surg. 2012;70:1459–63. https://doi.org/10.1016/J.JOMS.2011.05.003.
55. Hanna T, McKenzie W, Holmes J. Full-thickness skin graft from the neck for coverage of the radial forearm free flap donor site. J Oral Maxillofac Surg. 2014;72:2054–9. https://doi.org/10.1016/J.JOMS.2014.05.015.
56. Liang M, Swartz W, Jones N. Local full-thickness skin-graft coverage for the radial forearm flap donor site. Plast Reconstr Surg. 1994;93:621–5.
57. Van Der Lei B, Spronk CA, De Visscher JGAM. Closure of radial forearm free flap donor site with local full-thickness skin graft. Br J Oral Maxillofac Surg. 1999;37:119–22. https://doi.org/10.1054/BJOM.1997.0088.
58. Riecke B, Assaf A, Heiland M, Al-Dam A, Gröbe A, Blessmann M, et al. Local full-thickness skin graft of the donor arm—a novel technique for the reduction of donor site morbidity in radial forearm free flap. Int J Oral Maxillofac Surg. 2015;44:937–41. https://doi.org/10.1016/J.IJOM.2015.02.021.
59. Moreno-Sánchez M, González-García R, Ruiz-Laza L, de Zaldívar DMS, Moreno-García C, Monje F. Closure of the radial forearm free flap donor site using the combined local triangular full-thickness skin graft. J Oral Maxillofac Surg. 2016;74:204–11. https://doi.org/10.1016/J.JOMS.2015.08.003.
60. Bashir M, Fung V, Kernohan M, Ragbir M, Ahmed O. "Z-plasty" modification of ulnar-based fasciocutaneous flap for closure of the radial forearm flap donor defect. Ann Plast Surg. 2010;64:22–3. https://doi.org/10.1097/SAP.0B013E3181A13D8D.

61. Shoaib T, Van Niekerk WJC, Morley S, Ellabban MA, Soutar DS. The ulnar artery perforator based islanded V-Y flap closure of the radial forearm flap donor site. J Plast Reconstr Aesthetic Surg. 2009;62:421–3. https://doi.org/10.1016/J.BJPS.2008.05.038.
62. Jeng S, Wei F. The distally based forearm island flap in hand reconstruction. Plast Reconstr Surg. 1998;102:400–6. https://doi.org/10.1097/00006534-199808000-00017.
63. Hsieh C, Kuo Y, Yao S, Liang C, Jeng S. Primary closure of radial forearm flap donor defects with a bilobed flap based on the fasciocutaneous perforator of the ulnar artery. Plast Reconstr Surg. 2004;113:1355–60. https://doi.org/10.1097/01.PRS.0000112742.51430.A7.
64. Mashrah MA, Lingjian Y, Handley TP, Pan C, Weiliang C. Novel technique for the direct closure of the radial forearm flap donor site defect with a local bilobed flap. Head Neck. 2019;41:3282–9. https://doi.org/10.1002/HED.25839.
65. Hui K, Zhang F, Lineaweaver W. Z-plasty closure of the donor defect of the radial forearm free flap. J Reconstr Microsurg. 1999;15:19–21. https://doi.org/10.1055/S-2007-1000066.
66. Akyürek M, Safak T. Direct closure of radial forearm free-flap donor sites by double-opposing rhomboid transposition flaps: case report. J Reconstr Microsurg. 2002;18:33–6. https://doi.org/10.1055/S-2002-19707.
67. Potet P, De Bonnecaze G, Chabrillac E, Dupret-Bories A, Vergez S, Chaput B. Closure of radial forearm free flap donor site: a comparative study between keystone flap and skin graft. Head Neck. 2020;42:217–23. https://doi.org/10.1002/HED.25977.
68. Shimbo K, Okuhara Y, Yokota K. The use of ipsilateral skin grafts or local flaps for the closure of a free radial forearm flap donor site: a systematic review. J Plast Surg Hand Surg. 2021;55(5):261–7. https://doi.org/10.1080/2000656X.2021.1883631.
69. Richardson D, Fisher S, Vaughan E, Brown J. Radial forearm flap donor-site complications and morbidity: a prospective study. Plast Reconstr Surg. 1997;99:109–15. https://doi.org/10.1097/00006534-199701000-00017.
70. Dediol E, Uglešić V, Knežević P, Lemac D. Donor-site outcomes for the osteocutaneous radial forearm free flap. J Reconstr Microsurg. 2018;33:e3–4. https://doi.org/10.1055/S-0038-1635087.
71. Dean N, Wax M, Virgin F, Magnuson J, Carroll W, Rosenthal E. Free flap reconstruction of lateral mandibular defects: indications and outcomes. Otolaryngol Head Neck Surg. 2012;146:547–52. https://doi.org/10.1177/0194599811430897.
72. Virgin F, Iseli T, Iseli C, Sunde J, Carroll W, Magnuson J, et al. Functional outcomes of fibula and osteocutaneous forearm free flap reconstruction for segmental mandibular defects. Laryngoscope. 2010;120:663–7. https://doi.org/10.1002/LARY.20791.

# Nonvascularized Bone Harvest and Transfer

# 16

Aurora G. Vincent and Spenceer R. Anderson

## Introduction

Nonvascularized autologous bone grafting (NVABG) is commonly employed to reconstruct a wide array of bony defects [1–5], including craniofacial, upper, and lower extremity reconstructions. NVABG can be used alone to augment native bone, to fill in short bony gaps up to 6 cm, and to augment osteotomy sites of vascularized bone flaps. NVABG donor sites can include the cranium, iliac crest, tibia, fibula, and radius. Donor site selection often depends on multiple factors, including the recipient site location, intraoperative patient positioning, and, importantly, graft volume. NVABG is a reliable method for reconstruction because of its inherent osteoconductive, osteoinductive, and osteogenic potential [6–8] when compared to nonautologous modalities. Additionally, NVABG can be routinely obtained without significant donor site compromise.

Identifying appropriate patients for NVABG is integral to overall successful graft take and outcome. NVABG relies solely on the quality of the recipient site soft tissue and vascularity for nutritional support leading to successful incorporation and union. Therefore, NVABG is at high risk of failure and is not recommended to be used in wound beds that have been previously irradiated or otherwise suffered vascular compromise. In these scenarios, vascularized tissue would be warranted.

A. G. Vincent (✉)
Eisenhower Army Medical Center, Fort Gordon, GA, USA
e-mail: aurora.g.vincent.mil@health.mil

S. R. Anderson
Division of Plastic and Reconstructive Surgery, Wright State University Boonshoft School of Medicine, Dayton, OH, USA



F. Sokoya, A. G. Vincent (eds.), *Manual of Head and Neck Reconstruction*,
https://doi.org/10.1007/978-3-031-65999-7_16

The iliac crest is traditionally the most common donor site utilized when a large volume of grafting material is required [6], and it is considered the gold standard [8] among potential donor sites because of ease of access, opportunity for cortical and/or cancellous bone harvest, and sufficient local soft tissue for donor site coverage. This chapter will focus on iliac crest NVABG, highlighting the harvest technique, intraoperative pearls, and postoperative considerations for patients undergoing reconstruction.

## Iliac Crest Nonvascularized Bone Harvest

### Preoperative Considerations

The patient's profession and activity level are important to consider before harvest; the harvest site and scar location can be visible with certain types of bikinis, can make the wear of a heavy belt uncomfortable, and can lead to prolonged hip pain with walking. In cases in which harvest may significantly interfere with postoperative activity and return to work, then alternative sites can be considered. Bony landmarks at the hips can often be palpated even in obese individuals, so patient BMI is often not a prohibitory factor to harvest. Previous abdominal surgery would rarely preclude iliac crest harvest as a nonvascularized graft, but the harvest site should be inspected for previous scars or injuries nonetheless.

### Steps of Harvest

1. Mark the apex of the anterior–superior iliac spine (ASIS) to a point approximately 5 cm anterior along the rim. This mark is for reference.
2. Mark the intended incision approximately 2 cm inferior to the marked apex (Fig. 16.1).

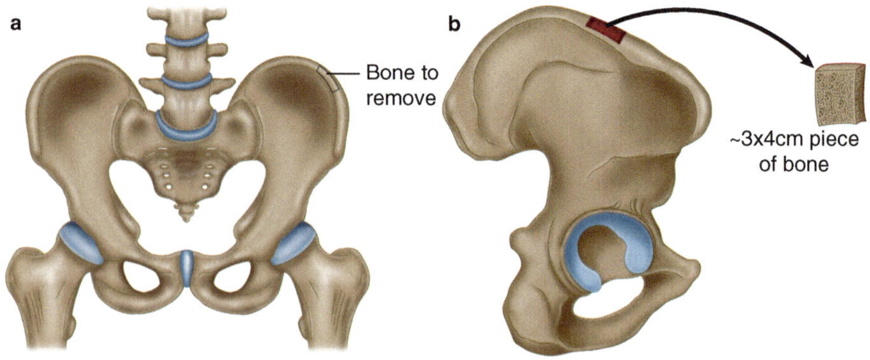


**Fig. 16.1** Harvest of a solid, solitary piece of bone from the deep iliac crest

3. Roll the skin superiorly so the intended incision is directly overlying the ASIS, and incise.
   (a) The skin is rolled until it's directly overlying the spine for ease of dissection. The incision is not made directly over the ASIS when the skin is in its resting position, as this can contribute to worsened postoperative pain and irritation. Also, incisions over the ASIS are more likely to be visible with the wear of swim apparel or low-cut pants, whereas lower-placed incisions are more hidden.
4. Dissect with monopolar cautery to the bony spine, then dissect in a subperiosteal fashion medial to the ilium, along its medial face, to remove muscle and expose the medial bony surface.
5. Place a Taylor Retractor (Fig. 16.2) into the wound pocket with the retractor tip curled laterally to protect and retract muscular tissue while exposing the iliac bone.
6. Under copious irrigation, use a reciprocating saw to make anterior and posterior vertical cuts into the bone, the width of the desired amount of bone to harvest (typically 2–3 cm). Cuts should be extended 5 mm deeply into the ilium, or roughly the width of the reciprocating saw blade itself.
7. Connect the cuts superiorly across the apex of the bone with the reciprocating saw.
8. Use a broad osteotome to deepen the apex incision and release bone from superior to inferior. A single sheet of bone, typically 3 × 4 cm, can be released.

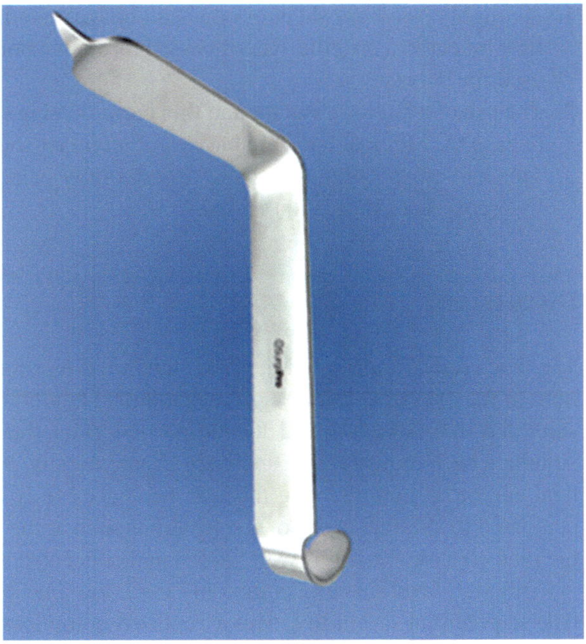

**Fig. 16.2** Taylor retractor. The important feature of this retractor is the tip that flares outward. During harvest, the tip can be placed against the medial aspect of the ilium. This will provide adequate and stable retraction of abdominal contents while also preserving an appropriate working space for bone harvest

## Wound Closure

1. Irrigate the wound with copious amounts of normal saline.
2. Place a sheet of gelfoam over the harvest area.
3. Bipolar cautery can be employed to achieve hemostasis, but there typically is minimal bleeding after the bony wound bed is covered with gelfoam.
4. Close the skin and subcutaneous tissues in layers. The authors prefer to use interrupted 3-0 vicryls for a deep closure, subcuticular running monocryl, then skin glue over the surface.

## Postoperative Considerations

1. Patients may walk, shower, and engage in regular activities as appropriate, given restrictions for other surgical procedures.
2. A drain is not necessary to be placed in the wound bed, and the risk of significant postoperative bleeding at the harvest site is minimal so long as hemostasis is observed after gelfoam is applied to the bony wound.
3. Patients may experience some pain and discomfort at the incision site, but this is typically lessened (and irritated less by clothing) when the incision is inferior to the ASIS.

## Pearls

1. A roughly 3 × 4 cm sheet of bone can be harvested. As necessary, the sheet can later be cut to a specific size or passed through a bone mill; the bone pate is then used for harvest.
2. The use of a Taylor retractor and thin reciprocating saw blade are important tools to ease the efficient and safe harvest of an intact sheet of bone.
3. This harvest techniques leads to no externally-palpable defects and only a short (3–4 cm) scar inferior to the ASIS.

## Discussion

The iliac crest is considered the gold standard donor for NVABG-based reconstruction. In the operative setting, gross anatomical landmarks simplify donor site exposure, and due to anatomical location, often grant the opportunity for a two-team simultaneous reconstructive approach. Anatomically, the iliac crest yields both cortical and/or cancellous bone that can be successfully harvested in larger amounts compared to alternative donor site locations such as the radius or tibia. Aesthetically, the iliac crest donor site is well hidden and concealed at the level of the waist.

Although favorable and commonly used, the iliac crest donor site is not without risk or potential morbidity. Minor reported complications include temporary gait disturbance, skin hypersensitivity, surgical site infection, and most commonly, acute pain [5]. Major complications, although rare, include possible donor site fracture or abdominal hernia [5]. Katz et al. specifically evaluated outcomes of iliac crest bone harvest in the elderly population. Their study found that although the volume of bone graft harvested was associated with a longer hospital stay, the overall procedure is safe for both the young and the aged.

Despite rare occurrences of fracture post iliac crest harvest, biomechanical analyses have been performed to identify risk factors for possible donor site fracture. Schmitz et al. reported three factors for consideration to reduce the risk or prevent donor site fracture. First, harvesting below the peak of the iliac crest ridge preserves structure integrity and more adequately balances mechanical stress along the bone. Second, ensuring a proper balance of length versus depth of harvest should be considered for biomechanical purposes. Lastly, harvesting bone approximately 2 cm posterior to the anterior superior iliac spine can minimize the risk of fatigue fracture.

In conclusion, the iliac crest is a reliable, viable donor site for NVABG harvest employed for bone defects requiring reconstruction. The iliac crest donor site offers simplicity and efficiency of harvest, minimal morbidity, and therefore, should be considered an integral part of the reconstructive surgeon's armamentarium.

## References

1. Agrawal A, Mehrotra D, Mohammad S, Singh R, Kumar S, Pal U. Randomized control trial of non-vascularized fibular and iliac crest graft for mandibular reconstruction. J Oral Biol Craniofac Res. 2012;2(2):90–6.
2. Marasli M, Kibar B, Cavit A. Comparison of the functional and radiological outcomes of vascularized and non-vascularized bone graft options in the treatment of scaphoid nonunion. Jt Dis Relat Surg. 2021;32(3):736–43.
3. Omeje K, Efunkoya A, Amole I, Akhiwu B, Osunde D. A two-year audit of non-vascularized iliac crest bone graft for mandibular reconstruction: technique, experience and challenges. J Korean Assoc Oral Maxillofac Surg. 2014;40:272–7.
4. Hirche C, Xiong L, Heffinger C, et al. Vascularized versus non-vascularized bone grafts in the treatment of scaphoid non-union: a clinical outcome study with therapeutic algorithm. J Orthop Surg. 2017;25(1):1–6.
5. Katz M, Ooms M, Heitzer M, et al. Postoperative morbidity and complications in elderly patients after harvesting of iliac crest bone grafts. Medicina (Kaunas). 2021;57:759.
6. Wortman D, Klein-Nulend J, van Ruijven L, Schortinghuis J, Vissinkn A, Raghoebar G. Incorporation of anterior iliac crest or calvarial bone grafts in reconstructed atrophied maxillae: a randomized clinical trial with histomorphometric and micro-CT analyses. Clin Implant Dent Relat Res. 2021;23:492–502.
7. Azi M, Aprato A, Santi I, Kfuri M Jr, Masse A, Joeris A. Autologous bone graft in the treatment of post-traumatic bone defects: a systematic review and meta-analysis. BMC Musculoskelet Disord. 2016;17:465.
8. Schmitz P, Neumann C, Neumann C, Nerlich M, Dendorfer S. Biomechanical analysis of iliac crest loading following Cortico-cancellous bone harvesting. J Orthop Surg. 2018;13(1):108.

# Part V

# Facial Reanimation

# Masseteric Nerve Transfer for Facial Reinnervation

# 17

Marc H. Hohman and Aurora G. Vincent

## Introduction

The nerve to the masseter muscle is a branch of the mandibular division of the trigeminal nerve and, as such, provides a conveniently located donor motor nerve that can be used to replace or supplement the function of the facial nerve. While both nerves provide motor control to muscles within the face, there are important practical differences between the two. The first is that the use of the masseteric nerve for smile rehabilitation will initially require patients to bite down to produce oral commissure excursion, but with postoperative physical therapy and practice, many will learn to smile without needing to clench the jaw. Some patients, particularly children, will develop a spontaneous smile via the masseteric nerve, but most adults lack this degree of neuroplasticity [1]. The second is the basal firing rate, which is relatively high in the facial nerve and relatively low in the masseteric nerve. The facial nerve's high resting tone prevents facial droop in repose, whereas the masseteric nerve's low resting tone helps prevent bruxism.

The masseteric nerve is commonly used for zonal reinnervation of the midface, specifically for smile rehabilitation, but it can be used to replace the main trunk of

M. H. Hohman
Baghdad Diplomatic Support Center, Baghdad, Iraq

Department of Surgery, Uniformed Services University of the Health Sciences, Bethesda, MD, USA
e-mail: marc.h.hohman.mil@health.mil

A. G. Vincent (✉)
Eisenhower Army Medical Center, Fort Gordon, GA, USA
e-mail: aurora.g.vincent.mil@health.mil


F. Sokoya, A. G. Vincent (eds.), *Manual of Head and Neck Reconstruction*,
https://doi.org/10.1007/978-3-031-65999-7_17

the facial nerve as well; in those cases, it may not provide sufficient facial muscle tone at rest. The masseteric nerve contains approximately 3000 axons, fewer than half as many as the 7000 fibers within the main trunk of the facial nerve, but more than the 900 typically found in a recipient buccal branch [2]. When the proximal facial nerve is not available for grafting, for example in a patient with a skull base lesion or in a patient with type 2 neurofibromatosis who is likely to develop a skull base lesion in the future, the masseteric nerve may be transferred and coapted end-to-end with the main trunk of the facial nerve. In those cases, additional static suspension of the brow, nasal base, nasolabial fold, and oral commissure may provide supplemental resting facial tone. Alternatively, an end-to-side facial to hypoglossal nerve transfer may be preferable as an option for providing resting facial tone, with the masseteric nerve employed specifically for smile rehabilitation [3]. In addition to replacing the facial nerve, the masseteric nerve may be used to innervate functional free muscle flaps as well as to reinnervate the zygomaticus major muscle in cases of either chronic flaccid or spastic facial paralysis [4, 5]. When employed for reinnervation in patients with spasticity, concomitant selective neurectomy of synkinetic facial nerve branches may improve outcomes [6].

Locating the masseteric nerve is technically less challenging in cases of flaccid paralysis because maintaining the integrity of the nearby facial nerve branches is of minimal clinical concern; when performed in patients with residual facial tone, however, frontal, zygomatic, and buccal branches may all be injured during dissection. The method of isolating the masseteric nerve described herein is based upon measurements from the tragal cartilage, the zygomatic arch, and the parotidomasseteric fascia, which is the most reliable technique in the authors' experience [2]. Once located, the masseteric nerve can be transferred into the buccal facial nerve branch that controls the zygomaticus major to rehabilitate the smile. This recipient buccal branch is typically located during exposure to the masseteric nerve, but its identity should be verified with surface landmarks and electrical stimulation [7].

## Buccal Branch Identification

Ensure that no long-acting paralytic agents will be used during induction of general anesthesia, and inject the face with plain epinephrine for hemostasis, avoiding any local anesthetic to prevent loss of nerve stimulation. Add 1 mL of 1:1000 (1 mg/mL) epinephrine to a 100-mL bag of normal saline to produce plain 1:101,000 epinephrine. Mark the letter "P" on the paralyzed side of the face to avoid confusion while the patient remains under general anesthesia.

1. Make an abbreviated preauricular Blair incision, running from within the temporal hair tuft down to the lobule (Fig. 17.1), and raise a sub-SMAS (superficial musculoaponeurotic system) flap extending approximately 6 cm anterior to the tragus. Facial nerve branches will become apparent, running along the masseteric fascia beyond the anterior border of the parotid gland.
2. Locate the buccal branch (Fig. 17.2) that primarily controls the zygomaticus major muscle at Zuker's point, halfway along a line between the root of the helix

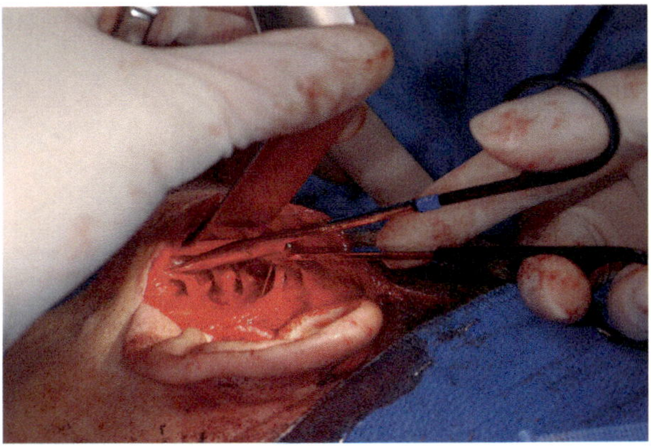

**Fig. 17.1** Abbreviated preauricular blair incision

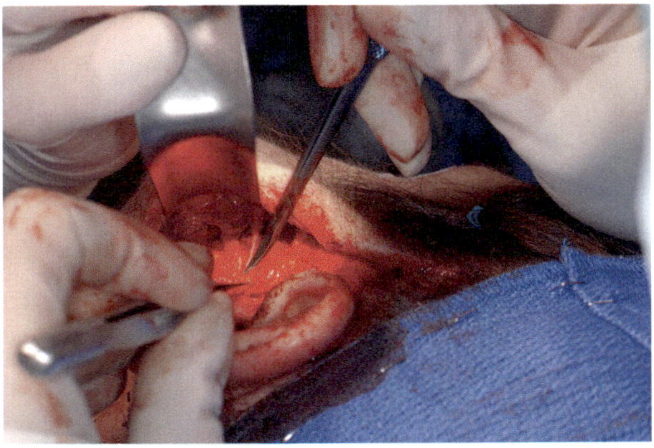

**Fig. 17.2** Buccal branch of the facial nerve

and the oral commissure; confirm its function via electrical stimulation. This nerve will lie superior to and in the same plane as the transverse facial vessels and Stensen's duct, as well as one or two other large buccal branches. Dissect this branch proximally until it branches and then mobilize it circumferentially in preparation for coaptation to the masseteric nerve.

## Masseteric Nerve Identification

1. Mark a point on the parotidomasseteric fascia 3 cm anterior to the anterior border of the tragal cartilage and 1 cm inferior to the inferior margin of the zygomatic arch (Fig. 17.3). This point is usually within 1 cm of the buccal branch previously identified. Incise the fascia vertically and dissect bluntly between the fibers of the masseter muscle. If the face is flaccidly paralyzed, the muscle can be incised aggressively for better exposure; if the patient has facial tone, dissection should proceed more carefully to avoid injury to facial nerve branches in the area.

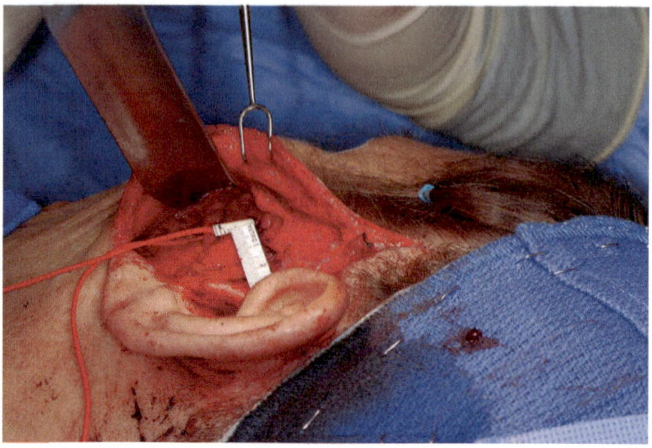

**Fig. 17.3** Estimation of masseteric nerve location

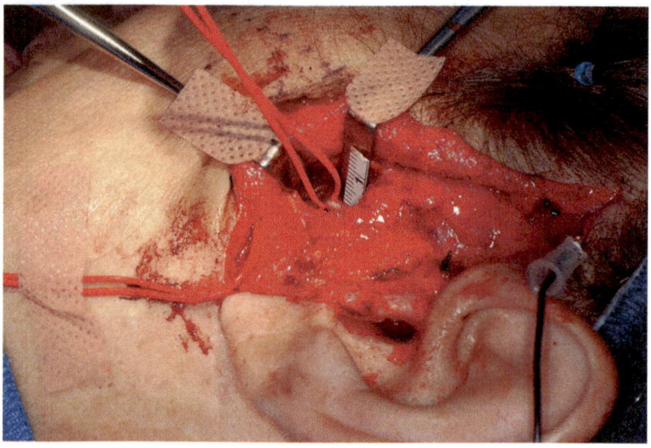

**Fig. 17.4** Masseteric nerve identification

2. The masseteric nerve (Fig. 17.4) will run roughly parallel to the muscle fibers and will lie beneath a tendious layer, close to the ramus of the mandible, roughly 1.5 cm deep to the parotidomasseteric fascia. A vein will closely accompany the nerve. Once the nerve has been located, verify its identity with electrical stimulation.
3. Retract the masseter fibers anteriorly and posteriorly, and dissect the nerve distally until it branches. Then, dissect the nerve as proximally as possible, toward the sigmoid notch of the mandible. Mobilize the nerve (Fig. 17.5) circumferentially using a McCabe dissector or small right-angle clamp. Visualization with an operating microscope may be helpful at this stage because the nerve is only 1–2 mm in diameter.

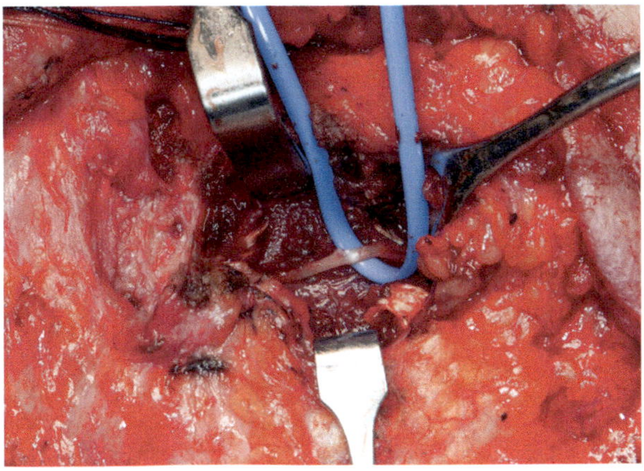

**Fig. 17.5** Masseteric nerve exposure

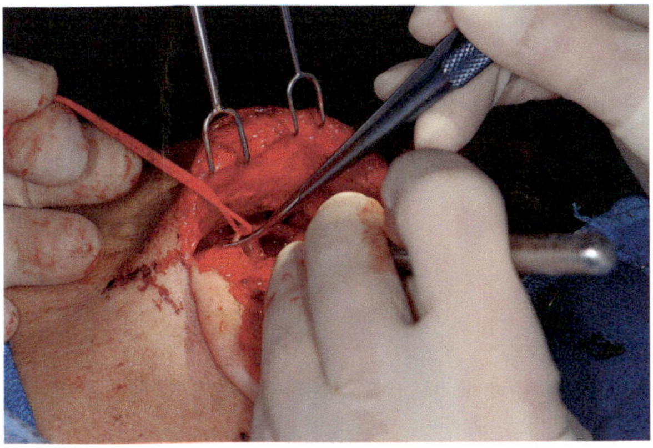

**Fig. 17.6** Transection of the buccal nerve

## Nerve Transfer

1. Transect the mobilized buccal nerve (Fig. 17.6) as proximally as possible, but do not include additional branches.
2. Transect the masseteric nerve (Fig. 17.7) as distally as possible, also prior to its branch point.
3. Reflect the masseteric nerve out of the masseter muscle belly to the greatest extent possible; it may not reach all the way out of the cavity. Reorient the distal stump of the transected buccal branch toward the masseteric nerve in preparation for neurorrhaphy (Fig. 17.8).

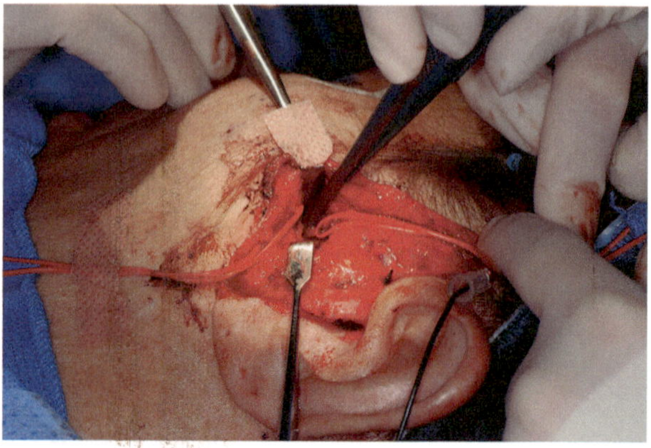

**Fig. 17.7** Transection of the masseteric nerve

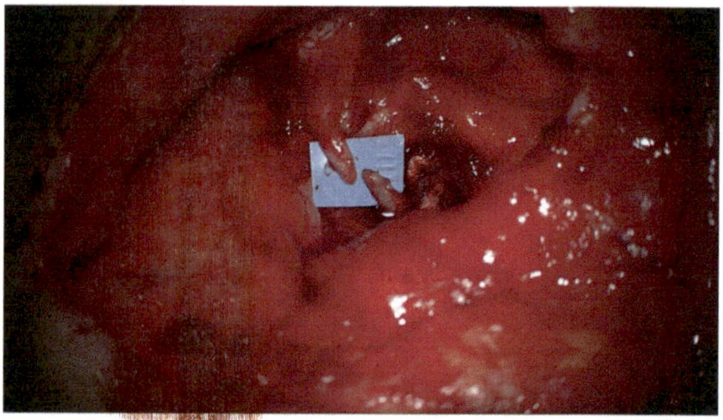

**Fig. 17.8** Nerve reorientation for neurorrhaphy

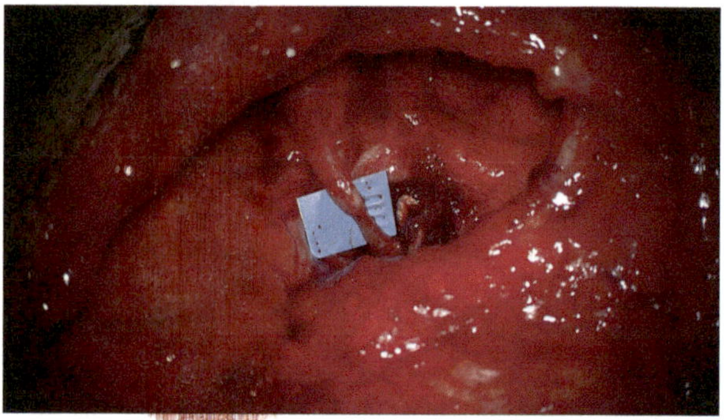

**Fig. 17.9** Coaptation of the buccal branch and masseteric nerve

4. Coapt the nerves (Fig. 17.9) in an end-to-end fashion using fine sutures, such as 10-0 nylon, on a cutting needle. Only two or three interrupted stitches are usually required, placed into the epineurium. Avoid overtightening and impacting or herniating the fascicles through the neurorrhaphy. Consider the application of fibrin glue and/or a nerve protection sheath over the coaptation site.

## Pearls

- Insist on the use of no long-acting paralytics during intubation for patients undergoing masseteric nerve transfer or, indeed, any facial nerve procedure. Loss of stimulability of trigeminal and facial nerve branches during these cases may increase the risk of iatrogenic injury.
- Avoid local anesthetic use in this procedure. The rate of metabolism of these agents varies tremendously among patients, and stimulability of the relevant nerve branches may be lost for hours following injection.
- Exposure of the masseteric nerve is more challenging in patients with synkinesis than with flaccid paralysis because care must be taken to avoid injury to facial nerve branches in the vicinity of the masseteric nerve when there is residual mimetic function.
- Masseter muscle atrophy after masseteric nerve transfer is common, but frequently resolves over several months. It does not usually affect mastication because of redundant function in the temporalis and medial pterygoid muscles, but it may cause noticeable facial asymmetry; counsel patients accordingly during the preoperative visit.
- Transect the masseteric nerve as distally as possible to maximize the chance of reflecting the cut end out of the cavity in the masseter muscle, which in turn will facilitate the neurorrhaphy.

## References

1. Dusseldorp JR, van Veen MM, Guarin DL, Quatela O, Jowett N, Hadlock TA. Spontaneity assessment in dually innervated gracilis smile reanimation surgery. JAMA Facial Plast Surg. 2019;21(6):551–7.
2. Borschel GH, Kawamura DH, Kasukurthi R, Hunter DA, Zuker RM, Woo AS. The motor nerve to the masseter muscle: an anatomic and histomorphometric study to facilitate its use in facial reanimation. J Plast Reconstr Aesthet Surg. 2011;65(3):363–6.
3. Pepper JP. Dual nerve transfer for facial reanimation. JAMA Facial Plast Surg. 2019;21(3):260–1.
4. Hohman MH, Hadlock TA. Microneurovascular free gracilis transfer for smile reanimation. Oper Tech Otolaryngol Head Neck Surg. 2012;23(4):262–7.
5. Miller MQ, Hadlock TA. Beyond Botox: contemporary management of nonflaccid facial palsy. Fascial Plast Surg Aesthet Med. 2020;22(3):65–70.
6. Vincent AG, Bevans SE, Robitschek JM, Wind GG, Hohman MH. Masseteric nerve transfer and selective neurectomy for rehabilitation of the synkinetic smile. JAMA Facial Plast Surg. 2019;21(6):504–10.
7. Dorafshar AH, Borsuk DE, Bojovic B, Brown EN, Manktelow RT, Zuker RM, Rodriguez ED, Redett RJ. Surface anatomy of the middle division of the facial nerve: Zuker's point. Plast Reconstr Surg. 2013;131(2):253–7.

# 18 Outpatient Periocular Reanimation

Marc H. Hohman and Aurora G. Vincent

## Introduction

The vast majority of patients with acute facial paralysis can be managed exclusively with conservative therapy and oral medications. Bell's palsy accounts for over 80% of acute facial paralysis, and very few of these patients require operative intervention because 73–93% will return to premorbid facial function, or very close to it, over the course of a year [1, 2]. The patients most in need of periocular procedures are those who are anticipated to recover slowly or who will later require more definitive reinnervation or reanimation procedures. This group includes patients with medical comorbidities or advanced age and complete hemifacial infectious paralysis (Bell's palsy, Ramsay Hunt syndrome, Lyme disease, etc.), patients with poor Bell's phenomena or corneal anesthesia, and patients with known transection of the facial nerve. Periocular procedures are also indicated in patients with milder presentations who nevertheless are unable to maintain ocular health and comfort with drops, lubricant, taping, and eyelid stretching [3].

Multiple periocular procedures have been designed to improve eye closure, among them upper eyelid loading and lower eyelid tightening. There are several ways of performing both of these operations as well. Herein, the pretarsal approach to eyelid weight placement is described, along with the lateral tarsal strip

M. H. Hohman
Baghdad Diplomatic Support Center, Baghdad, Iraq

Department of Surgery, Uniformed Services University of the Health Sciences, Bethesda, MD, USA
e-mail: marc.h.hohman.mil@health.mil

A. G. Vincent (✉)
Eisenhower Army Medical Center, Fort Gordon, GA, USA
e-mail: aurora.g.vincent.mil@health.mil


F. Sokoya, A. G. Vincent (eds.), *Manual of Head and Neck Reconstruction*,
https://doi.org/10.1007/978-3-031-65999-7_18

canthoplasty. While preseptal placement of an upper eyelid weight may provide a superior aesthetic result in many patients, the more inferior location of the weight resulting from a pretarsal placement increases the mechanical advantage, particularly at night when the patient is supine and makes eye closure more complete. The choice of implant will depend on surgeon preference and patient factors. Platinum has a lower tissue reactivity rate than gold and has a lower profile under the skin because of its slightly higher density, and chains are less likely to cause clinically significant astigmatism than solid weights but are more likely to extrude in the long run [4, 5]. Ideally, one would apply adhesive weights of varying masses to the patient's affected eyelid to determine the ideal size of the implant preoperatively, but a good starting place for most patients is 1.2 g. In most cases, there will not be an ideal mass that permits complete eye closure without causing any blepharoptosis; therefore, the weight selected should balance the two competing factors.

Lateral tarsal strip canthoplasty is also a straightforward clinic procedure sufficient for alleviating most cases of minor paralytic ectropion, particularly when performed under local anesthesia in the same session as upper eyelid loading. Medial canthopexy and lower lid suspension can be added for more severe cases, particularly in older patients with chronic flaccid paralysis, but these procedures are typically performed under general anesthesia because of the extent of surgery and care necessary to avoid damage to the lacrimal system.

## Pretarsal Upper Eyelid Weight Placement

1. While the patient is upright, mark the upper eyelid crease incision (Fig. 18.1), roughly the length of the weight and centered just lateral to the medial limbus or wherever the lagophthalmos is greatest. In patients with multiple creases, choose one roughly 8 mm above the lash line. Inject local anesthetic with epinephrine just under the skin to avoid a hematoma; place a substantial amount medially because the infratrochlear nerve is often under-anesthetized, and this frequently causes the patient discomfort during surgery. Prep the skin with 5% povidone-

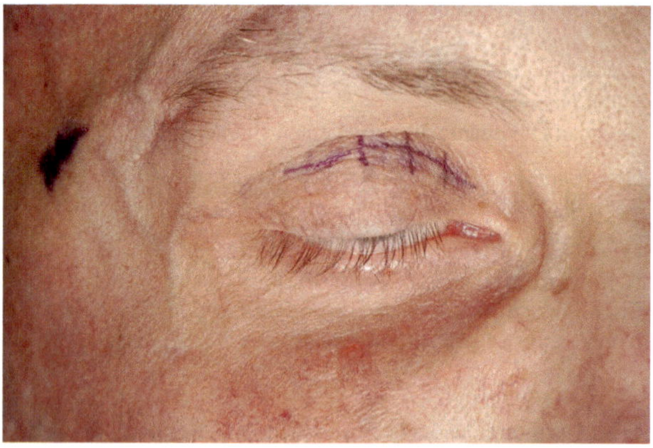

**Fig. 18.1** Eyelid marking

iodine solution, taking care to avoid disrupting the surgical markings. Below, the medial and lateral vertical lines are the anticipated medial and lateral extents of the incision, and the central vertical line is where the lagophthalmos is most pronounced.

2. Incise through the skin with a #15 blade (Fig. 18.2), stopping at the surface of the orbicularis oculi muscle.
3. Dissect sharply with fine scissors through the orbicularis oculi (Fig. 18.3), angled inferiorly toward the tarsal plate, avoiding dissection superior to the tarsal plate, which can injure the aponeurosis of the levator palpebrae superioris muscle.
4. Identify and skeletonize the tarsal plate (Fig. 18.4), extending the dissection medially and laterally as necessary to allow placement of the weight roughly 2 mm superior and parallel to the lash line. Obtain hemostasis with bipolar electrocautery on a low setting, such as 10–12 watts.

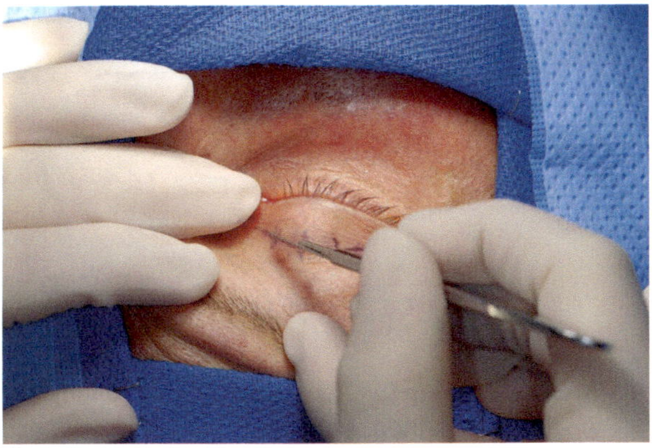

**Fig. 18.2** Eyelid incision

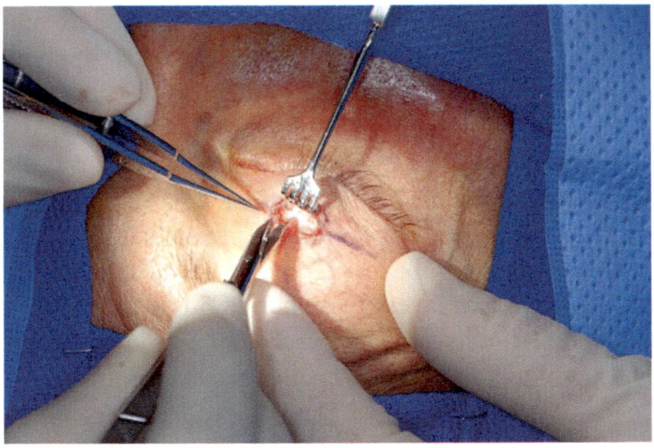

**Fig. 18.3** Sharp dissection through orbicularis oculi

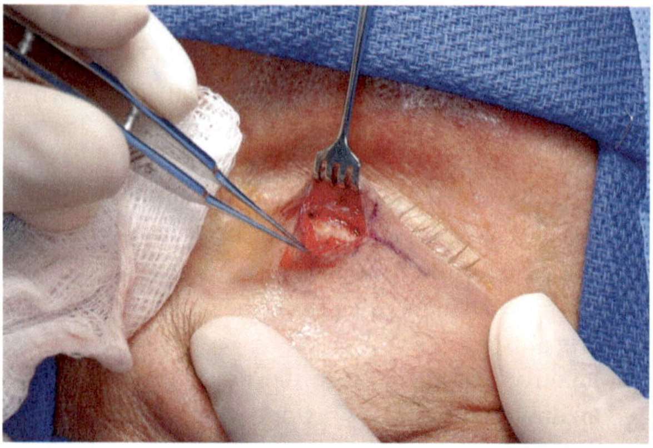

**Fig. 18.4** Tarsal plate

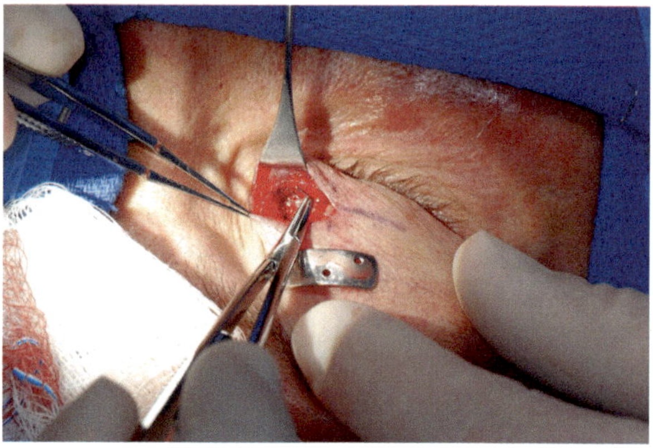

**Fig. 18.5** Securing the implant with a partial-thickness suture through the tarsal plate

5. After confirming that the pocket is large enough to accommodate the weight in the desired position, suture it to the tarsal plate using a clear 6-0 nonabsorbable monofilament suture (Fig. 18.5). The needle should only be passed partial thickness through the tarsal plate to avoid injuring the cornea either during surgery or afterwards if the suture material were to cause an abrasion. Displace the eyelid off the globe prior to passing the suture by applying tension as the patient looks downwards. The assistant should provide confirmation that the needle has not violated the conjunctiva by examining the everted eyelid while the needle is still in the tarsal plate (Fig. 18.6). Place the sutures at the inferior border of the weight first and then the superior border. Take care to ensure the knots pass perpendicularly across the edges of the plate so that there is no slack in the sutures so that the weight will be less likely to shift postoperatively.
6. Close in two layers, with buried 5-0 absorbable sutures in the orbicularis oculi and 6-0 interrupted absorbable sutures in the skin (Fig. 18.7). Apply ophthalmic antibiotic ointment and a cold pack.

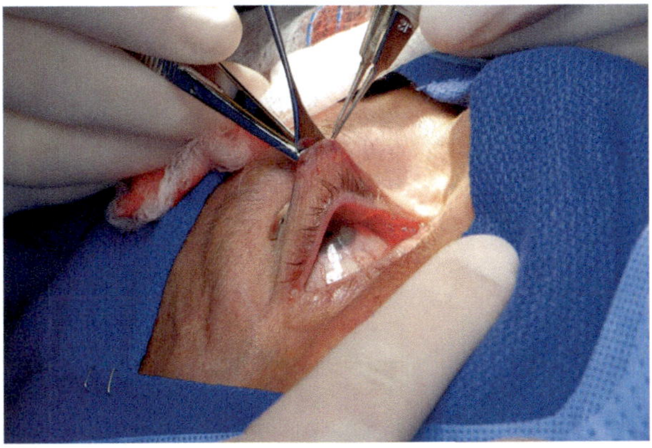

**Fig. 18.6** Checking to make sure the suture has not violated the conjunctiva before pulling it through

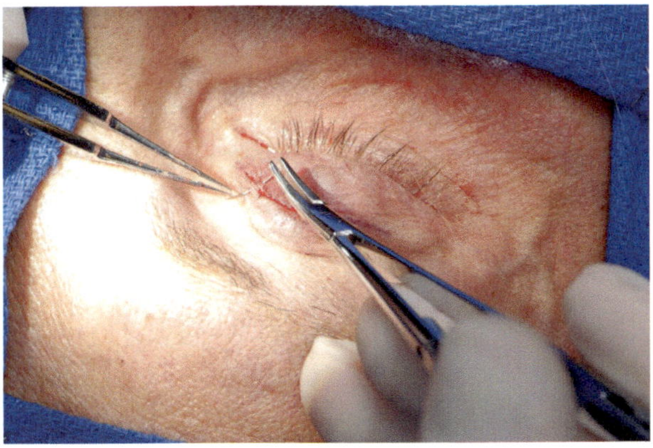

**Fig. 18.7** Suture closure

## Lateral Tarsal Strip Canthoplasty

1. Perform a lateral canthotomy with fine scissors out to the lateral orbital rim (Fig. 18.8), using a crow's foot wrinkle, if practical.
2. Retract the lateral lower eyelid and perform a complete inferior cantholysis (Fig. 18.9), dividing all of the palpable inferior fibers of the lateral canthal ligament.
3. Make a back-cut incision in the lateral lower eyelid (Fig. 18.10) just below the inferior border of the inferior tarsal plate, roughly 5 mm long and 4 mm below the lash line.
4. Denude the gray line parallel to the back cut (Fig. 18.11).
5. Elevate the skin and orbicularis oculi muscle off the tarsal strip (Fig. 18.12).
6. Scrape the conjunctiva off the tarsal strip with a #15 blade (Fig. 18.13).
7. Place a lateral canthal reapproximation suture (Fig. 18.14) using a 5-0 absorbable suture running parallel to the gray line, with the knot oriented laterally, then

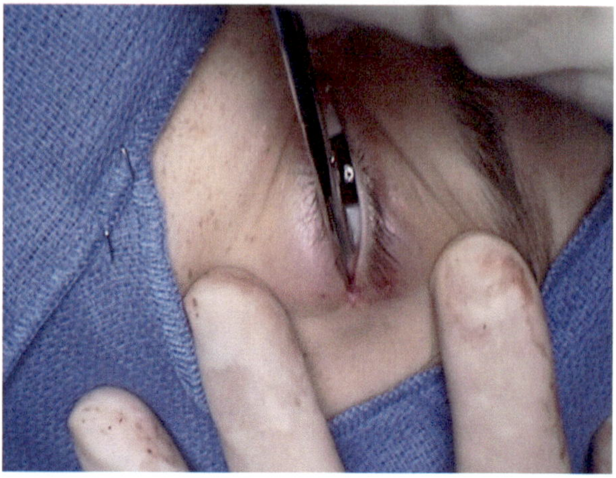

**Fig. 18.8** Lateral canthotomy

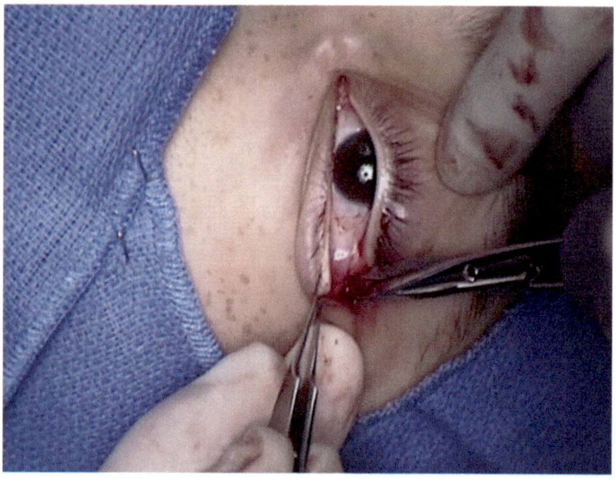

**Fig. 18.9** Inferior cantholysis

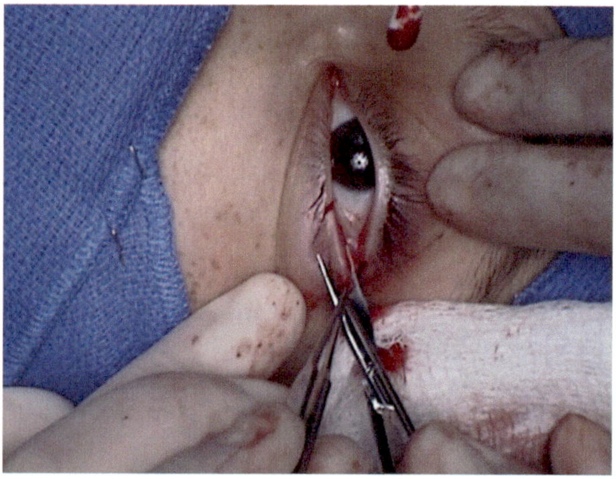

**Fig. 18.10** Back cut of the lower eyelid

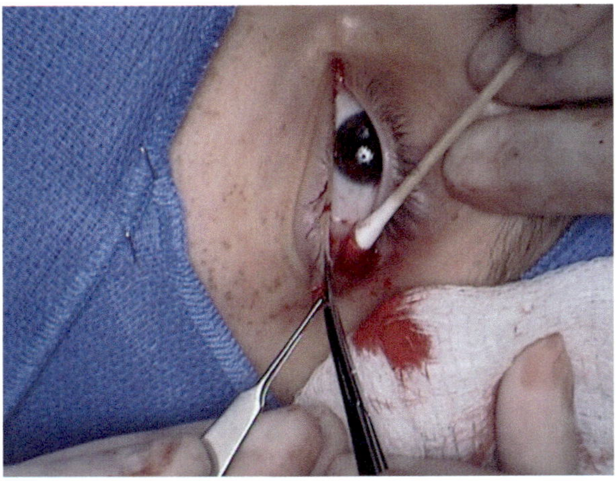

**Fig. 18.11** Denuding the gray line

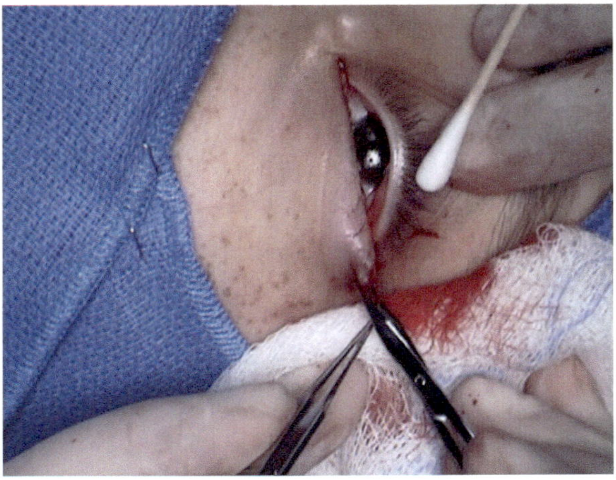

**Fig. 18.12** Elevation of the skin and orbicularis oculi

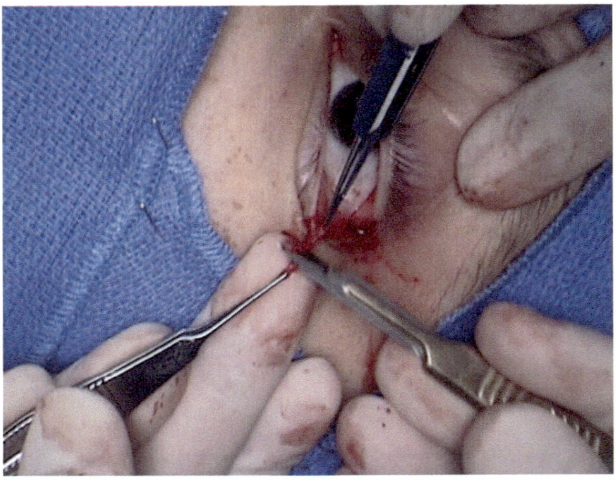

**Fig. 18.13** Scraping off the conjunctiva

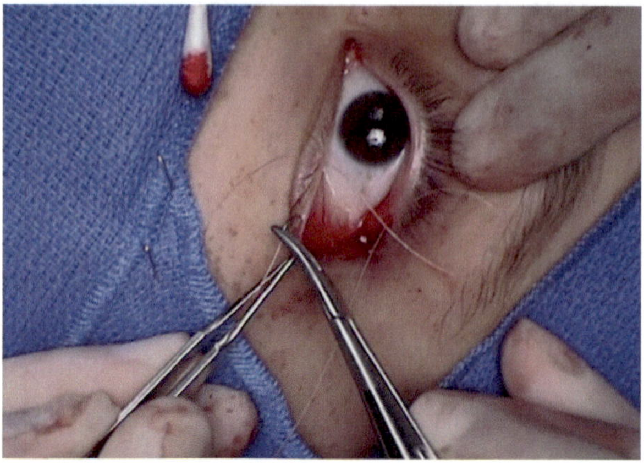

**Fig. 18.14** Lateral canthal reapproximation suture

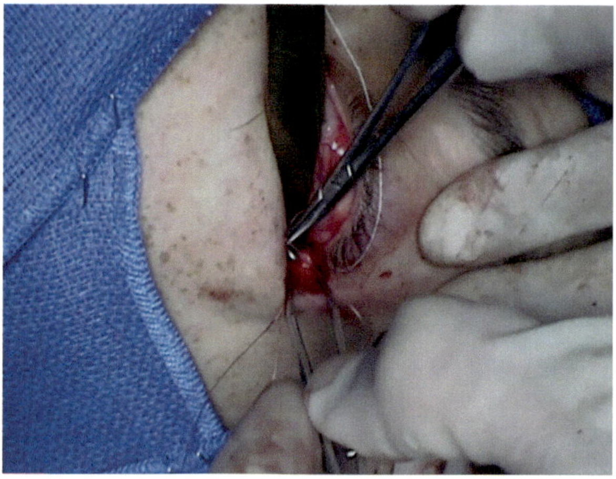

**Fig. 18.15** Lateral tarsal strip suture placement

reflect the suture medially with a clamp; this stitch is placed prior to suspending the tarsal strip because it is more challenging to place afterwards.

8. Place a double-armed 4-0 polyester suture (Fig. 18.15) into the lateral aspect of the tarsal strip with both needles passing deep to superficial, one superior to the other. Then, displacing the globe medially with an empty scalpel handle or a malleable retractor, pass the needles deep to superficial through the periorbita roughly 2 mm superior to the level of the medial canthus, keeping the needles and suture passes parallel to each other. Tie the suture tightly enough to overcorrect by 10–20%.
9. Tie down the lateral canthal reapproximation suture to create a sharp, natural-appearing canthus (Fig. 18.16), and then close in layers, using the remnant of the canthus suture to close the orbicularis oculi and 6-0 interrupted absorbable suture for the skin. Trim any excess lower eyelid skin as necessary.

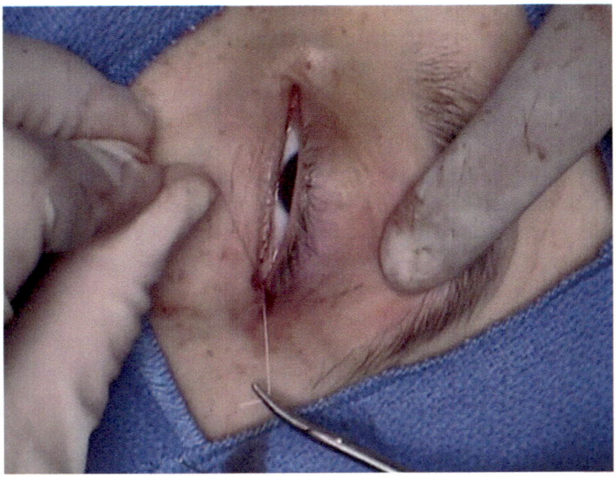

**Fig. 18.16** Tying down the canthal sutures

## Pearls

- There is no perfect weight that will produce complete eye closure without blepharoptosis, so counsel patients accordingly. The correct eyelid weight will minimize or eliminate the requirement for eyedrops and ointment without causing bothersome blepharoptosis, but patients will still often notice incomplete eye closure on windy days or when washing their hair in the shower. When in doubt, a 1.2 g weight works in most cases.
- Avoid dissection superior to the tarsal plate, as this can injure the levator aponeurosis and cause blepharoptosis.
- To avoid corneal abrasions, confirm that the sutures used to secure the weight are placed only in partial thickness through the tarsal plate.
- Place the lateral canthal approximation suture prior to suspending the tarsal strip to save time and effort.
- Reduce the risk of producing bradycardia via the oculocardic reflex by minimizing time spent applying pressure to the globe when suspending the tarsal strip.
- Ensure patients plan to be driven home, even if the operation is performed under local anesthesia, because operated eyes will likely be swollen and blurry by the time of discharge.

## References


1. Escalante DA, Malka RE, Wilson AG, Nygren ZS, Radcliffe KA, Ruhl DS, Vincent AG, Hohman MH. Determining the prognosis of Bell's palsy based on severity at presentation and electroneuronography [published online ahead of print March 30, 2021]. Otolaryngol Head Neck Surg. 2022;166(1):151–7.

2. Sullivan FM, Swan IC, Donnan PT, Morrison JM, Smith BH, McKinstry B, Davenport RJ, Vale LD, Clarkson JE, Hammersley V, Hayavi S, McAteer A, Stewart K, Daly F. Early treatment with prednisolone or acyclovir in Bell's palsy. N Engl J Med. 2007;357(16):1598–607.
3. Hohman MH, Hadlock TA. Etiology, diagnosis, and management of facial paralysis: 2000 patients at a facial nerve center. Laryngoscope. 2014;124(7):e283–93.
4. Silver A, Lindsay R, Cheney M, Hadlock T. Thin profile platinum eyelid weighting: a superior option in the paralyzed eye. Plast Reconstr Surg. 2009;123(6):1697–703.
5. Pausch NC, Kunht CP, Halam D. Upper-eyelid weight implants for patients with lagophthalmos-comparison of rigid and flexible implants. J Craniomaxillofac Surg. 2018;46(10):1843–9.

# Static Facial Suspension with Fascia Lata 19

Marc H. Hohman and Aurora G. Vincent

## Introduction

Facial paralysis affects multiple different aspects of mimetic function, including smile symmetry and resting oral commissure position, nasolabial fold depth and orientation, and external nasal valve patency [1]. While the majority of facial paralysis will either resolve spontaneously or ultimately result in hypertonicity, tumor resection and nerve transection will often result in long-term flaccid facial palsy [2]. The gold standard for these patients should be dynamic reanimation with functional muscle; however, not all patients are appropriate candidates for lengthy microvascular procedures. When multiple medical comorbidities, anatomical considerations, or patient preferences contraindicate muscle transfer, static suspension may be an acceptable alternative. Additionally, static suspension may be employed to augment results obtained with functional muscle transfer [3].

Common materials used for facial suspension include fascia lata, expanded polytetrafluoroethylene, and nonabsorbable suture; these can all be employed at multiple locations within the face, including the oral commissure, the nasolabial fold, and the nasal base. While addressing all three of these targets simultaneously may be an attractive option for a patient who requires a minimally-invasive facial

M. H. Hohman
Baghdad Diplomatic Support Center, Baghdad, Iraq

Department of Surgery, Uniformed Services University of the Health Sciences, Bethesda, MD, USA
e-mail: marc.h.hohman.mil@health.mil

A. G. Vincent (✉)
Eisenhower Army Medical Center, Fort Gordon, GA, USA
e-mail: aurora.g.vincent.mil@health.mil



F. Sokoya, A. G. Vincent (eds.), *Manual of Head and Neck Reconstruction*, https://doi.org/10.1007/978-3-031-65999-7_19

reanimation solution, suspension of the nasal base and/or the nasolabial fold may provide additional improvement of resting symmetry for patients undergoing dynamic reanimation, such as sterno-omohyoid free muscle transfer for smile rehabilitation.

There are myriad approaches to suspension of the nasal base, nasolabial fold, and oral commissure; herein, a limited-access technique is described, involving a short alar groove incision, percutaneous stab incisions at the nasolabial fold, and an abbreviated Blair preauricular incision. An alternative method employing a full-length nasolabial fold skin excision is also detailed. Similarly, there are several methods of harvesting fascia lata; the open harvest is presented here, as it provides optimal exposure and visualization, but a variant that uses short transverse incisions is discussed as well [4].

## Fascia Lata Harvest

1. Mark the groove on the lateral thigh that runs between the quadriceps and hamstring muscles (vastus lateralis and biceps femoris) roughly halfway down the thigh. Making the incision too far superiorly will expose the tensor fasciae latae muscle rather than the desired fascia itself. If the incision is made longitudinally, it will be 8–10 cm in length to permit harvest of 12–14 cm of fascia, as shown. If incisions are made to limit incision length (dashed black lines) transversely, they should be separated by 12–14 cm to allow harvest of a sufficient length of tissue (Fig. 19.1).
2. Dissect down to the fascia lata through fat and a thin band of fascia (Fig. 19.2). The true fascia lata will be a very apparent white, fibrous layer. Use a sponge to wipe the fat off its surface and expose the necessary amount of fascia. If performing three-level suspension, a piece 14 cm long by 8 cm wide should suffice for most patients. If suspending the nasal base, a 1.5 cm wide piece is required; 4 cm of width is adequate for the nasolabial fold, and 2 cm suffices for the oral commissure.

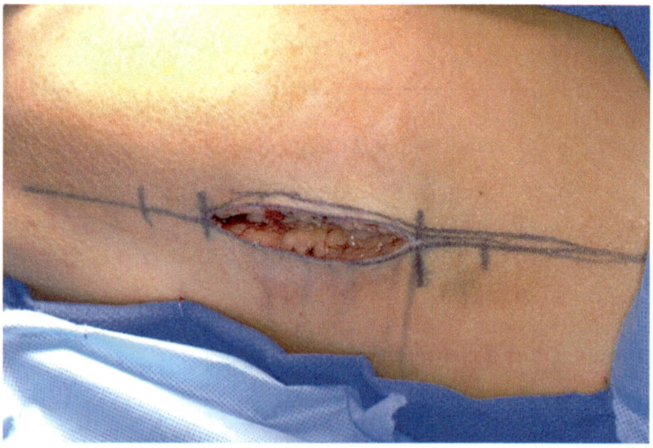

**Fig. 19.1** Incision markings, both transverse (black dashed lines) and longitudinal (marker) approaches

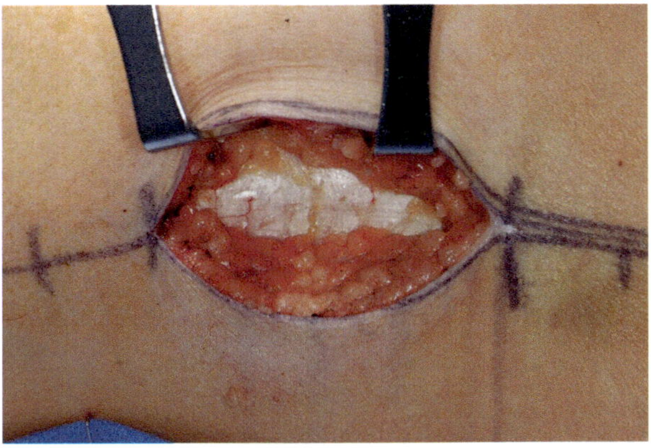

**Fig. 19.2** Exposure of fascia lata

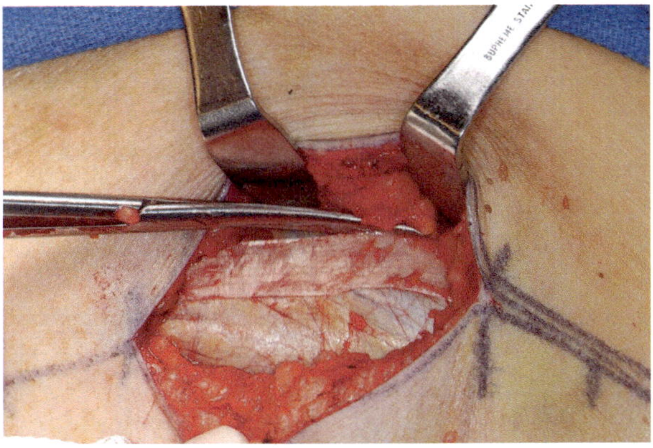

**Fig. 19.3** Incision through fascia lata completed with blunt-tipped scissors

3. Make a stab incision with a #15 blade parallel to the fibers of the fascia, and then complete the incision with blunt-tipped scissors to avoid injuring the underlying muscle (Fig. 19.3). Make the posterior incision first. Otherwise, the vastus lateralis will herniate through the incision and displace the fascia posteriorly, which will impede access.
4. Mobilize the deep surface of the fascia (Fig. 19.4) from the underlying muscle with a finger sweep and then make the transverse incisions to complete the harvest. A right-angled scissor, like a Jorgensen, can help ensure an even cut. Apply tension to the fascia when making the final incision to prevent retraction and harvest of a shorter piece than planned.
5. Obtain hemostasis and close in layers. If only a narrow strip of fascia lata was harvested, it may be possible to close the fascia and prevent muscle herniation. Take care to close the dead space and consider suction drain placement, although a drain is not usually necessary if hemostasis is adequate and a pressure dressing is applied. Divide the fascia into ribbons of appropriate width: 1.5 cm for nasal base suspension, 4 cm for nasolabial fold suspension, and 2 cm for oral commissure suspension (Fig. 19.5).

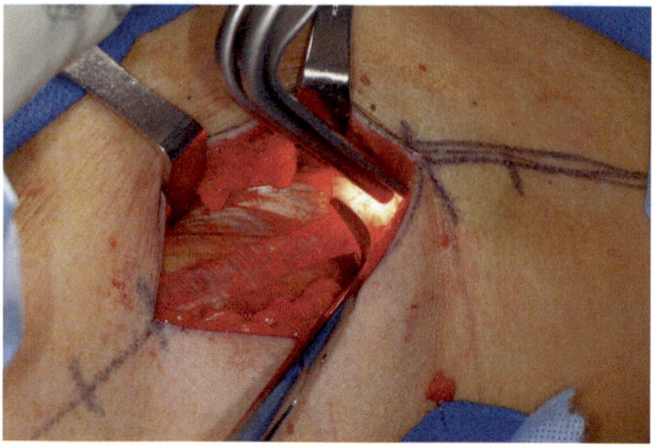

**Fig. 19.4** Deep mobilization of the fascia

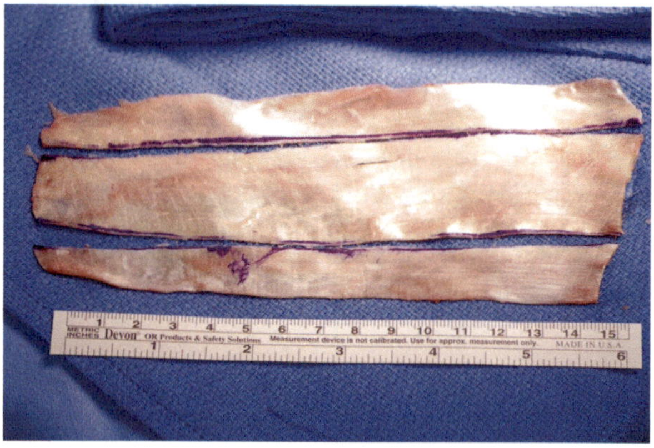

**Fig. 19.5** Harvested fascia lata cut into appropriate strips

## Static Facial Suspension

1. Mark the alar-facial incision (Fig. 19.6) just lateral to the alar-facial junction, meeting the superior aspect of the nasolabial fold to create a naturally-appearing nasofacial isthmus. The nasolabial fold should be marked preoperatively while the patient is upright. Roughly 2 mm anterior to the nasolabial fold, 10–12 percutaneous stab incisions should be marked as well. Mark the letter "P" on the paralyzed side of the face to avoid confusion while the patient remains under general anesthesia.
2. Make an abbreviated preauricular Blair incision, running from high within the temporal hair tuft down to the lobule, and raise a sub-SMAS (superficial musculoaponeurotic system) flap (Fig. 19.7) extending to the nasolabial fold and the modiolus of the oral commissure, where the zygomaticus major muscle inserts onto the orbicularis oris muscle.
3. Make the nasolabial fold stab incisions with a #11 blade, then tailor the 4 cm wide band of fascia lata with a gentle curve on the anterior edge to parallel the nasolabial fold (Fig. 19.8). Place the fascia under the facial flap and insert it into

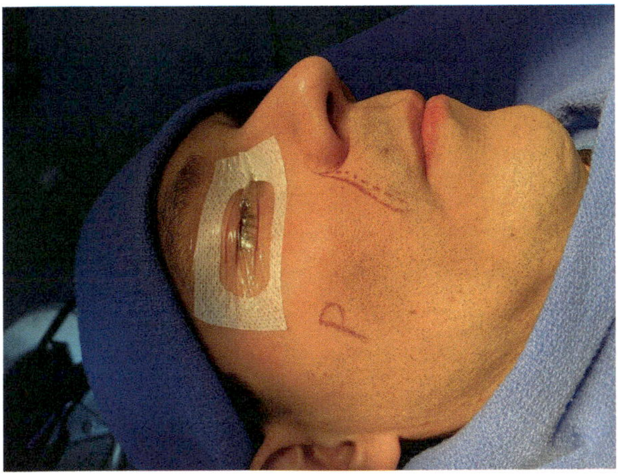

**Fig. 19.6** Alar-facial incision marking

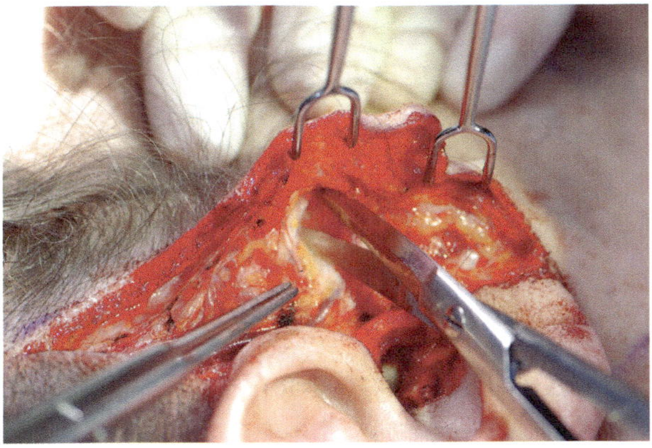

**Fig. 19.7** Sub-SMAS elevation

the nasolabial fold using 3-0 polypropylene sutures with double-armed straight needles as follows: the first needle is passed through the stab incision into the facial wound; the second needle is then passed from the first stab incision through the dermis and into the adjacent stab incision, where it is retrieved, reloaded on the needle driver, and then passed through the stab incision and into the facial wound (Fig. 19.9). Repeat with each of the stab incisions. The number of sutures required is $n$–1, in which $n$ is the number of stab incisions; for 10 stab incisions, 9 sutures (18 needles) are required. It is critical to keep all of the needles in order and avoid twisting the sutures. Placing the needles point down into a suture booklet may be helpful. Once the sutures have all been passed through the stab incisions, the needles can be passed through the fascial band at regular intervals along its anterior edge, and the fascia advanced into the facial wound until its edge rests immediately subjacent to the dermis of the nasolabial fold. The sutures are then tied with the knots buried under the fascia. Do not overtighten the knots, or the skin will dimple unnaturally. The tension on the fascia itself will create the nasolabial fold, not the tension on the knots.

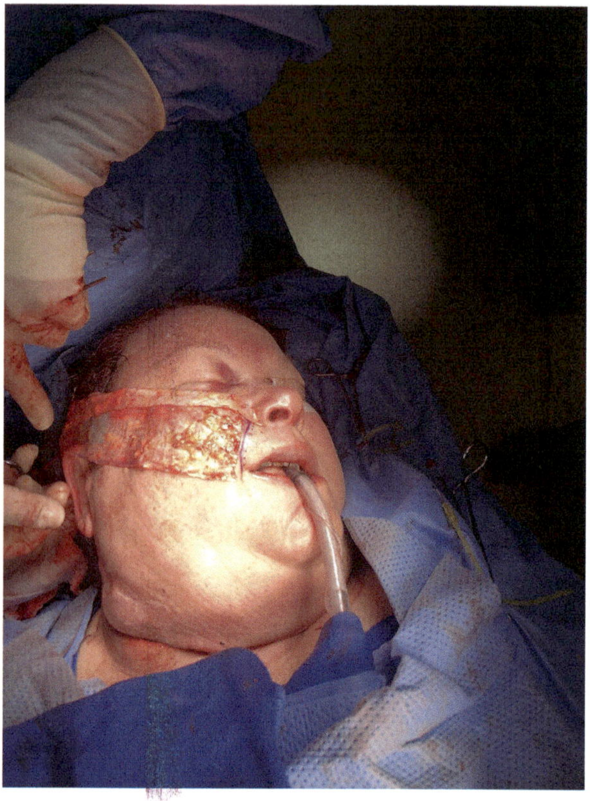

**Fig. 19.8** Fascia lata tailoring to fit the face. This patient is undergoing nasolabial fold and alar base suspension in addition to sterno-omohyoid functional free muscle transfer

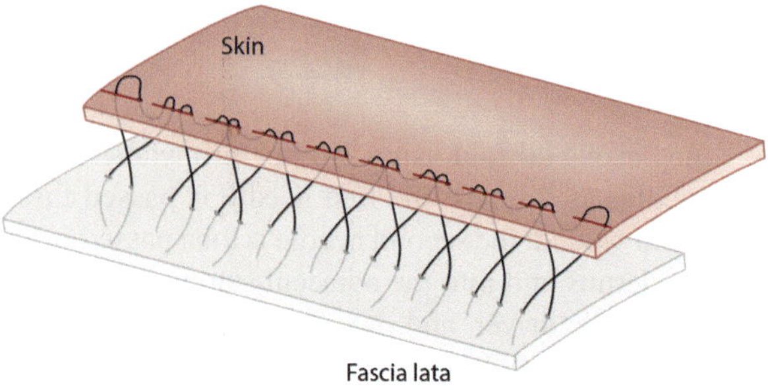


**Fig. 19.9** Illustration of the suture topology. Placing the sutures through stab incisions allows them to bury while avoiding a noticeable scar. The knots are tied beneath the fascia lata to prevent them from becoming palpable

4. Alternatively, an incision can be made directly in the nasolabial fold and a triangular section of dermis inferomedial to it deepithelialized (Fig. 19.10); this inferiorly-based dermal tab is affixed to the fascia lata with buried 3-0 nonabsorbable sutures, and the fascia then passed into the facial wound (Fig. 19.11). The fascia lata should be sutured to the undersurface of the dermal tab, with the knots located deep to the fascia to prevent them from being palpable. This method leaves a visible scar but is technically more straightforward than the minimally invasive technique described previously.

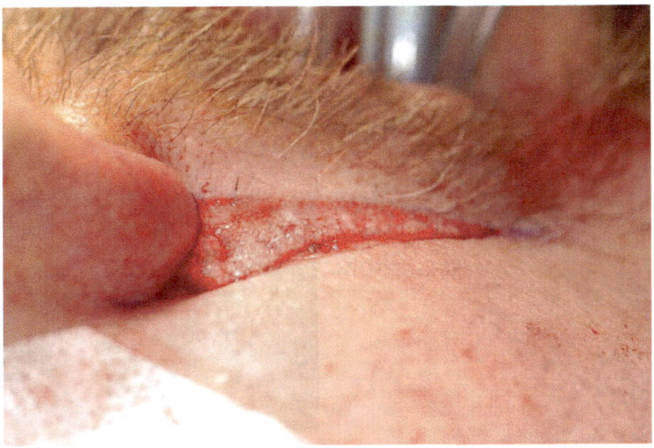

**Fig. 19.10** Alternative direct nasolabial fold incision

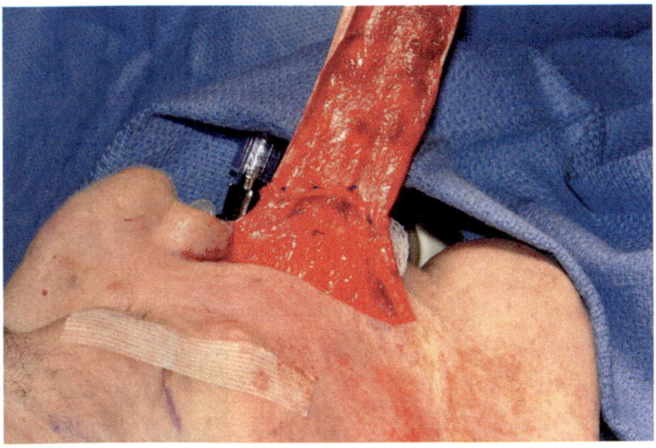

**Fig. 19.11** Affixed fascia lata graft to be passed into the face. (Photograph courtesy of Tessa A Hadlock, MD)

5. Make the alar-facial incision and tailor the 1.5 cm wide fascial ribbon to parallel the curve of the alar-facial junction (Fig. 19.12). Secure the fascia to the deep fibrous tissue and sesamoid cartilages of the ala using 3-0 nonabsorbable suture while the fascia is draped across the contralateral side of the face. This arrangement will bury the knots once the fascia is passed into the face.
6. Secure the 2 cm wide fascial ribbon to the modiolus of the oral commissure with 3-0 nonabsorbable suture, taking care to place the knots deep into the fascia. Figure 19.13 depicts the inset of all three ribbons of fascia lata via a nasolabial incision, and Fig. 19.14 depicts the final position in the face. If no nasolabial incision is used, the oral commissure and nasolabial ribbons will be located under the facial flap. Using a long clamp, tunnel from the facial incision to the alar-facial incision and pass the nasal base fascial ribbon back under the flap, taking care to avoid twisting it. Close the alar-facial incision with 6-0 absorbable suture prior to applying tension to the fascia. Otherwise, the incision invaginates and becomes very challenging to suture.
7. Apply tension and tack the fascia lata strips to the temporalis fascia with 2-0 nonabsorbable suture (Fig. 19.15), starting with the oral commissure ribbon just

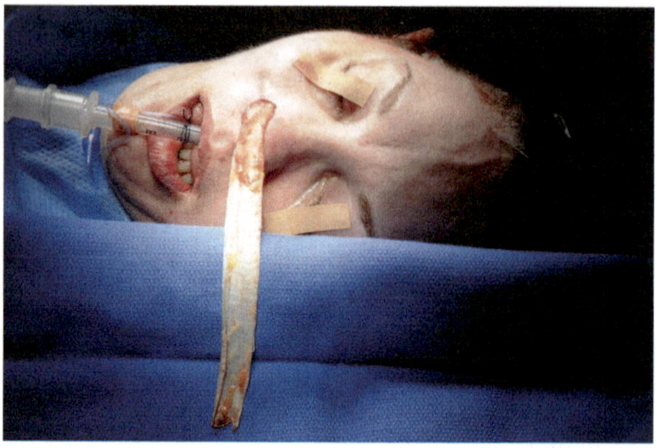

**Fig. 19.12** Estimation of fascia lata position through alar-facial incision

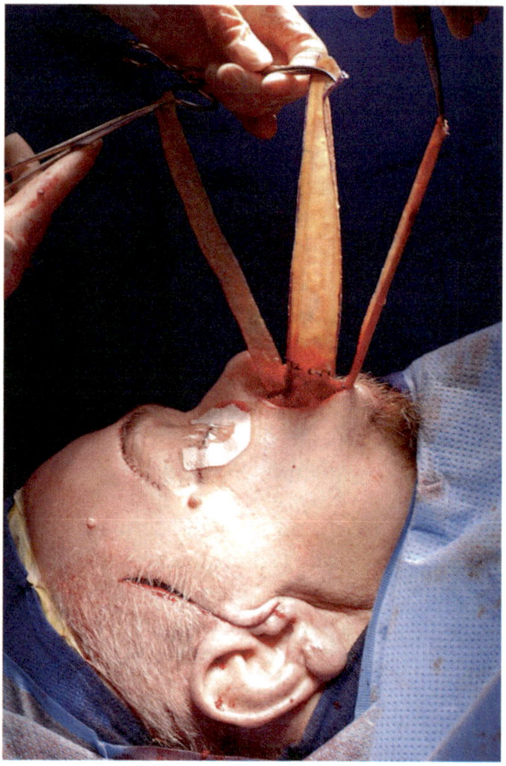

**Fig. 19.13** Inset of all three ribbons of fascia lata via a nasolabial incision

superior to the auricle, then the nasolabial fold ribbon superior to that, and then the nasal base ribbon in the most superior position. Overcorrect by approximately 20% to avoid loss of suspension in the early postoperative period. Close in layers over a drain and apply a pressure dressing unless a fresh microvascular anastomosis is present.

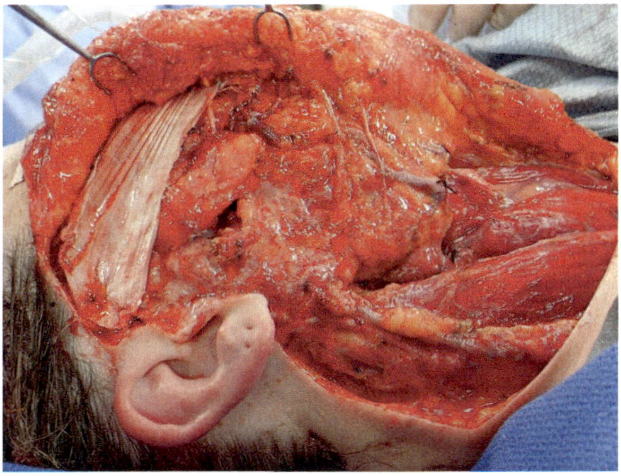

**Fig. 19.14** Fascia lata (blue arrow) in place overlying a sterno-omohyoid free muscle flap

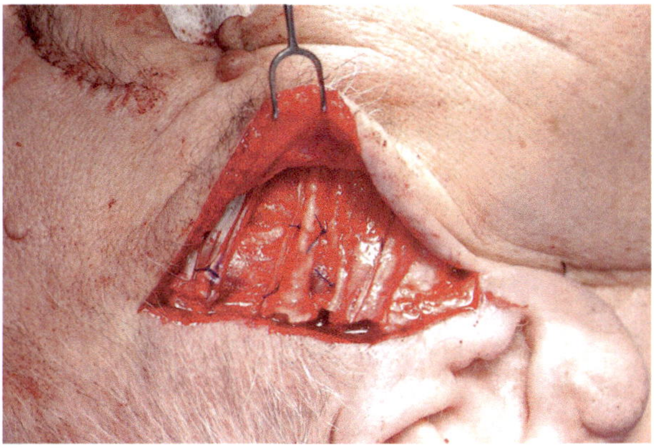

**Fig. 19.15** Tacking of fascia lata to temporalis fascia

## Pearls

- Mark the nasolabial fold on the paralyzed side preoperatively with the patient sitting upright, using the nasolabial fold on the unaffected side as a template.
- Make the posterior fascia lata harvest incision before the anterior one to prevent vastus lateralis herniation from obstructing the view of the fascia.
- Bury all knots underneath the ribbons of fascia lata to prevent them from becoming palpable.
- Close the alar-facial incision prior to applying tension to the fascia in order to save time and effort.
- When performing a minimally invasive nasolabial fold suspension, do not overtighten the knots that secure the fascia lata to the dermis, as this will cause dimpling in the skin.
- Overcorrect facial suspension by roughly 20% and counsel patients accordingly in order to prevent postoperative dissatisfaction.

- If periocular procedures are performed concomitantly with nasal base suspension, anticipate prolonged infraorbital edema due to interruption of lymphatic drainage by the fascia lata.
- If performing static suspension and muscle transfer, place the fascial ribbons superficial to the transferred muscle to act as a glide plane under the skin and prevent muscle tethering to the dermis.

## References

1. Hadlock TA, Greenfield LJ, Wernick-Robinson M, Cheney ML. Multimodality approach to management of the paralyzed face. Laryngoscope. 2006;116(8):1385–9.
2. Hohman MH, Bhama PK, Hadlock TA. Epidemiology of iatrogenic facial neve injury: a decade of experience. Laryngoscope. 2014;124(1):260–5.
3. Kiefer J, Braig D, Thiele JR, Bannasch H, Stark GB, Eisenhardt SU. Comparison of symmetry after smile reconstruction for flaccid facial paralysis with combined fascia lata grafts and functional gracilis transfer for statis suspension or gracilis transfer alone. Microsurgery. 2018;38(6):634–42.
4. Faris C, Heiser A, Jowett N, Hadlock T. Minimal nasolabial incision technique for nasolabial fold modification in patients with facial paralysis. JAMA Facial Plast Surg. 2018;20(2):148–53.

# Functional Sterno-omohyoid Free Muscle Transfer for Facial Reanimation

# 20

Marc H. Hohman and Aurora G. Vincent

## Introduction

When patients with chronic facial paralysis of greater than 1–2 years in duration desire dynamic rehabilitation, the mimetic muscles have typically atrophied and are no longer able to accept reinnervation for these patients and for patients with congenital facial palsy who were born with deficient mimetic musculature, replacement of the muscles as well as their motor nerves is required. Additionally, patients with severe synkinesis may be candidates for functional free muscle transfer, which can provide improved function and cosmesis by bypassing the injured facial nerve [1].

The choice of donor muscle is determined by patient requirements and goals, anatomical considerations, and surgeon preference; numerous options are available. The latissimus dorsi can provide a substantial amount of bulk, as well as overlying skin, if necessary. The pectoralis minor is substantially slimmer and is very popular but has a notoriously variable venous outflow pattern. The gracilis muscle, first reported as a facial reanimation option in 1976, is the most commonly used donor muscle for functional free tissue transfer in North America, because of its anatomical consistency and the ease with which it can be harvested while facial surgery is ongoing [2].

M. H. Hohman
Baghdad Diplomatic Support Center, Baghdad, Iraq

Department of Surgery, Uniformed Services University of the Health Sciences, Bethesda, MD, USA
e-mail: marc.h.hohman.mil@health.mil

A. G. Vincent (✉)
Eisenhower Army Medical Center, Fort Gordon, GA, USA
e-mail: aurora.g.vincent.mil@health.mil



F. Sokoya, A. G. Vincent (eds.), *Manual of Head and Neck Reconstruction*,
https://doi.org/10.1007/978-3-031-65999-7_20

Despite its reliability, the gracilis lacks two major features possessed by native facial muscles: low volume and the ability to contract rapidly. It is a large postural muscle, and when transferred to the face, it must first undergo substantial debulking to avoid adding noticeable excess subcutaneous volume. Aggressive debulking removes the muscle's fascial layer and potentially increases the chance of dermal tethering; more importantly, debulking risks denervating the muscle and compromising its contractility. The speed with which facial muscles contract is one of their defining characteristics however. Histologically, facial muscles have low mitochondrial counts and comprise largely type II "fast twitch" fibers, in contrast to the gracilis' high mitochondrial count "slow twitch" architecture [3]. Similar to the facial muscles, the anterior cervical strap muscles are also made up primarily of type II fibers, and they have the advantage of being comparatively slim without requiring debulking.

The other advantage provided by strap muscles is that more than one belly can be harvested based on the same nerve and vascular pedicle. Transferring the sternohyoid and omohyoid together permits replacement of the zygomaticus major and levator labii superioris simultaneously, providing a more natural, dentate smile than can be achieved with methods that replace only the zygomaticus major muscle, such as temporalis or traditional gracilis transfer [4]. More recently, the gracilis has been divided into multiple individual slips of functional muscle in order to provide multiple vectors of facial movement, but doing so risks denervation and requires a large volume of muscle [5, 6]. Likewise, the serratus anterior muscle is naturally configured with multiple slips that correspond to different ribs; however, like the gracilis, it is much larger than native facial muscles [7]. The ability of the sterno-omohyoid flap to produce dual-vector smile reanimation using slim, fast twitch muscles is a major advantage. Lastly, the neural input to the strap muscle flap is the ansa cervicalis, which is long and possesses two major branches for input; both can be coapted to the masseteric nerve to maximize reliability of the flap, or one end of the ansa may be sutured to the masseteric nerve and the other to a cross-face nerve graft, which potentially improves spontaneity and symmetry of the smile [8]. Loss of the ansa cervicalis along with two strap muscles from one side of the neck has not resulted in any reports of postoperative speech or swallowing difficulties.

Despite seeming like an ideal reconstructive option, the strap flap does have two notable disadvantages. The first is that because it is harvested ipsilaterally to the facial paralysis, simultaneous harvest and recipient site preparation is challenging. The second is that the vascular anatomy is variable, and while the superior thyroid artery is generally reliably located, the venous outflow is highly variable as it is with the pectoralis minor flap. Outflow typically drains through the vena comitans of the superior thyroid artery, the superior thyroid vein, the middle thyroid vein, or a ranine vein. Herein, the technique of sterno-omohyoid harvest and inset as well as sural nerve harvest and cross-face nerve graft placement are detailed. For a description of masseteric nerve dissection for innervation of the strap flap, please see Chap. 17.

## Recipient Site Preparation

Ensure that no long-acting paralytic agents will be used during induction of general anesthesia, and inject the face with plain epinephrine for hemostasis, avoiding any local anesthetic in order to prevent loss of nerve stimulation. Add 1 mL of 1:1000 (1 mg/mL) epinephrine to a 100 mL bag of normal saline to produce plain 1:101,000 epinephrine. Mark the letter "P" on the paralyzed side of the face to avoid confusion while the patient remains under general anesthesia.

1. Make a modified Blair incision, running from within the temporal hair tuft down to the lobule and then down the lateral neck, joining a transverse skin crease to travel to the midline, approximately 2 cm superior to the clavicle. Then, raise a sub-SMAS (superficial musculoaponeurotic system) flap (Fig. 20.1) extending to the oral commissure and around the upper lip, exposing the orbicularis oris muscle; continue the flap elevation in a subplatysmal plane 2–3 cm past the midline of the neck.
2. Identify and isolate the recipient vessels (Fig. 20.2), preferably the distal facial artery and vein superior to the inferior margin of the mandible. The superficial temporal vessels and/or the external jugular vein are viable alternatives.
3. Place a 6-hole titanium miniplate at the inferior orbital rim via a preseptal, transconjunctival approach.
   (a) Incise the conjunctiva 2–3 mm below the inferior margin of the tarsal plate, from the punctum medially out to the lateral canthus. Carry the incision through the capsulopalpebral fascia (Fig. 20.3).
   (b) Place a tension suture through the capsulopalpebral fascia and retract it over the cornea with a hemostat, then continue the dissection, separating the orbicularis oculi muscle from the orbital septum (Fig. 20.4) until the infraorbital rim is reached.
   (c) Expose the maxilla and place the 6-hole titanium miniplate just inferior to the infraorbital rim (Fig. 20.5), but do not tighten the screws completely, leaving room for needle and suture passage later in the operation.

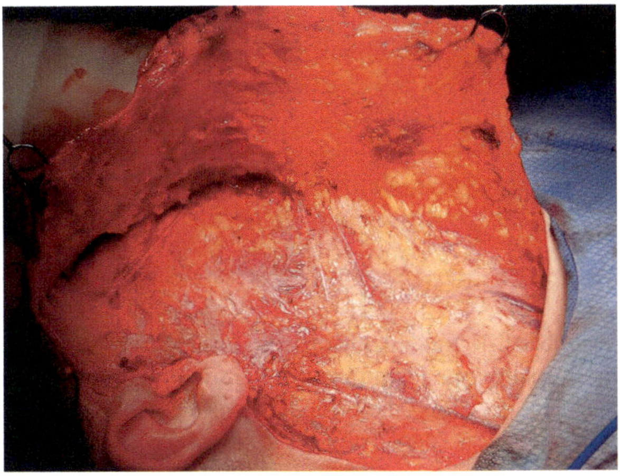

**Fig. 20.1** Flap elevation

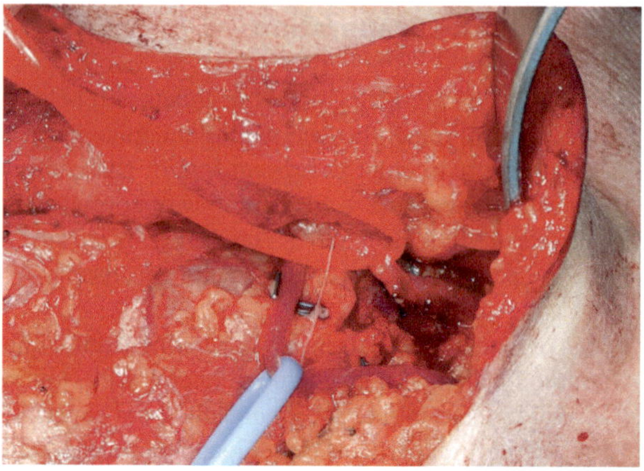

**Fig. 20.2** Recipient vessel isolation

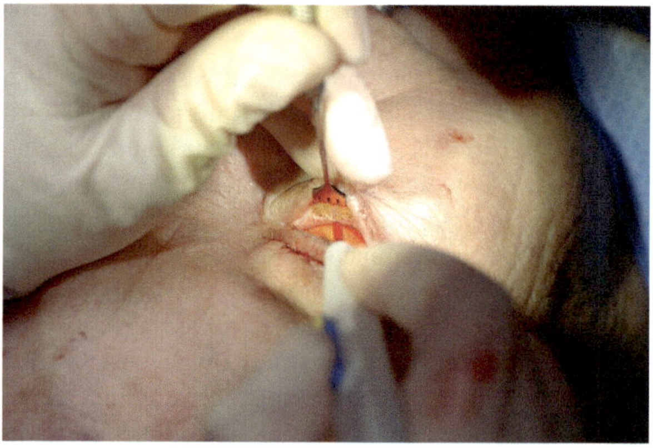

**Fig. 20.3** Incision through conjunctiva and capsulopalpebral fascia

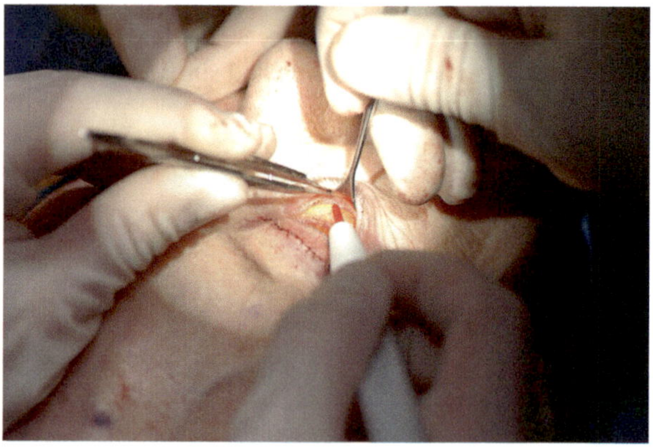

**Fig. 20.4** Dissection between orbicularis oculi and orbital septum to orbital rim

4. Place 2-0 braided, absorbable inset sutures: one at the modiolus of the oral commissure, one just inferior to it, and one just superior to it, then two more farther medially along the orbicularis oris muscle of the upper lip. Apply superolateral

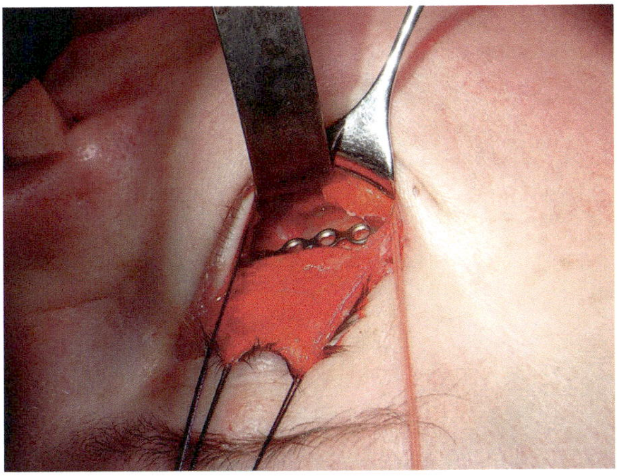

**Fig. 20.5** Titanium plate placement

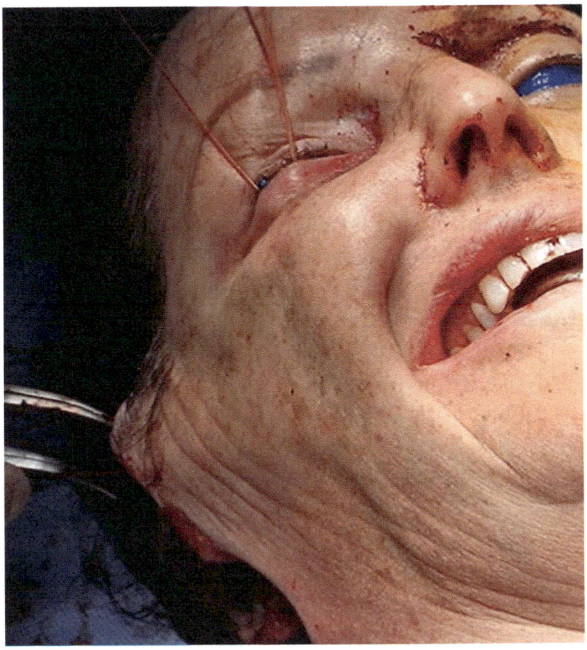

**Fig. 20.6** Adjustment of suture placement until the appearance of the smile is appropriate and there is neither unnatural dimpling of the skin nor eversion of the lip

tension to the three lateral sutures towards the superior margin of the auricular helix while applying tension to the two medial sutures over the infraorbital mini-plate; adjust suture placement until the appearance of the smile is appropriate and there is neither unnatural dimpling of the skin nor eversion of the lip (Fig. 20.6).

5. Identify and isolate the masseteric nerve, as described in Chap. 17 (Fig. 20.7).

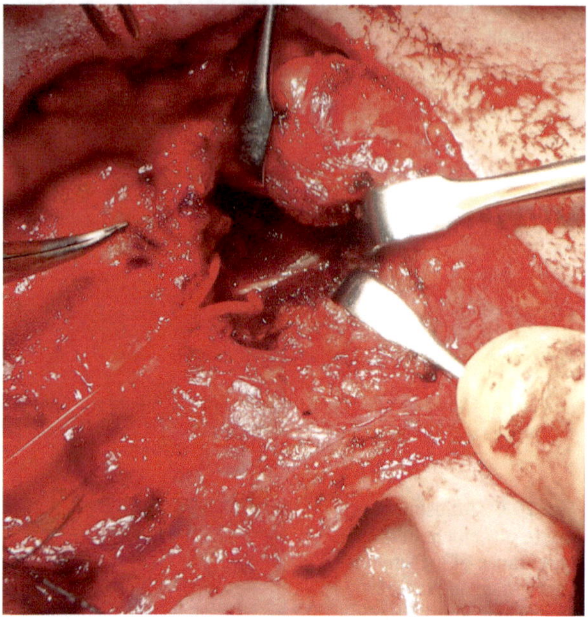

**Fig. 20.7** Identification of the masseteric nerve

## Optional: Sural Nerve Harvest and Cross-Face Nerve Grafting for Dual Innervation of the Flap

### Sural Nerve Harvest

1. Make a transverse incision 1 cm superior and 1 cm posterior to the lateral malleolus of the ankle and identify the lesser saphenous vein within the wound . Retract the vein and isolate the underlying sural nerve (Fig. 20.8).
2. Divide the sural nerve as inferiorly as possible, but superior to its branch point, and then pass the nerve through a tendon stripper (Fig. 20.9). Maintain tension on the nerve while advancing the stripper, gently twisting back and forth. Resistance will be encountered when the nerve branches over the gastrocnemius muscle. Once the stripper has been advanced roughly 30 cm up the leg, it can be twisted sharply to divide the nerve; alternatively, a stab incision over the end of the stripper will provide access to the sural nerve for transection.
3. Retrieve the stripper and leave a hemostat on the inferior/distal end of the nerve (Fig. 20.10).

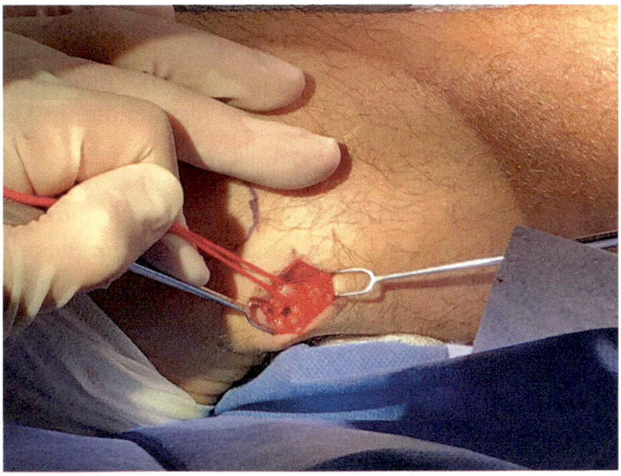

**Fig. 20.8** Isolation of the sural nerve

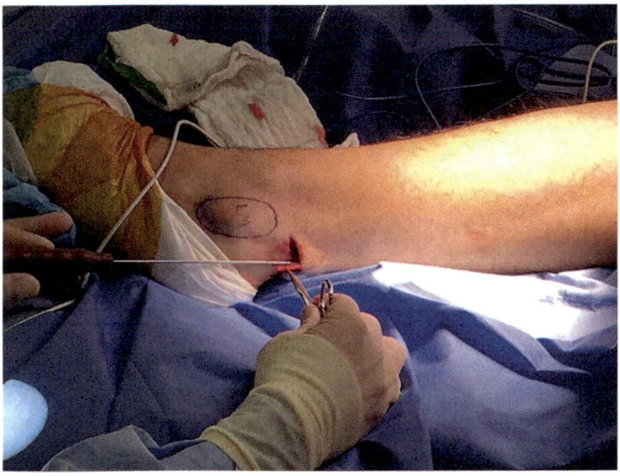

**Fig. 20.9** Tendon-stripper-assisted harvest of the sural nerve

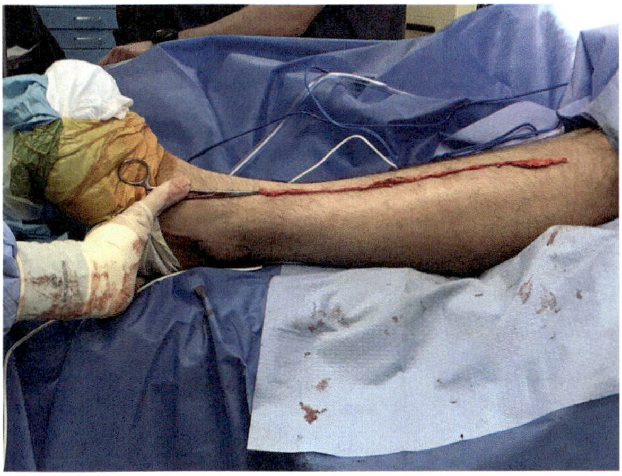

**Fig. 20.10** Harvested sural nerve with hemostat identifying the distal end

## Cross-Face Nerve Grafting

1. Isolate the primary branch to the zygomaticus major on the non-paralyzed side (Fig. 20.11), according to the instructions in Chap. 17, section on "Buccal Branch Identification".
2. Make a stab incision in the superior gingivolabial sulcus, superior to the canine, and advance a Wright fascia passer needle through it and into the wound on the non-paralyzed side of the face, then suture the proximal end of the sural nerve graft to the tip of the needle and retract the end of the nerve out through the stab wound (Fig. 20.12).

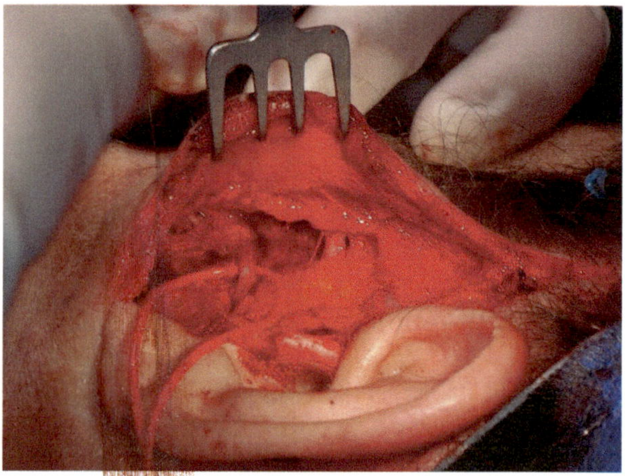

**Fig. 20.11** Buccal branch isolation

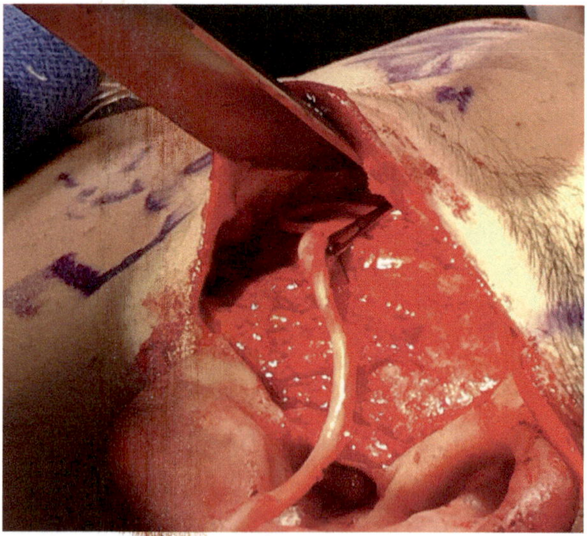

**Fig. 20.12** Passing the sural nerve across the face

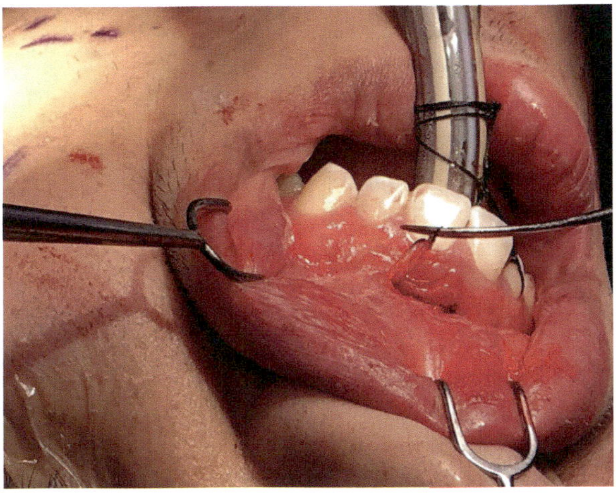

**Fig. 20.13** Passing the sural nerve through the gingiva

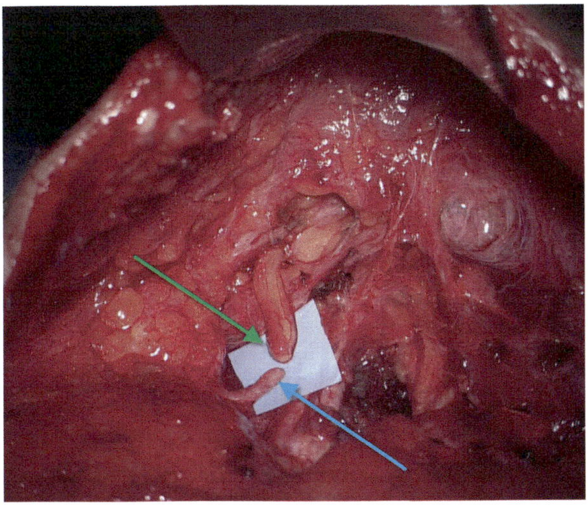

**Fig. 20.14** Completion of sural nerve transfer to the contralateral face. *The distal end of the sural nerve graft (green arrow) is left near the proximal end of the primary buccal branch (blue arrow) on the non-paralyzed side in preparation for neurorrhaphy*

3. Repeat the process with a stab incision over the contralateral canine and retract the proximal end of the nerve graft into it (Fig. 20.13).
4. Repeat once more, passing the Wright needle from the wound on the paralyzed side into the gingivolabial sulcus stab incision and retracting the proximal end of the nerve graft into the wound (Fig. 20.14).

## Sterno-omohyoid Muscle Flap Harvest

1. Retract the sternocleidomastoid muscle laterally to expose the internal jugular vein, then skeletonize the internal jugular vein in order to expose the ansa cervicalis (Fig. 20.15), whose apex should lie deep to the omohyoid. Skeletonize as

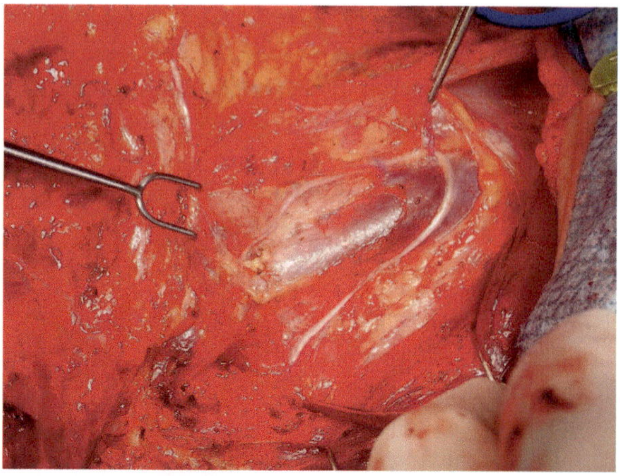

**Fig. 20.15** Ansa cervicalis relationship to internal jugular vein

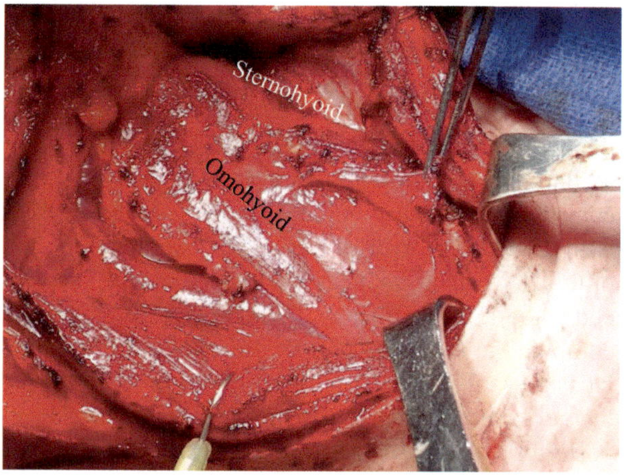


**Fig. 20.16** Sternohyoid and Omohyoid identification in the neck

much of the ansa cervicalis as possible, following the anterior limb to the hypoglossal nerve and the posterior limb to the cervical rootlets. Identify the inferior branches off the apex of the ansa to the omohyoid and sternohyoid; after stimulation, divide the remaining branches off the ansa to permit mobilization.

2. Divide the omohyoid inferiorly, roughly 2 cm beyond the inferior ansa branches, through the tendon as it joins the lateral belly of the muscle. Follow the superficial surface of the omohyoid to reach the sternohyoid, then divide that at the level of the clavicle (Fig. 20.16). Follow the medial border of the sternohyoid superiorly to the hyoid bone. If available, include an anterior jugular vein in the flap for outflow. Separate the superior ends of the sternohyoid and omohyoid muscles from the hyoid bone.
3. Divide the ansa cervicalis as superiorly as possible and mobilize it completely, taking care to avoid injury to any veins or branches of the superior thyroid artery. Elevate the sterno-omohyoid flap along the superficial surface of the deep strap muscles in order to maintain the blood supply within the fascia. Identify and

preserve the superior laryngeal nerve. Divide the branches of the superior thyroid artery and vein that supply the thyroid gland and the larynx. Dissect the superior thyroid artery medially toward the flap, taking care to keep its vena comitans intact. Include the superior thyroid artery vena comitans or superior thyroid vein in the harvest; include any associated ranine veins as well. Ligate the superior thyroid artery as it emerges from the external carotid artery to complete flap harvest (Fig. 20.17).

## Sterno-omohyoid Muscle Flap Inset

1. Run a locked 2-0 braided, absorbable suture along the cut edges of the sternohyoid muscle. These sutures will constitute "neo-tendons" to help retain the inset sutures and prevent them from pulling through the muscle once tension is applied. Pass the two upper lip inset sutures through the tendon at the inferior edge of the omohyoid muscle and the three oral commissure inset sutures through the inferior cut edge of the sternohyoid muscle, behind the neo-tendon, tying the knots on the deep surfaces of the muscles (Fig. 20.18).

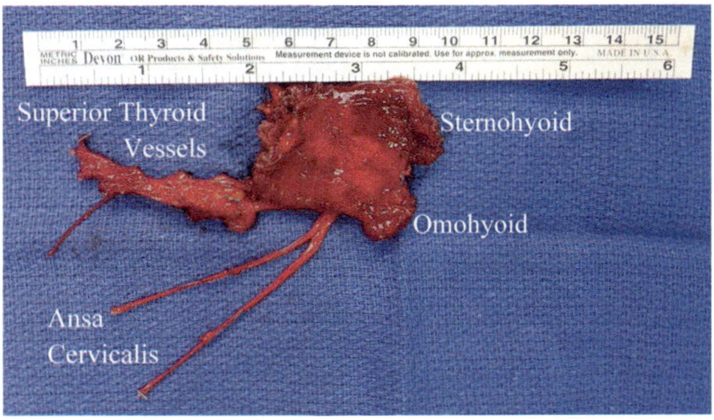


**Fig. 20.17** Harvested sterno-omohyoid flap

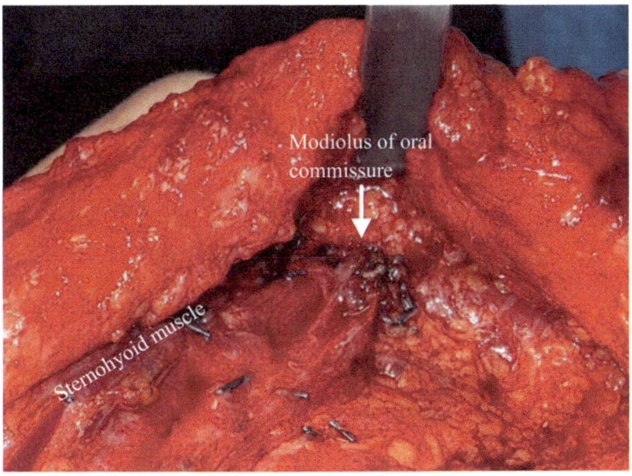


**Fig. 20.18** Flap neo-tendon placement in the face with the modiolus

2. Perform the microvascular anastomosis between the superior thyroid artery and the facial artery, ideally. Observe venous outflow from the flap and select the most appropriate vein for anastomosis to the facial vein. Consider coupling a second outflow vein from the flap to the external jugular vein as well (Fig. 20.19). Implantable Doppler probes may be useful for flap monitoring in the immediate postoperative period.
3. Trim the cut ends of the ansa cervicalis and the masseteric nerve, then perform the microsurgical neurorrhaphy (Fig. 20.20). Coapt the nerves in an end-to-end fashion using fine suture, such as 10-0 nylon, on a cutting needle. Only two or three interrupted stitches are usually required at each site. Avoid overtightening and impacting or herniating the fascicles through the neurorrhaphy. If a cross-face nerve graft is included, trim the sural nerve ends and the buccal branch, and then perform the second and third neurorrhaphies. If no cross-face graft is planned, both ends of the ansa cervicalis should be coapted to the masseteric nerve, and this may be facilitated with a collagen nerve wrap.
4. Fold the omohyoid to bury the upper 40%, nearest the orbit, underneath the rest of the muscle in order to shorten it and improve contractility. Pass two 2-0 braided,

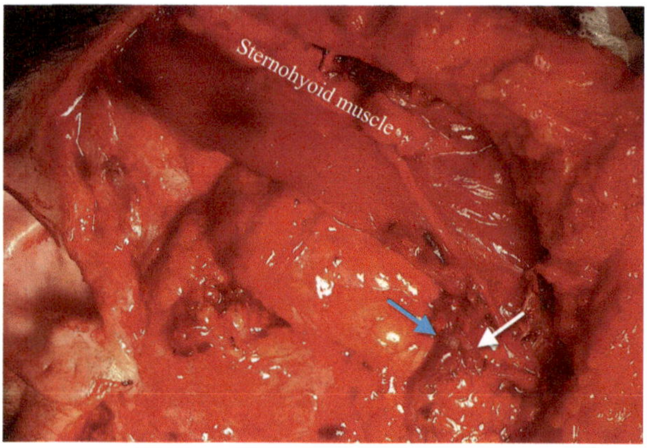


**Fig. 20.19** Microvascular anastomosis in the face. The blue arrow indicates the venous anastomosis, performed with a coupler, and the white arrow indicates the arterial anastomosis, which was sutured with 9-0 nylon

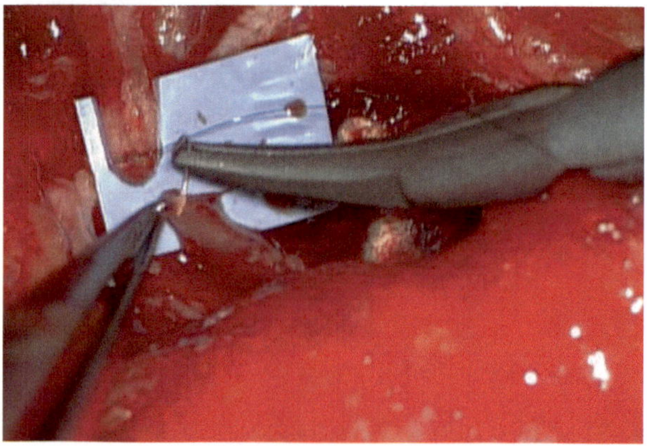

**Fig. 20.20** Neurorrhaphy in the face

absorbable sutures through the fold and secure them to the infraorbital miniplate, then screw down the plate completely. Stretch the sternohyoid muscle and using 2-0 nonabsorbable sutures, tack the free end of the sternohyoid muscle to the temporalis fascia in a vector directed just superior to the apex of the helix (Fig. 20.21).
5. Optionally, place any additional static suspension slings at this juncture, taking care not to overtighten them and risk compromising perfusion to the flap (Fig. 20.22). Fascia lata ribbons should be located superficial to the sterno-omohyoid flap in order to prevent dermal tethering and provide a glide plane for muscle contraction.
6. Close the incisions in layers. The facial wound on the non-paralyzed side should not require a drain if hemostasis is adequate and there is no parotid gland injury, but the wound on the paralyzed side will require one or two suction drains, as a pressure dressing should not be applied over fresh microvascular anastomoses. Figure 20.23 depicts the final flap position beneath the superficial structures of the face.

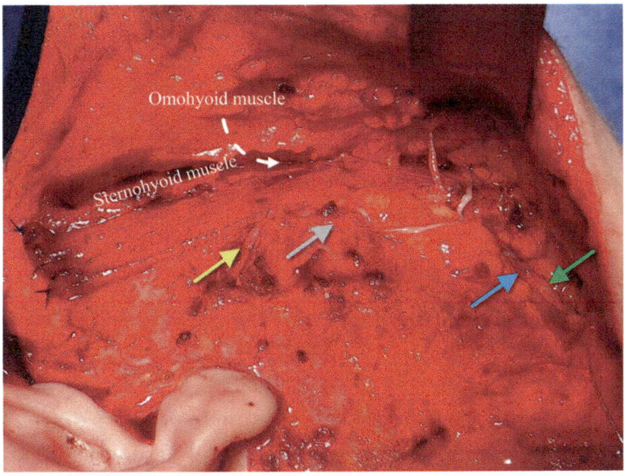


**Fig. 20.21** The sternohyoid muscle has been inset; the omohyoid muscle is buried beneath the skin flap, situated medially in the face and inferior to the orbit. The masseteric nerve is indicated by the yellow arrow, the cross-face nerve graft by the gray arrow, the venous outflow by the blue arrow, and the arterial inflow by the green arrow

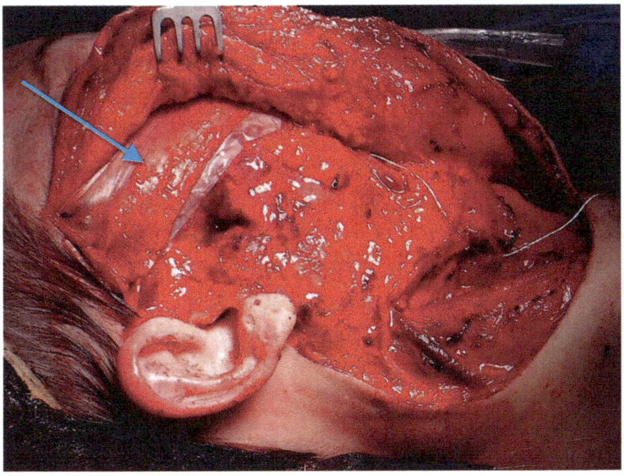

**Fig. 20.22** A band of fascia lata (blue arrow) was placed to suspend the nasolabial fold

**Fig. 20.23** Final Flap position beneath the face

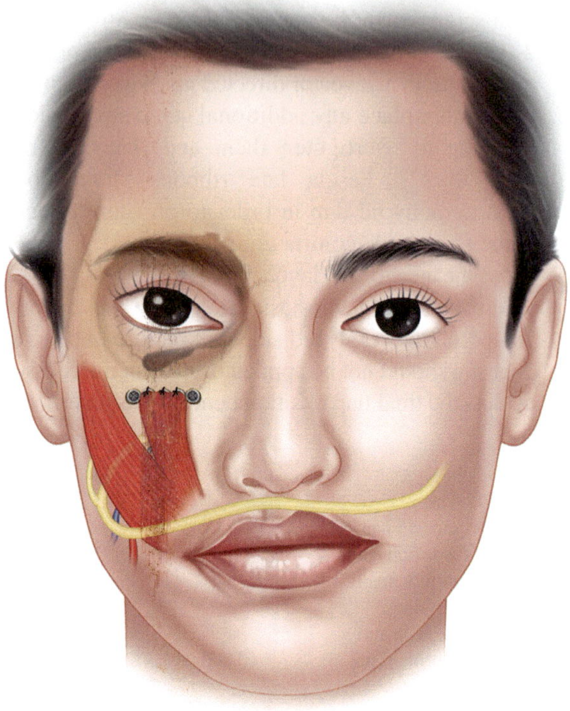

## Pearls

- Insist on the use of no long-acting paralytics during intubation for patients undergoing sterno-omohyoid functional free muscle transfer, or indeed any facial nerve procedure. Loss of stimulability of trigeminal and facial nerve branches during these cases increases the risk of iatrogenic injury.
- Avoid local anesthetic use in this procedure. The rate of metabolism of these agents varies tremendously among patients, and stimulability of the relevant nerve branches may be lost for hours following injection.
- Sacrifice of the primary motor branch to the zygomaticus major on the non-paralyzed side for cross-face nerve grafting does not typically result in any noticeable change in the appearance of the smile; if it were to weaken the smile subtly, however, it would serve to improve overall facial symmetry.
- Cross-face nerve grafting may be employed as an alternative to nerve transfer, but due to the low axon count (300–900 fibers), is better used for zonal facial reinnervation than hemifacial reinnervation, and outcomes are superior in younger patients due to their higher axon counts.

- Reversing the direction of the sural nerve graft, as described above, helps to reduce axonal loss by preventing axonal growth out of the graft via microbranches.
- When harvesting the flap, remember that the branches that control the sternohyoid and omohyoid come off the very bottom of the ansa cervicalis, so extreme care should be taken when dissecting in this area in order to avoid denervating the flap.
- Include two or three veins in the flap if possible; the best outflow can be selected after arterial anastomosis is complete by determining which vein bleeds most briskly.
- The flap inset described is the ideal situation; however, vascular considerations may necessitate adjustment of the surgical plan. Short vascular pedicles or the use of the superficial temporal artery may mandate reorientation of the flap. It does not matter which muscle is used for which vector.
- Because the flap is buried, monitoring will be performed using palpation and Doppler signals. The face and flap will swell over the first several days, but the flap should remain supple if it is viable. Duplex ultrasonography may be performed on postoperative day 1 to confirm flap perfusion and outflow.

## References

1. Lindsay RW, Bhama P, Weinberg J, Hadlock TA. The success of free gracilis muscle transfer to restore smile in patients with nonflaccid facial paralysis. Ann Plast Surg. 2014;73(2):177–82.
2. Harii K, Ohmori K, Torii S. Free gracilis transplantation with microneurovascular anastomoses for the treatment of facial paralysis. A preliminary report. Plast Reconstr Surg. 1976;57(2):133–43.
3. Alam DS. The sternohyoid flap for facial reanimation. Facial Plast Surg Clin North Am. 2016;23(1):61–9.
4. Vincent AG, Bevans SE, Robitschek JM, Groom KL, Herr MW, Hohman MH. Sterno-omohyoid free flap for dual-vector facial reanimation. Ann Otol Rhinol Laryngol. 2020;129(2):195–200.
5. Boahene KO, Owusu J, Ishii L, Ishii M, Desai S, Kim I, Kim L, Byrne P. The multivector gracilis free functional muscle flap for facial reanimation. JAMA Facial Plast Surg. 2018;20(4):300–6.
6. Ein L, Hadlock TA, Jowett N. Dual-vector gracilis muscle transfer for smile reanimation with lower lip depression. Laryngoscope. 2021;131(8):1758–60.
7. Sakuma H, Tanaka I, Yazawa M, Shimizu Y. Multivector functioning muscle transfer using superficial subslips of the serratus anterior muscle for longstanding facial paralysis. J Plast Reconstr Aesthet Surg. 2019;72(6):964–72.
8. Dusseldorp JR, van Veen MM, Guarin DL, Quatela O, Jowett N, Hadlock TA. Spontaneity assessment in dually innervated gracilis smile reanimation surgery. JAMA Facial Plast Surg. 2019;21(6):551–7.

# Part VI

# Reconstruction of Congenital Defects

# Unilateral Cleft Lip Repair

# 21

Arya Namin and Ryan F. Brown

## Introduction

Cleft lip deformity is due to failure of the fusion of the paired medial nasal prominences and paired maxillary prominences during the sixth and seventh weeks of embryonic development to form the upper lip [1]. Routine use of prenatal ultrasonography has led to antepartum diagnosis, which can be made as early as 18 weeks gestation [2]. Cleft lip has a male predominance, with a 2:1 ratio [1]. Cleft lip afflicts Asians and Native Americans most commonly (1 in 500 births), while it afflicts Africans (1 in 2500 births) least commonly [1]. Cleft lip deformity has been described since ancient times, and unfortunately, these individuals were treated poorly due to a lack of understanding of embryology and superstitions of the times [3]. In the sixteenth century, an embryologic etiology of the cleft was suggested, and our understanding of this deformity has continued to evolve since that time [3]. One of the first documented cleft lip repairs was undertaken in China around 400 A.D. when a physician stitched the edges of the defect together and required strict dietary restrictions and voice rest for 100 days postoperatively [4]. Efforts at repairing cleft lips were again reported beginning in the fifteenth and sixteenth centuries, which were largely described as sacrificing the margins of the cleft and suturing them together [3]. This typically resulted in a vertical scar and shortening of the lip [3]. This technique prevailed until the mid-nineteenth century when various techniques utilizing flaps were described to improve the outcomes of cleft lip surgery [5].

A. Namin
Department of Otolaryngology and Facial Plastic Surgery Associates, Fort Worth, TX, USA

R. F. Brown (✉)
Department of Head and Neck Surgery/Facial Plastic Surgery, The Permanente Medical Group, Santa Rosa, CA, USA
e-mail: Ryan.f.brown@kp.org



F. Sokoya, A. G. Vincent (eds.), *Manual of Head and Neck Reconstruction*,
https://doi.org/10.1007/978-3-031-65999-7_21

In the 1940s and 1950s, various techniques utilizing lateral tissue flaps were described and gained popularity [6–8]. The introduction of the rotation-advancement repair of the cleft lip deformity by Dr. Millard in 1955 offered a new technique that preserved the three-fourths of a normal Cupid's bow, one philtral column, and the philtral dimple on the medial side of the cleft [9]. Dr. Millard's technique has been modified by himself and many other surgeons since its original description and is the most popular method of repair today [9]. Mohler described his modification of the rotation-advancement flap in which he placed the back cut into the columellar base with the goal of creating a mirror image of the philtral column on the noncleft side [10]. Similar to Mohler's objective in preserving the philtral column of the noncleft side, the anatomic subunit approximation technique also sought to preserve the non-cleft phitral column and reconstruct a mirror image of this anatomy [11].

## Anatomy

Lip development occurs during 4–8 weeks of embryonic development [1]. Cleft lip deformity is due to failure of the fusion of the paired medial nasal prominences and paired maxillary prominences during the sixth and seventh weeks of embryonic development to form the upper lip [1]. The primary palate forms from the fusion of the paired medial nasal processes by 6 weeks gestation, giving rise to the premaxilla [1]. Unilateral cleft lip presents with a wide spectrum of severity ranging from complete to more subtle incomplete clefts. Incomplete cleft lips have cutaneous continuity between the medial and lateral lip segments. These lesser-form cleft lips have been subdivided into three subgroups: minor-form cleft extends 3 mm or more above the normal Cupid's bow peak, microform cleft is characterized by a notched vermilion junction with Cupid's bow peak elevated less than 3 mm above the normal side, and mini-microform cleft is characterized by a discontinuous vermilion without elevation of the Cupid's bow peak and a hypoplastic mucosal free margin [12]. Bilateral cleft lip similarly presents with a spectrum of severity, with the complete bilateral cleft lip representing about 54% of these cases [12]. Patients with symmetrical incomplete cleft lip account for 22% of cases, and patients with asymmetrical cleft lip account for 23% of cases [12]. In bilateral complete cleft lip, the premaxilla grows independently of the maxilla on either side and subsequently may protrude considerably [1]. The columella is considerably shorter, the nasal tip is broad and flat, and the alar bases are overly wide [13]. The protrusive premaxilla necessitates preoperative dentofacial orthopedics to allow for optimal results in a single-staged repair [13].

In unilateral cleft lip, the premaxilla is outwardly rotated and projecting, while the lateral maxillary segment is retropositioned and medially displaced [14]. The nose has characteristic deformities in unilateral cleft lip. The caudal septum and nasal spine are displaced into the noncleft nostril, and there is unilateral shortness of the columella [14]. The lateral crura of the lower lateral cartilage is flattened, the alar base is displaced laterally, inferiorly, and posteriorly, and the vestibular lining is deficient [14]. The orbicularis oris muscle in the lateral lip inserts into the alar wing, and the muscle in the medial lip between the midline and the cleft is hypoplastic [14]. The curves of the normal upper lip have been likened to the shape of Cupid's bow throughout history [15]. In the normal lip, the cutaneous vermillion junction, or white roll, appears to be histologically related to the pars marginalis of the orbicularis oris [15]. The philtral columns are histologically related to decussating orbicularis oris muscle fibers with musculocutaneous insertions [15]. In patients with cleft lip, the pars marginalis of the orbicularis oris is underdeveloped; therefore, the white roll is not present around the cleft [15].

## Indications

Treatment of cleft lip requires surgical repair. This typically involves a multidisciplinary team and can involve a course in presurgical orthopedics. The timing of surgical repair and the decision of whether to address the nasal deformity at the time of cleft lip repair is something that is debatable and influenced by surgeon preference and case-specific variables [1, 16–18]. In regards to the timing of repair, the rule of 10s has been proposed [19]. This requires the patient to weigh 10 pounds, have a hemoglobin of 10 mg/ dL, a white blood cell count of less than 10,000/$m^3$, and an age of 10 weeks [1, 19]. Worldwide, it has been found that 66% of surgeons repair cleft lip when the patient is 3–6 months of age, while 33% of surgeons repair the cleft lip when the patient is less than one month old [16]. The advantages of waiting until 3–6 months of age include allowing for a course of presurgical orthopedics and also to allow for additional growth. While some argue that anesthetic risks are decreased, others argue that the anesthetic risk is not different between a 3-month-old child and a healthy full-term newborn [1, 16, 20]. Multiple groups have reported good aesthetic outcomes with cleft lip repair during the first month of life in healthy full-term babies and have argued for the benefits of improved feeding and improved psychological effects for the family [16, 20].

During the first part of the twentieth century, repair of the cleft lip nasal deformity was delayed for fear of disturbing growth. However, over the past several decades, the safety and efficacy of primary rhinoplasty during the cheiloplasty have been well reported on [18, 21, 22]. With the advent of nasoalveolar molding and postoperative nasal stenting, long-term aesthetic results have improved beyond what primary rhinoplasty alone could achieve. In a retrospective study examining nostril height and width ratios at 5 years of age after primary rhinoplasty, nasoalveolar molding, or nasoalveolar molding and primary rhinoplasty, it was found that patients who underwent both nasoalveolar molding and primary rhinoplasty with overcorrection of nostril height had improved outcomes [23]. Managing the bilateral cleft nasal deformity is particularly challenging, and the utility of presurgical orthopedics in these patients has been described as well [17, 24].

## Preoperative Planning

Patients with cleft lips should be under the care of a multidisciplinary team, including a pediatrician, dietician, feeding/speech specialist, orthodontist, and social worker. Weight gain should be carefully monitored in the preoperative period. Patients with syndromes or comorbidities should be under the care of appropriate pediatric specialists.

Efforts to minimize the cleft lip deformity preoperatively with the goals of improving the ease of repair and hopefully long-term outcomes have long been attempted [25–28]. It was noted that the cleft lip nasal deformity was largely due to deformity of the lower lateral cartilage and nasal base and that auricular deformities could be successfully managed in a nonoperative fashion in neonates [28]. Subsequently, nasal molding was undertaken to partially correct the nasal deformity prior to definitive repair. Lip taping and adhesion were also described in attempts to narrow wide clefts [25, 26]. While lip adhesion did narrow the cleft width, the disadvantages of lip adhesion being a separate general anesthetic and the potential for scarring that would potentially impair or limit definitive repair have led this technique to be utilized less frequently during the current era [25]. Lip taping did not require an anesthetic but did not have an effect on the nasal form or alveolar deformity. Lip taping is commonly utilized with nasoalveolar molding. The objectives to improve the nasal, lip, and alveolar deformity prior to definitive repair eventually led to the description and more widespread use of nasoalveolar molding.

An important consideration in preoperative planning is presurgical orthopedics and, more specifically, nasoalveolar molding, which was introduced by Grayson in the late 1990s [27, 29]. It was found that molding techniques could improve the nasal deformity in cleft lip prior to repair and, therefore likely improve the long-term outcome [28]. In nasoalveolar molding, an orthodontic device is made to mold to the alveolar segments that narrow the gap and also have a nasal component that extends from the alveolar device on a wire to mold the shape of the lower lateral cartilage and nasal base [29–31]. The Grayson and Figueroa techniques are the two most commonly utilized techniques in nasoalveolar molding, and a study comparing the outcomes of these techniques found no significant differences in the long-term postsurgical outcomes [29]. The vast majority of studies support that nasoalveolar molding improves the outcomes of cleft lip repair and that better outcomes can be achieved in more severe deformities [27, 30, 31]. The nasolabial deformity in the bilateral complete cleft lip is particularly challenging to address, and patients who have undergone preoperative nasoalveolar molding were found to have significantly improved columellar length and require significantly less secondary nasal surgery [32].

## Instruments/Equipment

- Bipolar electrocautery
- Skin hooks

- Forceps (Adson, 0.5 mm, Bishop-Harmon, etc.)
- Fine-tipped dissecting scissors (tenotomy, converse, curved iris, etc.)
- Frazier tip suction
- Caliper
- Needle driver
- Elevator (Cottle, Freer)
- Dissolvable sutures

## Surgical Technique

### Marking

The surgical procedure begins with the marking of the anatomical landmarks with a Caliper. Methylene Blue can be used, but the authors like to use a 25- or 27-gauge needle and stab the tip of the needle into the tip of a blue marking pen. This tends to run less than Methylene Blue. The needle can then be used to mark the lip landmarks and tattoo the dermis. If the tip of the needle penetrates the dermis of the skin, then the surgical prep will not remove the markings.

The markings (see Fig. 21.1) that are made include:

1. The depth of cupid's bow (1).
2. The height of cupid's bow on the noncleft side (2).
3. Then, use the distance between the depth of the cupid's bow on the non-cleft side and then mark the same distance from the cupid's bow on the cleft side (3).
4. Measure the height of the philtral column on the noncleft side (4 to 2). Then measure the philtral column on the cleft side (5 to 3).** The difference between these two philtral columns will be the length/width of the C-flap.
5. Mark 1 mm up on the columella, 3/5th of the way on the columella away from the cleft. (The cutting line will be from 3 to 6).
6. Mark the back cut from the point marked on the columella at a 90-degree angle (point 7). The length of the back cut will be the length of the C-flap measured in step #4. (If there is a large asymmetry and a long C-flap is needed, the back cut should not cross the philtral column, but once the philtral column is reached, the cut should follow the philtral column inferiorly.)
7. Take the measurement from the noncleft side philtral column (4 to 2), and with the caliper, find a point medial to the alar base and vermillion on the cleft side and mark that and the point on the cleft-side vermillion that equals that measurement (8 to 9).
8. Measure the visible lip where the cut through the red lip will happen on the cleft and noncleft sides and try to have them match.
9. The flaps in the surgery can be marked. The authors prefer to use the above points and make dots, as they find it less messy and does not smear as much. But flaps can be drawn out once the above points have been marked. The C-flap will be skin only and is lateral to the 3–6 philtral column cut and does not include lip

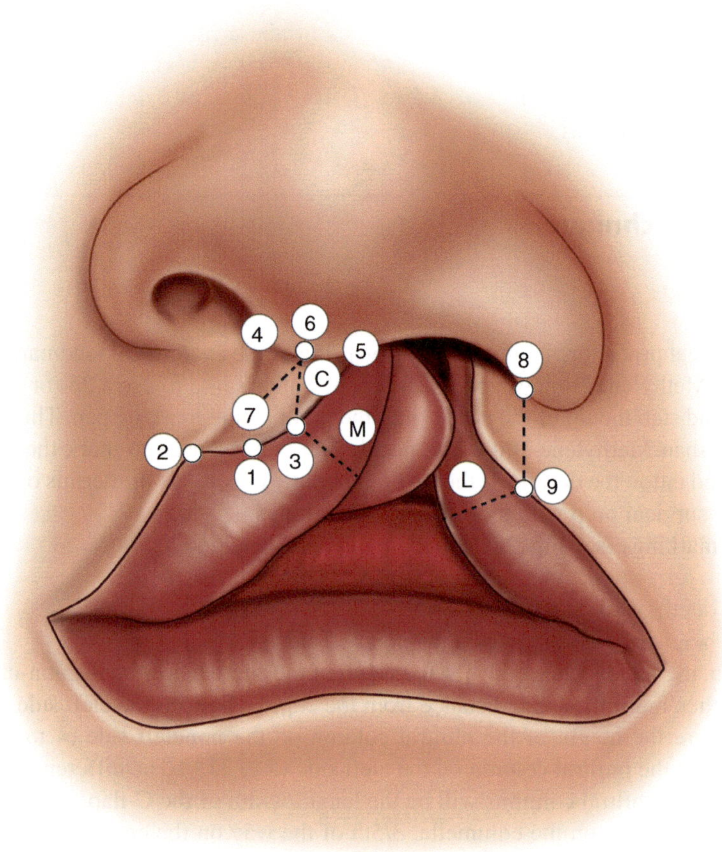


**Fig. 21.1** Markings for unilateral cleft lip repair

mucosa. It should be based just posterior to the cleft-side medial crura in the nose. The M-flap is the lip mucosa and vermillion just inferior to the C-flap skin on the noncleft side. It is a superiorly based flap. The M-flap (medial flap) can be used to help repair the nasal floor in a wide cleft. But it is best to save all tissue until you are sure that it is not needed. The L-flap (lateral flap) is the lip vermillion and mucosa just medial to the planned philtral column cut on the cleft side (8 to 9). It is a superiorly based flap and is always used to add tissue underneath the nostril rim, so that the ala can be curved on the cleft side. It can also be used to repair a nasal floor defect.

The lip is then injected with local anesthetic with epinephrine to decrease bleeding. The authors like to use a mixture of 1% lidocaine with 1:100,000 epinephrine and 0.25% plain Marcaine. The face is then prepped, and the patient is draped in the usual sterile fashion (See Fig. 21.2).

## Surgical Steps/Incisions

1. Incise from the height of Cupid's bow on the cleft side to the point marked on the columella and then cut the measured length of the back cut (3 to 6). The authors like to use an 11 blade to be able to make nice straight cuts along the planned incision lines.
2. Cut along the vermillion lateral from the 3 to 6 cut (do not include any) and raise the C-flap. Keep the C-flap thick so that it is well-vascularized. Extend the elevation of the flap to just posterior to the footplate of the medial crura in the cleft-side nostril.
3. Raise the M-flap. If it is a complete cleft lip, then the M flap can be continued posteriorly into the nose and onto the septum. This can be used to close a wide nasal floor defect. Elevation of the septal flap is best done with a caudal or freer elevator and should be elevated right on top of the cartilage.
4. Make the cut along the cleft-side that was marked 8 to 9. Once you reach the vermillion it is possible to save a V shape of extra vermillion that can be used to plump up the central lip.

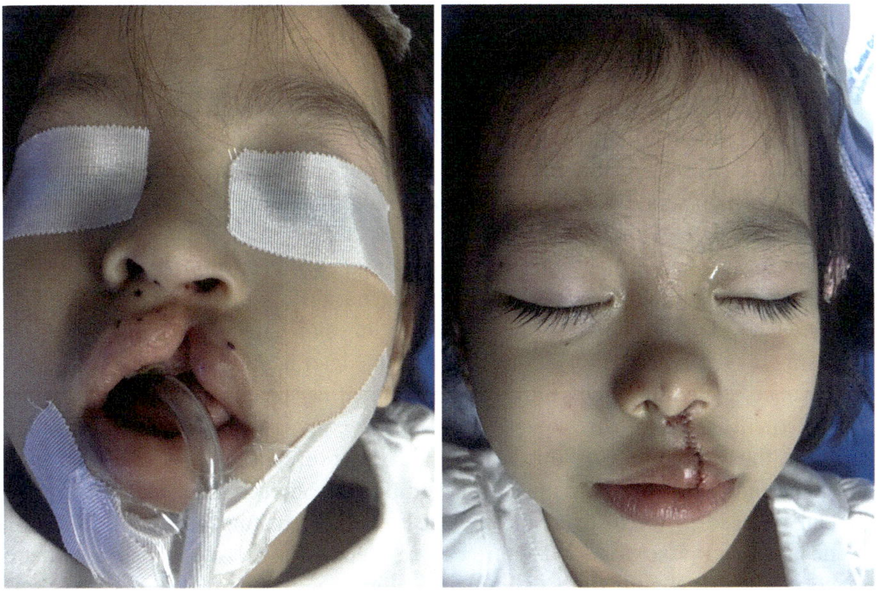

**Fig. 21.2** Pre-op markings and post-op result

5. Cut along the upper gingival buccal sulcus of the cleft side. Then, elevate the soft tissue that overlies the maxilla. The width of the cleft will determine how aggressive you need to be in this elevation. It is best to put a finger on the eye because the distance is not far in infants. Care should be taken to not damage the infraorbital nerve. The authors prefer a supraperiosteal dissection.
6. Raise the L-flap. This is a mucosal flap. The superior cut of the flap will be cut right up to the superior lateral edge of the head of the inferior turbinate and the flap is based on the inferior turbinate. This cut should extend down to the piriform aperture and the soft tissue can be freed-up supraperiostally off of the maxilla and join the elevation that occurred through the upper gingival buccal sulcus incision. This should free up the cleft side lip so that it can be advanced without tension (See Fig. 21.3).
7. Using fine-tipped scissors (curved iris or converse), insert them between the medial crura and separate them. Then turn the scissors and come up over the domes and over the lower lateral cartilages. Separate the overlying skin from the cartilage. This will allow you to reposition the lower lateral cartilages more symmetrically. The cleft-side lower lateral cartilage, which is long and flattened, can finish being separated from the overlying skin by dissecting from the piriform and upper gingival-buccal sulcus cuts. A completely dissected tunnel should exist along the cleft side lower lateral cartilage and ala to break up abnormal attachments and allow it to be repositioned. All muscle attachments to the alar base on the cleft side should be removed.
8. Dissect free orbicular oris muscle pendants on both sides of the lip, but do not dissect past the philtral columns.

## Closing/Suturing

1. Inset the L-flap into the piriform aperture incision. This will provide extra tissue to be able to curve the ala. If the nasal floor has a defect, the L-flap can be inset into the piriform aperture incision but also bent over at its midpoint and attached to the M-flap/septal flap on the non-cleft side. If present, the nasal floor defect should be fixed with a combination of the M-flap/septal flap and L-flap, and any extra tissue should then be trimmed. Chromic or Vicryl suture can be used for this step. It is an important step to fill in the nasal floor defect, as it an area hard to reach in later cleft palate repair, and can leave an anterior fistula.
2. Using a 3-0 or 4-0 Vicryl suture, grab the lateral gingiva-buccal tissue and advance it medially and secure to the gingival periosteum. This will help take tension off of the repair.
3. Close the orbicularis oris muscle together. Make sure that you rotate and advance the lip and see where the muscle should line up on each side. Mattress sutures can be used to try to evert the muscle to aid in creating a philtral column if desired. Vicryl or Monocryl suture can be used. If the muscle is reapproximated correctly, this should almost completely align the cleft side ala.
4. Place a deep layer of dissolvable suture such as Vicryl or Monocryl.

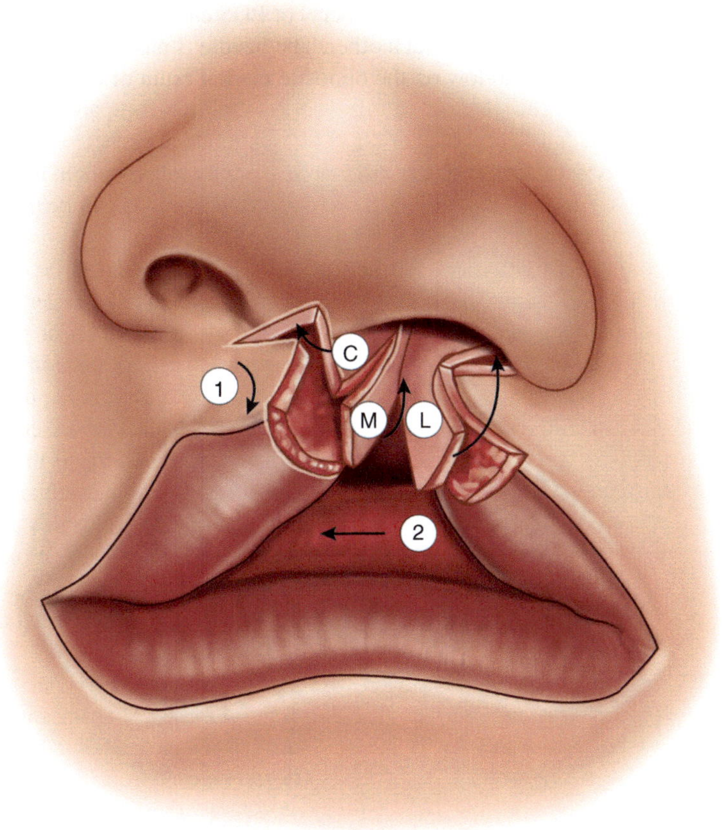


**Fig. 21.3** Appearance of lip after making initial surgical incisions. (1) Non-cleft side of lip will rotate down. (2) Cleft side of lip will advance forward. This is why it is called a rotation advancement procedure. Note that the rectangular defect at the base of columella will be filled by the "C flap". The "M flap" and the "L flap" will be used to close the nasal floor defect

5. Now inset the C-flap. With the noncleft side being rotated down, the 90-degree back cut should open to create a rectangular defect. The C-flap is inset in this defect, and the extra tip of the C-flap is trimmed.
6. Close the skin. Skin sutures should not provide any strength to the closure; there should be no tension on the closure from the deep sutures. The skin sutures are to align the skin and ensure that the skin on both sides of the repair is at the same level. Either permanent sutures or dissolvable fast-gut sutures can be used.

Permanent sutures will likely require another brief anesthetic to remove (see Figs. 21.4, 21.5, and 21.6).

A dissolvable suture such as a 4-0 Monocryl or PDS can be used to straighten the medial crura and reattach them to each other. The needle is passed from high on the noncleft side medial crura to low on the opposite medial crura of the cleft side, and

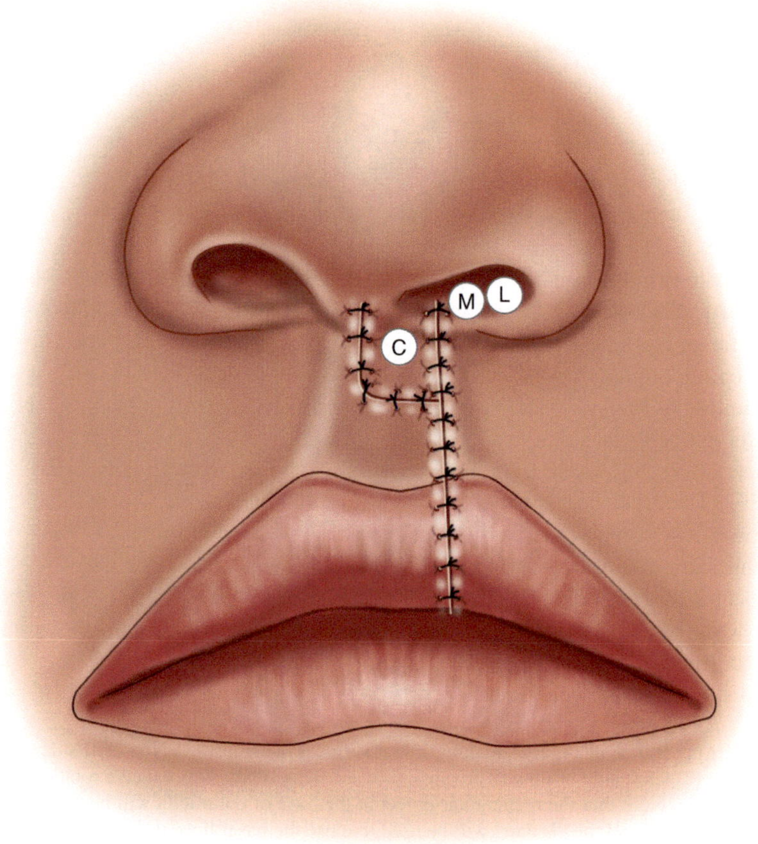


**Fig. 21.4** Appearance at the end of suturing. Note that the "C flap" has filled in the columellar defect. This hides the incisions within the base of the columella and avoids the non-anatomic curving incision of the traditional Millard repair. Note that no incisions have been made along the nasal ala on the cleft side which can create visible scars. The "M flap" and "L flap" are not seen from the outside, but are reconstructing the anterior nasal floor which will prevent an anterior fistula during the cleft palate repair which can be very hard to repair

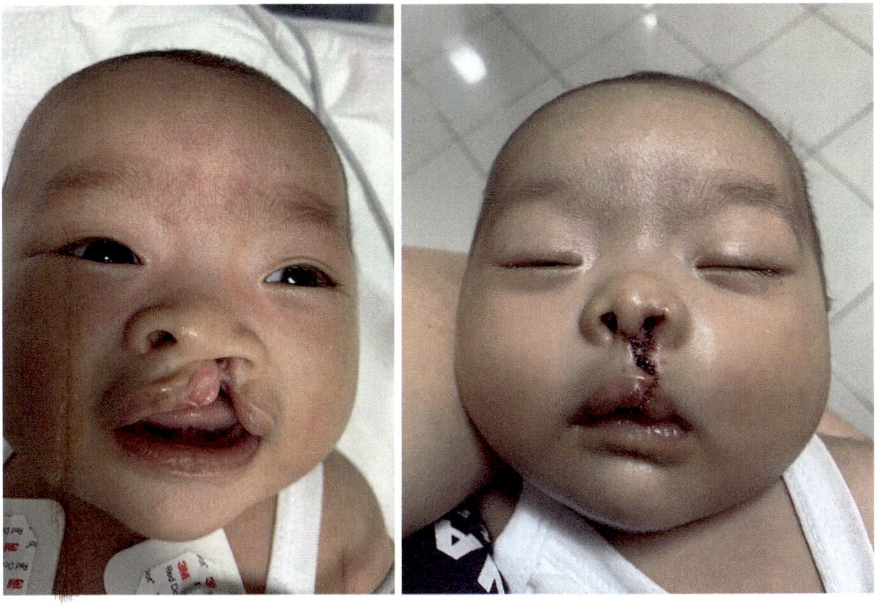

**Fig. 21.5** Pre and post-op photos for left-sided unilateral cleft lip

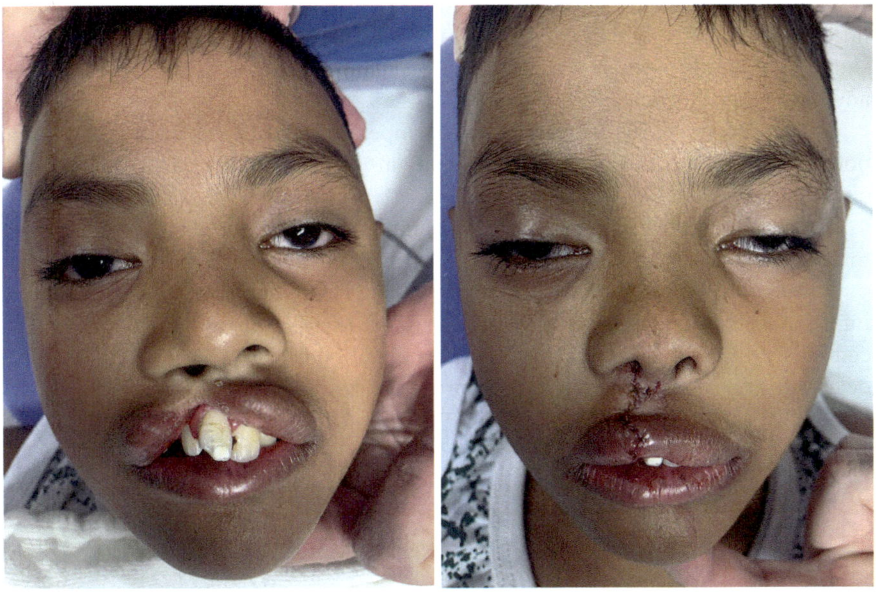

**Fig. 21.6** Pre and post-op photos for right-sided unilateral cleft lip

then back high on the cleft side and out high on the noncleft side and tied. If the cleft-side ala needs to be elevated at the end of the procedure, then dome elevation sutures can be placed. A Monocryl or PDS suture on a long, curved needle can then be passed from underneath the lower lateral cartilage on the non-cleft side, up over the tip, through the cleft-side lower lateral cartilage and into the cleft-side nostril. Then go back in from underneath the cleft-side lower lateral cartilage, over the domes, back through the upper cleft-side lower lateral cartilage and into the non-cleft side nostril. Tie this suture, and it will help elevate the flattened ala. This can be repeated as needed. The angle of turning the needle blindly over the tip is difficult but worth learning to improve the symmetry of the nostrils.

## Postoperative Management

Postoperative care includes routine incisional care of gently cleaning the incisions with saline every 2–6 hours, and then antibiotic ointment is applied to keep the incisions moist. It is important to show the parents how to clean the incision gently to avoid damaging the repair. Feeding begins when the baby desires. If an infant, then they can breastfeed, use a syringe or a soft-tipped bottle. Only breast milk or formula should be given. Pacifiers should not be used. If an older child, then very soft or pureed food should be given. Forks, straws, and other utensils should be avoided.

Parents should strongly be encouraged to use arm splints/restraints for 2–3 weeks in younger patients so that they cannot reach the lip repair and damage it. Infants should be placed to sleep on their backs to avoid the incision being rubbed against anything while sleeping.

Infants are typically discharged on postoperative day 1. Older children could potentially be performed as an outpatient depending on their health and circumstances.

Three to four weeks after surgery, Vitamin E oil or other products could be used to help improve scarring.

Postoperative nasal molding can be employed for up to 1 year postoperatively to improve the form of the lower lateral cartilage. Long-term follow-up into adolescence is important to assess aesthetic and functional results and identify patient desires for revisional procedures to improve the aesthetic outcome.

## References


1. Shkoukani MA, Chen M, Vong A. Cleft lip—a comprehensive review. Front Pediatr. 2013;1:53.
2. Jones MC. Prenatal diagnosis of cleft lip and palate: detection rates, accuracy of ultrasonography, associated anomalies, and strategies for counseling. Cleft Palate Craniofac J. 2002;39(2):169–73.
3. Bhattacharya S, Khanna V, Kohli R. Cleft lip: the historical perspective. Indian J Plast Surg. 2009;42(Suppl):S4–8.
4. Boo-Chai K. An ancient Chinese text on a cleft lip. Plast Reconstr Surg. 1966;38(2):89–91.
5. Perko M. The history of treatment of cleft lip and palate. Prog Pediatr Surg. 1986;20:238–51.

6. LeMESURIER AB. A method of cutting and suturing the lip in the treatment of complete unilateral clefts. Plast Reconstr Surg (1946). 1949;4(1):1–12.
7. Randall P. A triangular flap operation for the primary repair of unilateral clefts of the lip. Plast Reconstr Surg Transplant Bull. 1959;23(4):331–47.
8. Tennison CW. The repair of the unilateral cleft lip by the stencil method. Plast Reconstr Surg (1946). 1952;9(2):115–20.
9. Stal S, Brown RH, Higuera S, Hollier LH, Byrd HS, Cutting CB, et al. Fifty years of the Millard rotation-advancement: looking back and moving forward. Plast Reconstr Surg. 2009;123(4):1364–77.
10. Mohler LR. Unilateral cleft lip repair. Plast Reconstr Surg. 1987;80(4):511–7.
11. Fisher DM. Unilateral cleft lip repair: an anatomical subunit approximation technique. Plast Reconstr Surg. 2005;116(1):61–71.
12. Yuzuriha S, Oh AK, Mulliken JB. Asymmetrical bilateral cleft lip: complete or incomplete and contralateral lesser defect (minor-form, microform, or mini-microform). Plast Reconstr Surg. 2008;122(5):1494–504.
13. Mulliken JB, Wu JK, Padwa BL. Repair of bilateral cleft lip: review, revisions, and reflections. J Craniofac Surg. 2003;14(5):609–20.
14. Burt JD, Byrd HS. Cleft lip: unilateral primary deformities. Plast Reconstr Surg. 2000;105(3):1043–55; quiz 1056–7.
15. Mulliken JB, Pensler JM, Kozakewich HP. The anatomy of Cupid's bow in normal and cleft lip. Plast Reconstr Surg. 1993;92(3):395–403; discussion 404.
16. Jiri B, Jana V, Michal J, Jiri K, Dana H, Miroslav T, et al. Successful early neonatal repair of cleft lip within first 8 days of life. Int J Pediatr Otorhinolaryngol. 2012;76(11):1616–26.
17. Cutting C, Grayson B, Brecht L, Santiago P, Wood R, Kwon S. Presurgical columellar elongation and primary retrograde nasal reconstruction in one-stage bilateral cleft lip and nose repair. Plast Reconstr Surg. 1998;101(3):630–9.
18. Salyer KE. Early and late treatment of unilateral cleft nasal deformity. Cleft Palate Craniofac J. 1992;29(6):556–69.
19. Wilhelmsen HR, Musgrave RH. Complications of cleft lip surgery. Cleft Palate J. 1966;3:223–31.
20. McHeik JN, Sfalli P, Bondonny JM, Levard G. Early repair for infants with cleft lip and nose. Int J Pediatr Otorhinolaryngol. 2006;70(10):1785–90.
21. Salyer KE. Primary correction of the unilateral cleft lip nose: a 15-year experience. Plast Reconstr Surg. 1986;77(4):558–68.
22. McComb H. Primary correction of unilateral cleft lip nasal deformity: a 10-year review. Plast Reconstr Surg. 1985;75(6):791–9.
23. Chang C-S, Por YC, Liou EJ-W, Chang C-J, Chen PK-T, Noordhoff MS. Long-term comparison of four techniques for obtaining nasal symmetry in unilateral complete cleft lip patients: a single surgeon's experience. Plast Reconstr Surg. 2010;126(4):1276–84.
24. Lo L-J, Wong F-H, Mardini S, Chen Y-R, Noordhoff MS. Assessment of bilateral cleft lip nose deformity: a comparison of results as judged by cleft surgeons and laypersons. Plast Reconstr Surg. 2002;110(3):733–8; discussion 739–741.
25. Meijer R. Lip adhesion and its effect on the maxillofacial complex in complete unilateral clefts of the lip and palate. Cleft Palate J. 1978;15(1):39–43.
26. Pool R, Farnworth TK. Preoperative lip taping in the cleft lip. Ann Plast Surg. 1994;32(3):243–9.
27. Grayson BH, Garfinkle JS. Early cleft management: the case for nasoalveolar molding. Am J Orthod Dentofacial Orthop. 2014;145(2):134–42.
28. Matsuo K, Hirose T, Otagiri T, Norose N. Repair of cleft lip with nonsurgical correction of nasal deformity in the early neonatal period. Plast Reconstr Surg. 1989;83(1):25–31.
29. Chang C-S, Wallace CG, Pai BC-J, Chiu Y-T, Hsieh Y-J, Chen I-J, et al. Comparison of two nasoalveolar molding techniques in unilateral complete cleft lip patients: a randomized, prospective, single-blind trial to compare nasal outcomes. Plast Reconstr Surg. 2014;134(2):275–82.

30. Liou EJ-W, Subramanian M, Chen PKT, Huang CS. The progressive changes of nasal symmetry and growth after nasoalveolar molding: a three-year follow-up study. Plast Reconstr Surg. 2004;114(4):858–64.
31. Zheng J, He H, Kuang W, Yuan W. Novel three-dimensional coordinate system to analyze alveolar molding effects of pre-surgical nasoalveolar molding on infants with non-syndromic unilateral cleft lip and palate. J Craniofac Surg. 2020;31(3):653–7.
32. Lee CTH, Garfinkle JS, Warren SM, Brecht LE, Cutting CB, Grayson BH. Nasoalveolar molding improves appearance of children with bilateral cleft lip-cleft palate. Plast Reconstr Surg. 2008;122(4):1131–7.

# 22 Cleft Palate Repair

Adrian A. Ong, Ryan F. Brown, and Fiyin Sokoya

## Introduction

Cleft lip and/or palate is a common congenital malformation within the head and neck; the incidence of isolated cleft palate is ~1:2500 [1]. These orofacial clefts are most often an isolated finding but can be associated with syndromes or other comorbidities in 30–50% of cases [2]. Untreated, these patients may experience otologic diseases, speech and language problems, difficulty with oral feeding, velopharyngeal dysfunction, and psychosocial issues. Many surgical techniques have been developed and refined to address the various types of cleft palate, and surgical intervention is often tailored to the individual patient. Ultimately, the goal of cleft palate repair is to restore separation between the nasal and oral cavities to allow for oral feeding and improve verbal communication. Determining candidacy and the timing of repair for return to normal feeding, speech, and Eustachian tube function is then balanced with the impact of surgical intervention on maxillary growth [3].

## Anatomy

Understanding the normal anatomy of the palate is important to the repair of palatal clefts, which helps to separate the oral and nasal cavities (Fig. 22.1). The incisive foramen is an important landmark, and divides the primary palate consisting of the

A. A. Ong
Fort Worth, TX, USA

R. F. Brown
Department of Head and Neck Surgery/Facial Plastic and Reconstructive Surgery, Denver, CO, USA

F. Sokoya (✉)
Wellstar Health Systems, Atlanta, GA, USA


F. Sokoya, A. G. Vincent (eds.), *Manual of Head and Neck Reconstruction*,
https://doi.org/10.1007/978-3-031-65999-7_22

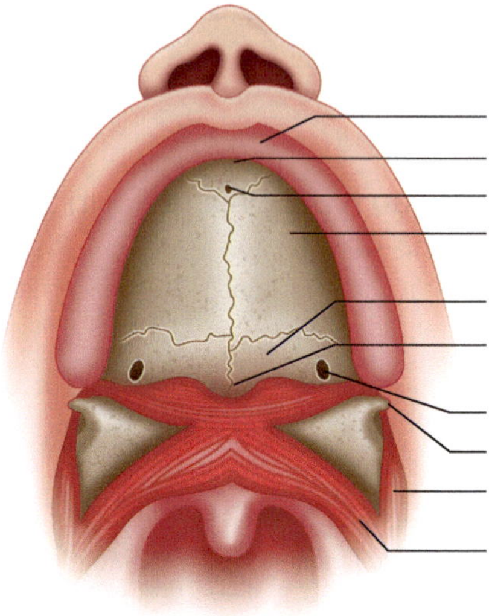


**Fig. 22.1** Normal anatomy of the palate

premaxilla anteriorly from the secondary palate consisting of the remainder of the hard palate and soft palate posteriorly.

The soft palate plays a key role in speech and swallowing function. The levator veli palatini muscle is the most significant structure within the soft palate. It is a paired muscle, which forms a sling from its origin at the base of the temporal bone to the midline. Together with its contralateral component, they elevate the soft palate to the posterior pharyngeal wall. In addition, the palatopharyngeus muscle aids in the elevation and posterior movement of the soft palate. The tensor veli palatini muscle originates from the medial pterygoid and inserts onto the palatine aponeurosis. It assists the levator veli palatini muscle in the elevation of the palate and helps maintain the normal function of the Eustachian tube. Finally, the uvularis muscle is a small muscle that originates from the palatine aponeurosis and inserts into the mucosa of the uvula. It shortens the uvula; however, it does not appear to play a significant role in speech.

The blood supply of the palate consists of the greater and lesser palatine arteries, which are distal branches of the maxillary artery. The greater palatine arteries are especially important as these contribute the main blood supply to the flaps used during cleft palate repair.

Clefts of the palate can consist of a combination of bony and soft-tissue abnormalities. Clefts of the secondary palate are typically midline, while clefts of the primary palate are asymmetric. In clefts of the secondary palate, the velar musculature is affected, with the levator veli palatini muscle oriented in a longitudinal direction with an anomalous insertion onto the bony cleft margin.

The most popular classification system for cleft palate is the Veau classification (Fig. 22.2), which describes cleft palates in four groups: Group I, defect of the soft palate only; Group II, defect involving both the hard and soft palate; Group III,

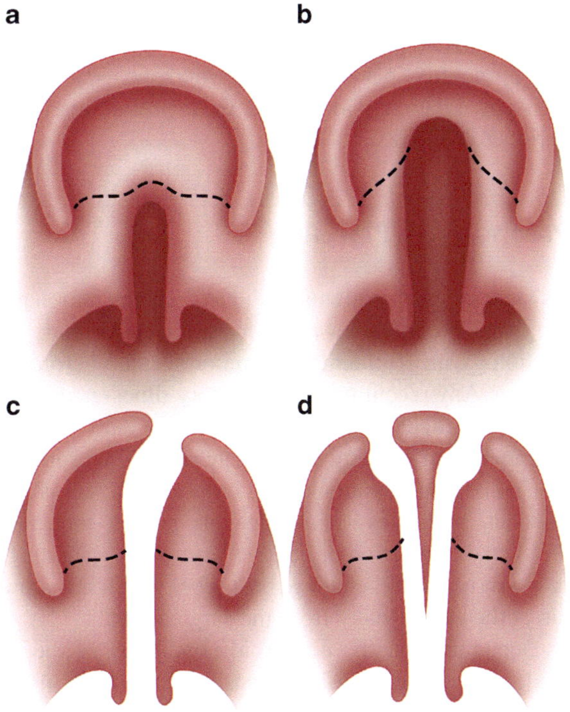


**Fig. 22.2** Veau classification. (**a**) Incomplete cleft involving the soft palate only; (**b**) cleft involving the hard and soft palate; (**c**) complete unilateral cleft involving the lip and palate; (**d**) complete bilateral cleft

defect involving the hard and soft palate and alveolus; and Group IV, bilateral complete cleft palate [4]. This classification can provide a framework for the appropriate type of repair.

## Indications/Contraindications

Nearly all patients will benefit from the repair of the cleft palate, and the question is not if but when. Repair of the cleft palate may have an effect on craniofacial skeletal growth, but this should be balanced with the development of proper speech and language [5]. The American Cleft Palate-Craniofacial Association currently recommends that the palate be closed by age of 18 months and preferably earlier when possible [6]. At most institutions, the cleft palate is repaired at 10–12 months of age [7, 8].

As many patients may have an associated syndrome and/or comorbidities, contraindications to cleft palate repair are related to those conditions and not the cleft palate itself. Life-threatening comorbidities, such as complex congenital heart disease, may require specialized care involving pediatric cardiology and pediatric anesthesiology to determine the safety of general anesthesia. In addition, surgery on patients with severe neurodevelopmental delay who are nonverbal and gastrostomy-tube dependent should be balanced with prognostic factors that portend improvement or worsening of their neurodevelopmental delay. In the immediate preoperative period, patients who have recently had an upper respiratory illness or hospitalization may benefit from postponing surgical intervention to decrease perioperative risks.

## Preoperative Planning

As stated earlier, patients with cleft palates may have significant comorbid conditions and preoperative assessment by the primary care provider with or without cardiology involvement is an important step before proceeding with surgical intervention. Any recent upper respiratory illnesses or hospitalizations are identified, as these may affect the timing of surgery.

Patients undergoing cleft palate repair are orotracheally intubated, and this may be challenging in patients with craniofacial anomalies. Cleft surgeons should communicate with anesthesia colleagues prior to induction, and discuss any significant physical examination or flexible laryngoscopy findings to maximize intubation success. An oral RAE endotracheal tube, which has a preformed bend, can be used to direct the circuit away from the surgical field.

Depending on the comorbid conditions of the patient, arrangements may be made for a bed in the intensive care unit, if close monitoring is required postoperatively.

Caregiver education is initiated during the preoperative visit to avoid any postoperative pitfalls. This is especially important for diet maintenance with options including squeeze bottles with tubing, traditional cups, syringe with tubings or spoon feeding with the goal of minimizing negative pressure in the oral cavity during feeding in the postoperative period [9].

## Instruments/Equipment Set

A head pad (either donut or horseshoe) is used to stabilize the patient's head and minimize movement throughout the duration of the case. A shoulder roll can also be placed if there are no contraindications to further cervical extension. Having the head and neck extended provides an easier view of the anterior palate, which can facilitate repair. The Dingman mouth retractor is commonly used during cleft palate repair. The teeth hooks can be adjusted during the case depending on the portion of the palate that requires exposure, and the lateral cheek retractors provide additional visualization. The use of a surgical headlight and loupe magnification are important for improved intraoperative visualization.

Periosteal elevation of the palatal flaps can be facilitated with a Joseph elevator or a #9 periosteal elevator. If additional pedicle length is required, the greater palatine artery can be carefully osteotomized. The authors find that a curved or 90-degree Beaver blade can help remove the fascia around the vascular pedicle if added freedom is needed of the flap. A curved elevator, such as a Woodson elevator, is needed to free off the nasal mucosa under the hard palate. The authors find that having fine-tipped dissecting scissors, such as longer tenotomy scissors, is helpful when freeing up the muscle from the hard palate and isolating the layers of the soft palate. During the closure, sutures with various types of suture needles may allow for improved placement intraorally, and it is up to the surgeon's preference. Typically, rounded tapered needles are helpful for the closure of the delicate and various palate flaps. Either monopolar or bipolar cautery can be used for hemostasis, with care taken to not over-cauterize the tissue flaps or endanger the vascular pedicle.

## Flap Design/Surgical Technique/Pearls

The type of palatoplasty is dependent on many factors, including the width of the hard and soft palatal clefts, width of the alveolar cleft, approximation of the soft palate cleft with the posterior pharyngeal wall, and presence of comorbidities [10]. The principles of an ideal palatoplasty include a separation of the nasal and oral cavities, tension-free and multilayer closure, establishing the correct anatomical orientation of the levator sling, and retro-positioning of the soft palate for appropriate velopharyngeal closure. The main palatoplasty techniques include (1) von Langenbeck palatoplasty, (2) two-flap palatoplasty (Bardach), (3) Furlow double-opposing Z-palatoplasty, and (4) the Children's Hospital of Philadelphia (CHOP) modification of the Furlow palatoplasty (Fig. 22.3).

To begin all palatoplasty techniques, the patient is placed supine on the operating room table in cervical extension if there are no contraindications. After orotracheal intubation, the mouth retractor is placed to expose the palate. Local anesthetic is infiltrated in the palate and assists in hydro-dissection in the region of the hard palate. It is important to give several minutes for the epinephrine component of the local anesthetic to work before making incisions so as to minimize bleeding. Care should be taken at every point in this process to avoid damage to the neurovascular bundle. Finally, an intravelar veloplasty is advised, which repositions the abnormally attached levator veli palatini muscles from the posterior edge of the hard palate to recreate the palatal muscular sling as it has been shown to improve speech outcomes in those undergoing palatoplasty [11].

### Von Langenbeck Palatoplasty

The palate is marked along the alveolar ridge and the medial aspect of the cleft edge. The lateral-releasing incisions near the alveolar ridge are performed first to create the anteriorly- and posteriorly-based flap. This incision can be carried laterally around the posterior extent of the alveolus if further mobilization is necessary. Next, the incisions of the medial cleft edge at the oral/nasal mucosal junction are brought

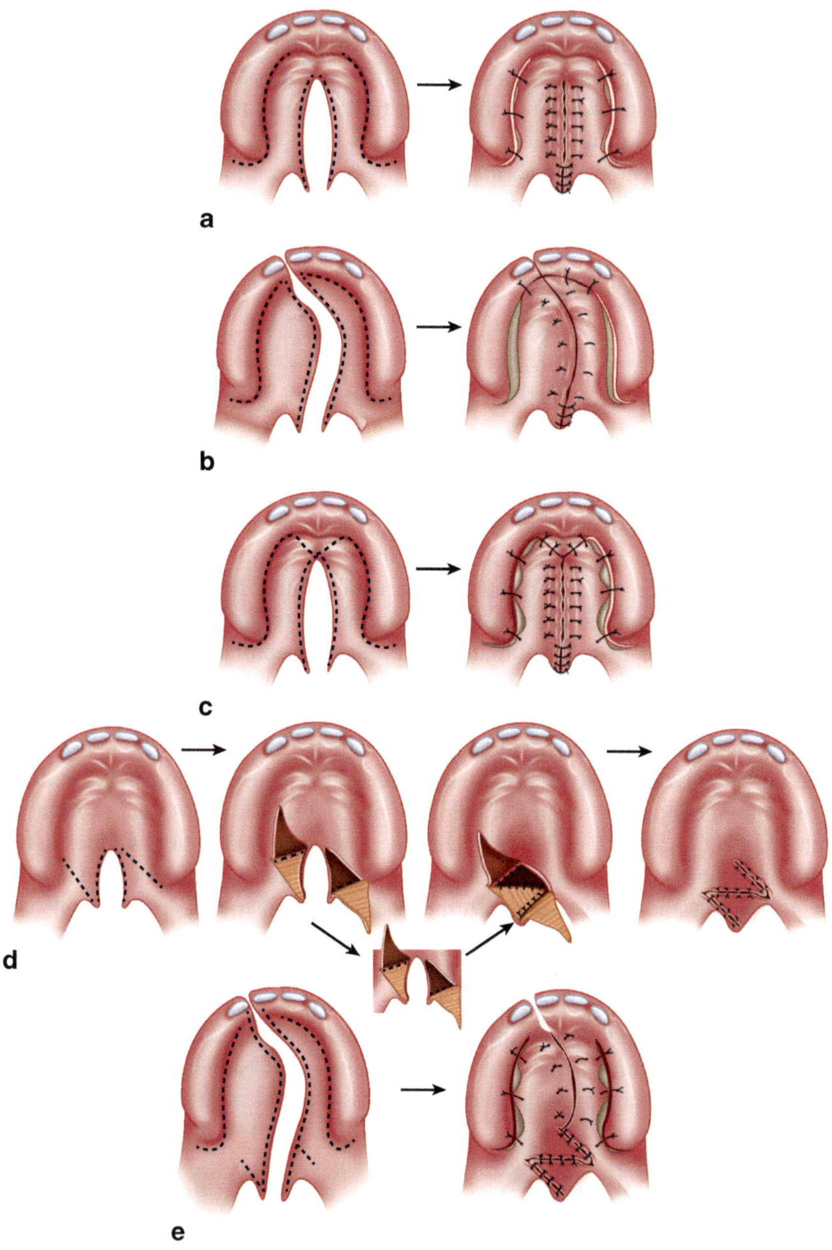


**Fig. 22.3** Types of cleft palate repair. (**a**) von Langenbeck palatoplasty; (**b**) two-flap palatoplasty (Bardach); (**c**) Furlow double-opposing Z-palatoplasty; (**d**) Children's Hospital of Philadelphia (CHOP) modification of the Furlow palatoplasty (**e**) Combined two-flap palatoplasty with Furlow doupole-opposing Z-palatoplasty at the soft palate

to the apex of the uvula. The mucosa overlying the vomer is incised and can provide additional flaps to achieve a tension-free closure.

Once all incisions are made, a subperiosteal dissection is carried from the lateral-releasing incision to the medial cleft edge. Blunt dissection to the posterior edge of the palate is carefully performed, and the greater palatine neurovascular bundle is identified. The greater palatine neurovascular bundle is circumferentially released, and additional length can be gained by releasing the pedicle using osteotomies in the bony canal.

Elevation of the nasal flaps is performed and can be carried to the lateral nasal wall as needed to provide tension-free closure. Once all flaps are elevated, attention is turned to the velar musculature to start the intravelar veloplasty. The levator veli palatini is released from its anomalous insertion onto the posterior edge of the hard palate. This can be elevated behind the greater palatine neurovascular bundle to provide additional length for the mucosal and muscle layers.

Nasal closure is performed with sutures placed in a mucosal-to-submucosal fashion such that the knots are along the nasal mucosal surface. The vomer flaps can be incorporated anteriorly to provide tension-free closure. Next, the intravelar veloplasty is completed. Interrupted or horizontal mattress sutures are used to reorient the levator veli palatini muscles and recreate the levator sling. Finally, the oral mucosa is closed with interrupted or running sutures in a posterior-to-anterior fashion. Sutures may be placed in the lateral-release incision for stabilization, but this is not often necessary.

## Two-Flap Palatoplasty (Bardach)

The two-flap palatoplasty is typically used in cases of complete cleft palate with adequate soft palate length. Similar to the von Langenbeck palatoplasty, the lateral-releasing incisions are marked; however, when incised, they are taken to the medial cleft margin edge. This connects the medial and alveolar incisions anteriorly creating a posteriorly based flap on the greater palatine neurovascular bundle. During subperiosteal dissection, the oral hard palate mucosa can be reflected posteriorly to identify and skeletonize the greater palatine neurovascular bundle. The vomer and nasal flaps are created. If the patient has a bilateral cleft palate, then bilateral vomer flaps can be used to help close the anterior nasal floor. Multilayer closure and intravelar veloplasty are performed similarly to the von Langenbeck palatoplasty. It is very common to have some gaps between the lateral and anterior alveolar ridge. It is important to place tacking sutures to hold the sutures in place and then surgical is placed over exposed bone. The cleft will be covered by the closure, and these new areas of exposed bone will re-mucosalize in a matter of days to weeks.

## Furlow Double-Opposing Z-Palatoplasty and Children's Hospital of Philadelphia Modification

The purpose of the double-opposing Z-palatoplasty is to reorient the levator veli palatini muscles into a horizontal sling position and to lengthen the soft palate [12]. The nasal and oral incisions do not overlap and theoretically decrease the risk of fistula formation. The hard palate is closed with vomer and nasal flaps for the nasal surface and oral mucoperiosteal flaps for the oral surface.

In the CHOP modification, the double-opposing Z-palatoplasty is used to treat the soft palate and hard palate, and lateral-releasing incisions or bipedicled flaps (von Langenbeck) are developed to treat the hard palatal defect [13]. The Z-palatoplasty incisions are shortened such that there is no intersection with the lateral-releasing incisions.

In the traditional Furlow repair, the hard palate mucoperiosteal flap is elevated from medial to lateral without lateral-releasing incisions. The greater palatine neurovascular bundle is identified, released circumferentially, and preserved. Next, the soft palate is dissected.

On the left, the mucosa is incised along the medial cleft edge and the planned Z-plasty incision to create a posteriorly based myomucosal flap. The anomalous fibers of the levator veli palatini muscle are released from the posterior edge of the hard palate and incorporated into the flap. This is dissected away from the undersurface of the nasal mucosa. A suture is placed at the apex of the left myomucosal flap to allow for retraction and access for nasal flap mobilization. On the right, an anteriorly based oral mucosal flap is elevated toward the hamulus and dissected in a submucoperiosteal plane once the lateral palatal shelf is reached.

On the right, a nasal myomucosal flap is then developed by incising the flap at the base of the oral mucosal flap and carried to the hamulus in an anterior-to-posterior direction. On the left, a nasal mucosal flap is created, beginning posteriorly and raised in an anterolateral direction toward the hamulus.

Once all flaps are developed, the nasal surface is closed by placing the right nasal posteriorly based myomucosal flap in its posteriorly transposed site. Sutures are placed initially at the base to allow for greater advancement of the flap and decreased tension in the closure. The left nasal anteriorly based mucosal flap is inset similarly. The left oral posteriorly based myomucosal flap is then overlayed onto its nasal compliment and sutured to reconstitute the levator sling. At this point, closure of the nasal surface of the hard palate is closed similar to the other types of palatoplasty. After nasal surface closure and reorientation of the levator muscles, the right oral anteriorly based mucosal flap is then transposed and inset. The oral hard palate mucosal closure is then performed in a posterior-to-anterior fashion.

The Furlow palatoplasty is commonly used to repair either a submucous cleft, isolated soft palate cleft, or velopharyngeal insufficiency caused by a short soft palate after primary cleft palate repair, as discussed below.

## Special Considerations

In patients with wide clefts (>20 mm), primary closure can be achieved with the previously mentioned palatoplasty techniques. Successful closure can be maximized with the extension of the lateral releasing incisions around the posterior alveolus onto the soft palate toward the retromolar trigone, release of the levator veli palatini muscles from both the oral and nasal mucosal flaps to increase flap mobility, and circumferential dissection and release of the greater palatine neurovascular pedicle with or without osteotomies. In those cases when excessive tension remains (primary wide clefts, revision cases with significant scar tissue), consideration can be given to the use of acellular dermal matrix. The use of acellular dermal matrix during palatoplasty when tension-free primary closure cannot be achieved may reduce fistula formation, with an overall fistula rate of 5.4% compared to 10.6% in those who did not undergo non-acellular dermal matrix palatoplasty [14].

A submucous cleft is characterized by dehiscence of the palatal musculature with intact overlying mucosa, causing difficulty in detection. Findings associated with a submucous cleft include midline notching of the hard palate, bifid uvula, and a zona pellucida (a bluish tint in the soft palate signifying lack of underlying musculature). Management of submucous clefts can include minimally invasive palatopharyngoplasty (MIPP), intravelar veloplasty, Furlow double-opposing Z-plasty, sphincter pharyngoplasty, and posterior pharyngeal flap. Currently, available data are mixed, and a Cochrane review on the management of submucous clefts showed no significant difference in outcome between MIPP versus MIPP with a pharyngeal flap or sphincter pharyngoplasty [15]. Calis et al. showed improved speech outcomes in patients undergoing submucous cleft repair with both Furlow double-opposing Z-plasty and pharyngeal flap combined with intravelar veloplasty; however, they suggested that pharyngeal flap repair be considered in patients with severe hypernasality [16].

## Postoperative Management

Depending on the surgeon's preference, a tongue stitch can be placed in the midline to assist with airway management in the post-anesthesia care unit and on the floor [17]. This can be removed once the patient is deemed safe from any potential airway obstruction. Patients are typically admitted for overnight observation to monitor for airway obstruction and provided liquid pain medication. Soft arm restraints can be used for those unable to follow commands to avoid disruption of the surgical site. Under close supervision, these should be released several times a day and range of motion exercises are encouraged. Patients are discharged once tolerating a pourable/pureed diet. Ideally, no straws or eating utensils are used during the healing period to prevent possible damage to the suture lines. During hospitalization, caregivers are educated on proper feeding, which is maintained until the first follow-up visit.

## Outcomes

The goals of palatoplasty include complete closure of the oral and nasal mucosa without the formation of a fistula, velopharyngeal competence with normal speech and feeding, minimal impact on facial skeletal growth, and improved Eustachian tube function. This is dependent on cleft size and shape, type of repair, and surgeon experience.

## Oronasal Fistula Rate

Oronasal fistula is a morbid complication resulting in hypernasality and nasal regurgitation. It is typically located at either the anterior hard palate or at the junction of the hard and soft palate repair. The incidence of oronasal fistula after primary cleft palate repair is approximately 8.6% [18]. Risk factors for the formation of an oronasal fistula include preoperative Veau classification (higher rate of fistula with class III/IV), cleft width (higher rate of fistula with cleft width of ~7.75 mm and greater), nutritional status of the patient, and surgeon volume (higher volume protective against fistula formation) [19–21]. The surgeon must pay special attention to the closure by careful development of robust tissue flaps and achieving a multilayer, tension-free closure. Acellular dermal matrix can be used as an adjunct to reduce the rate of oronasal fistula formation [14].

## Velopharyngeal Dysfunction

Velopharyngeal dysfunction (VPD) results from the inadequate closure of the velopharynx during speech causing air escape through the nose during oral consonant production. Symptomatically, patients develop hypernasal speech and nasal regurgitation during feeding. The estimated incidence of VPD following cleft palate repair has been reported to be between 15 and 30%, with older age at the time of repair (>2 years) being a risk factor for the development of VPD, resulting in poorer speech outcomes [22–24].

Management of VPD is complex and typically requires a multidisciplinary team, including a cleft surgeon, speech-language pathologist, and/or maxillofacial prosthodontist. Speech therapy may be used as a primary treatment or adjunct to prosthetic rehabilitation or surgical intervention. Some patients, especially those who are not surgical candidates, may benefit from an obturator or palatal lift fashioned by a maxillofacial prosthodontist. If surgical intervention is considered, it is individualized based on closure patterns identified on nasopharyngoscopy or fluoroscopy; surgical interventions include posterior pharyngeal wall augmentation, palatal lengthening, and/or alteration of the velopharynx (sphincter pharyngoplasty or posterior pharyngeal flap).

A prospective clinical trial compared the speech of two cohorts of patients with cleft palate undergoing either Furlow double-opposing Z-plasty or a two-flap palatoplasty (von Langenbeck) and found that the Furlow double-opposing Z-plasty resulted in better velopharyngeal function; however, the Furlow palatoplasty resulted in higher rate of fistula [25]. Intravelar veloplasty has been incorporated into cleft palate repair and has been shown to significantly improve postoperative speech outcomes, resulting in a decrease of secondary velopharyngeal rates from 10.2 to 4.6% [26].

## Facial Growth

There has been concern that cleft palate repair may inhibit facial growth, with a particular focus on the timing of repair. Liao et al. suggested that patients who underwent late hard palate repair had minimal adverse effects on the growth of the maxilla [3]. On the other hand, other studies have found late repair resulted in no impairments in maxillofacial growth, suggesting further research is necessary; however, late cleft palate repair resulted in higher rates of VPD and poorer speech outcomes [5, 24, 27]. Finally, some surgeons suggest less subperiosteal dissection of the hard palate to prevent maxillary growth impairments and advocate a two-stage approach to palatoplasty, in which the soft palate is repaired first, followed by delayed repair of the hard palate [28]. Ongoing research is needed to further define the effects of cleft palate repair on facial growth.

## Eustachian Tube Dysfunction

Eustachian tube dysfunction, including chronic otitis media with effusion, affects nearly all patients with cleft palate and is due to the anatomic disruption of the palatal muscular sling, causing an inability of the tensor veli palatini muscle to dilate the eustachian tube [29]. The resultant middle ear effusion manifests as conductive hearing loss, which can be improved with the placement of tympanostomy tubes, palatoplasty, and/or hearing amplification.

Most patients with cleft palate who undergo palatoplasty will achieve improved eustachian tube function by age 6 years [30]. Smith et al. showed that patients with cleft palate who underwent Furlow double-opposing Z-plasty had fewer sets of tympanostomy tubes postoperatively (1.8 sets of tympanostomy tubes) compared to those undergoing traditional two-flap palatoplasty (2.9 sets of tympanostomy tubes) [31]. In addition, intravelar veloplasty, which restores the palatal muscular sling, has been shown to improve eustachian tube function [32]. Despite eventual recovery of eustachian tube function after palatoplasty, patients with cleft palate remain at high risk for persistent hearing loss and for cholesteatoma, and these patients will continue to benefit from close otologic follow-up [33–35].

## References


1. Parker SE, Mai CT, Canfield MA, et al. Updated National Birth Prevalence estimates for selected birth defects in the United States, 2004-2006. Birth Defects Res A Clin Mol Teratol. 2010;88(12):1008–16.
2. Tolarová MM, Cervenka J. Classification and birth prevalence of orofacial clefts. Am J Med Genet. 1998;75(2):126–37.
3. Liao YF, Cole TJ, Mars M. Hard palate repair timing and facial growth in unilateral cleft lip and palate: a longitudinal study. Cleft Palate Craniofac J. 2006;43(5):547–56.
4. Allori AC, Mulliken JB, Meara JG, Shusterman S, Marcus JR. Classification of cleft lip/palate: then and now. Cleft Palate Craniofac J. 2017;54(2):175–88.
5. Liao YF, Mars M. Hard palate repair timing and facial growth in cleft lip and palate: a systematic review. Cleft Palate Craniofac J. 2006;43(5):563–70.
6. Parameters for evaluation and treatment of patients with cleft lip/palate or other craniofacial differences. Cleft Palate Craniofac J. 2017;55(1):137–156.
7. Dao AM, Goudy SL. Cleft palate repair, gingivoperiosteoplasty, and alveolar bone grafting. Facial Plast Surg Clin North Am. 2016;24(4):467–76.
8. Shaye D. Update on outcomes research for cleft lip and palate. Curr Opin Otolaryngol Head Neck Surg. 2014;22(4):255–9.
9. Bessell A, Hooper L, Shaw WC, Reilly S, Reid J, Glenny AM. Feeding interventions for growth and development in infants with cleft lip, cleft palate or cleft lip and palate. Cochrane Database Syst Rev. 2011;2011(2):CD003315.
10. Saothonglang K, Punyavong P, Winaikosol K, Jenwitheesuk K, Surakunprapha P. Risk factors of fistula following primary palatoplasty. J Craniofac Surg. 2021;32(2):587–90.
11. Téblick S, Ruymaekers M, Van de Casteele E, Nadjmi N. Effect of cleft palate closure technique on speech and middle ear outcome: a systematic review. J Oral Maxillofac Surg. 2019;77(2):405.e401–15.
12. Furlow LT Jr. Cleft palate repair by double opposing Z-plasty. Plast Reconstr Surg. 1986;78(6):724–38.
13. Kirschner RE, Wang P, Jawad AF, et al. Cleft-palate repair by modified Furlow double-opposing Z-plasty: the children's hospital of Philadelphia experience. Plast Reconstr Surg. 1999;104(7):1998–2010; discussion 2011–1994.
14. Aldekhayel SA, Sinno H, Gilardino MS. Acellular dermal matrix in cleft palate repair: an evidence-based review. Plast Reconstr Surg. 2012;130(1):177–82.
15. Nasser M, Fedorowicz Z, Newton JT, Nouri M. Interventions for the management of submucous cleft palate. Cochrane Database Syst Rev. 2008;(1):CD006703.
16. Calis M, Ustun GG, Ozturk M, Gunaydin RO, Kulak Kayikci ME, Ozgur F. Comparison of the speech results after correction of submucous cleft palate with Furlow palatoplasty and pharyngeal flap combined with intravelar veloplasty. J Craniofac Surg. 2018;29(1):e100–3.
17. Dorfman DW, Ciminello FS, Wong GB. Tongue suture placement after cleft palate repair. J Craniofac Surg. 2010;21(5):1601–3.
18. Hardwicke JT, Landini G, Richard BM. Fistula incidence after primary cleft palate repair: a systematic review of the literature. Plast Reconstr Surg. 2014;134(4):618e–27e.
19. Leu GR, Ebert BE, Roby BB, Scott AR. Cleft palate repair by otolaryngologist-head and neck surgeons: risk factors for postoperative fistula. Laryngoscope. 2021;131(6):1281–5.
20. Pollard SH, Skirko JR, Dance D, et al. Oronasal fistula risk after palate repair. Cleft Palate Craniofac J. 2021;58(1):35–41.
21. Yi CR, Kang MK, Oh TS. Analysis of the intrinsic predictors of oronasal fistula in primary cleft palate repair using intravelar veloplasty. Cleft Palate Craniofac J. 2020;57(8):1024–31.
22. Schuster T, Rustemeyer J, Bremerich A, Günther L, Schwenzer-Zimmerer K. Analysis of patients with a cleft of the soft palate with special consideration to the problem of velopharyngeal insufficiency. J Craniomaxillofac Surg. 2013;41(3):245–8.

23. Sullivan SR, Marrinan EM, LaBrie RA, Rogers GF, Mulliken JB. Palatoplasty outcomes in nonsyndromic patients with cleft palate: a 29-year assessment of one surgeon's experience. J Craniofac Surg. 2009;20(Suppl 1):612–6.
24. Zhao S, Xu Y, Yin H, et al. Incidence of postoperative velopharyngeal insufficiency in late palate repair. J Craniofac Surg. 2012;23(6):1602–6.
25. Williams WN, Seagle MB, Pegoraro-Krook MI, et al. Prospective clinical trial comparing outcome measures between Furlow and von Langenbeck palatoplasties for UCLP. Ann Plast Surg. 2011;66(2):154–63.
26. Sommerlad BC. A technique for cleft palate repair. Plast Reconstr Surg. 2003;112(6):1542–8.
27. Rohrich RJ, Rowsell AR, Johns DF, et al. Timing of hard palatal closure: a critical long-term analysis. Plast Reconstr Surg. 1996;98(2):236–46.
28. Liao YF, Yang IY, Wang R, Yun C, Huang CS. Two-stage palate repair with delayed hard palate closure is related to favorable maxillary growth in unilateral cleft lip and palate. Plast Reconstr Surg. 2010;125(5):1503–10.
29. Doyle WJ, Cantekin EI, Bluestone CD. Eustachian tube function in cleft palate children. Ann Otol Rhinol Laryngol Suppl. 1980;89(3 Pt 2):34–40.
30. Smith TL, DiRuggiero DC, Jones KR. Recovery of eustachian tube function and hearing outcome in patients with cleft palate. Otolaryngol Head Neck Surg. 1994;111(4):423–9.
31. Smith LK, Gubbels SP, MacArthur CJ, Milczuk HA. The effect of the palatoplasty method on the frequency of ear tube placement. Arch Otolaryngol Head Neck Surg. 2008;134(10):1085–9.
32. Hassan ME, Askar S. Does palatal muscle reconstruction affect the functional outcome of cleft palate surgery? Plast Reconstr Surg. 2007;119(6):1859–65.
33. Funamura JL, Lee JW, McKinney S, Bayoumi AG, Senders CW, Tollefson TT. Children with cleft palate: predictors of otologic issues in the first 10 years. Otolaryngol Head Neck Surg. 2019;160(5):902–10.
34. Harris L, Cushing SL, Hubbard B, Fisher D, Papsin BC, James AL. Impact of cleft palate type on the incidence of acquired cholesteatoma. Int J Pediatr Otorhinolaryngol. 2013;77(5):695–8.
35. Kappen IF, Schreinemakers JB, Oomen KP, et al. Hearing sensitivity in adults with a unilateral cleft lip and palate after two-stage palatoplasty. Int J Pediatr Otorhinolaryngol. 2017;94:76–81.

# Part VII

# Trauma Reconstruction

# Mandible Trauma Reconstruction

# 23

Arya Namin and Ugochukwu Umeh

## Introduction

In the current era, most mandibular fractures are sustained in motor vehicle collisions, although interpersonal violence is the most common etiology in some series [1, 2]. While the incidence of mandibular fractures has certainly increased with the advent of the motor vehicle, these injuries have been a challenge to humans for millennia. In ancient times, mandible fractures were considered untreatable and fatal injuries, likely due to infection and the functional impairment of untreated fractures [3]. Hippocrates is one of the first physicians to attempt the treatment of mandible fractures [3, 4]. Hippocrates described a method of closed reduction, interdental fixation with gold wires, and external leather straps to help keep the mandible in reduction [3, 4]. Little changed in the management of mandibular fractures until the eighteenth century when dental splints were first described in the management of mandibular fractures. The nineteenth century saw the advent of attempts at open reduction with internal fixation via wires as well as the first descriptions of maxillomandibular fixation [3, 5]. Thomas Gunning was amongst those who described maxillomandibular fixation through interdental splinting, and a modification of the Gunning splint is still an option in the management of edentulous patients today [6]. It was at the turn of the twentieth century that immobilization of mandibular fractures with plates and screws was first described [3, 5]. During the 1960s, widespread production of these plates and screws began, allowing for this technique to be more widely utilized [3, 5].

The objectives of mandibular trauma reconstruction are restoring the premorbid form and function of the mandible. This requires fracture reduction while in

A. Namin (✉)
Otolaryngology and Facial Plastic Surgery Associates, Fort Worth, TX, USA

U. Umeh
Medical University of Lublin, Lublin, Poland


F. Sokoya, A. G. Vincent (eds.), *Manual of Head and Neck Reconstruction*,
https://doi.org/10.1007/978-3-031-65999-7_23

premorbid occlusion with adequate fixation to allow for bone healing. Depending on patient characteristics, fracture location, concomitant craniomaxillofacial injuries, and severity of fracture displacement, the treatment required to achieve these goals can range from observation and soft diet to open reduction and internal fixation with load-bearing reconstructions. In this chapter, the various reconstructive options for condylar, ramus, angle, body, symphyseal, and parasymphyseal fractures will be discussed.

## Anatomy

The mandible consists of the condylar process, coronoid process, ramus, angle, body, symphysis, parasymphysis, and alveolar process [7–10]. The symphysis is the area of bone below the roots of the central incisors, and the parasymphysis is the area of bone below the roots of the lateral incisors and canines [8]. The mandibular body is the area of bone lateral to the canine and medial to the third molar [8]. The angle and ramus of the mandible extend from a vertical line behind the third molar to the outer mandibular angle posteroinferiorly and to the mandibular notch and bases of the condylar and coronoid processes superiorly [8]. The condylar head articulates with the glenoid fossa of the temporal bone. The condylar and coronoid processes are separated by the mandibular notch. The condylar process continues superiorly from the posterior border of the ascending ramus and can be broken down into the condylar head, neck, and base [9]. The lateral pterygoid inserts onto the pterygoid fovea of the condylar neck. The masseter and medial pterygoid muscles form a sling around the ramus and angle. The temporalis muscle inserts into the coronoid process of the mandible. On the medial surface of the ramus, the inferior alveolar neurovascular bundle enters the mandibular foramen. The mylohyoid groove begins immediately anterior to the mandibular foramen and then travels along the medial surface of the mandibular body. The mental foramen is found at the level of the second premolar or at the interspace of the premolars.

## Indications/Contraindications

### Symphysis and Parasymphysis

Symphyseal and parasymphyseal fractures typically require surgical treatment. In nondisplaced and immobile fractures, no-chew diet can be considered. Surgical treatment options for noncomminuted symphyseal and parasymphyseal fractures include closed reduction with maxillomandibular fixation, two-miniplate fixation, single thicker reconstruction plate fixation, lag screw fixation, and dynamic compression plate fixation (Fig. 23.1) [11]. Closed reduction with maxillomandibular fixation avoids the risks of internal fixation with open reduction. However, it does necessitate a prolonged period of immobilization, thus placing the patient at risk for malnutrition and temporomandibular joint dysfunction. When utilizing open

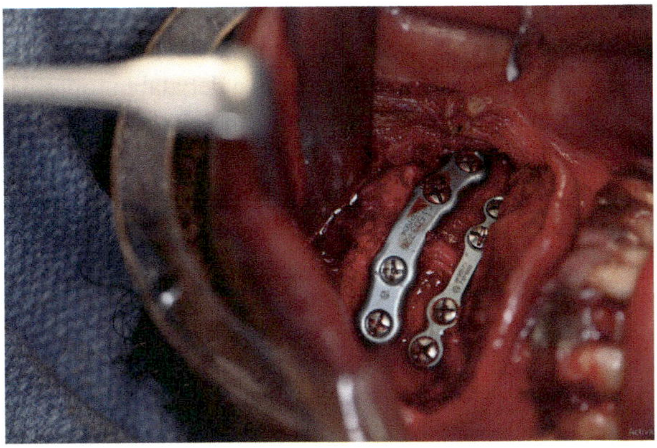

**Fig. 23.1** Symphyseal fracture fixated with a 2-mm thick locking plate along the inferior border of mandible with the two bicortical screws on each side of the fracture line and a miniplate superior to this with two monocortical screws on each side of the fracture line. The 2 mm thick plate along the inferior border was chosen due to the patient presenting 8 weeks after the initial injury with a concomitant infection that required treatment prior to the patient undergoing definitive repair

reduction internal fixation, the patient should be temporarily placed in maxillomandibular fixation to ensure premorbid occlusion. The advantages of miniplates are ease in bending the plates to the appropriate contour of the mandible and, therefore, improving the efficiency of the surgery. Excellent functional results with minimal complications have been obtained with the application of two 1-mm thick miniplates and monocortical screws in the treatment of noncomminuted symphyseal and parasymphyseal fractures [11]. Lee et al. recommends prescribing a soft diet for 6 weeks after treatment of symphyseal and parasymphyseal fractures with two miniplates and only leaving patients in maxillomandibular fixation if the presence of other craniomaxillofacial injuries necessitated this [11]. Locking plates provide potential advantages of less screw loosening, greater stability, and less precise bending of the plate because of the internal/external fixator principle [12]. However, locking plates are more expensive, and a prospective trial comparing locking plates to standard plates did not find any significant difference in short-term complication rates [12]. Lag screw fixation has been found to have similar outcomes as plate fixation; however, this technique is associated with more intraoperative challenges in obtaining proper fixation [13].

## Body

Mandibular body fractures commonly require treatment. In nondisplaced and immobile fractures, a soft diet can be considered. Surgical treatment options for mandibular body fractures include closed reduction with maxillomandibular fixation, two-miniplate fixation, single thicker reconstruction plate fixation, and dynamic compression plate fixation. The application of a miniplate inferiorly with bicortical screws and a miniplate superiorly with monocortical screws offers a stable repair obviating the need for postoperative maxillomandibular fixation [14]. The plate thickness and need for bicortical screws is a debatable topic. However, a prospective study has found equivalent rates of fracture healing in patients treated with thicker plates and bicortical screws and patients treated with thinner plates and monocortical screws [15]. In sagittally and obliquely oriented fractures of the mandibular body and ramus, lag screws can offer a good option for repair. If lag screws are utilized, at least two need to be placed in order for the repair to be stable. Compression plate fixation is less commonly utilized due to the unforgiving nature of these plates. However, they have been successfully used in atrophic mandibles, for which they were originally described [16]. In comminuted fractures and fractures with devitalized bone, a load-bearing reconstruction must be undertaken with at least three bicortical screws on each side of the fracture (Figs. 23.2 and 23.3) [17]. In cases where the devitalized bone is removed, resulting in an intervening gap, cellular bone matrix (ViviGen® Cellular Bone Matrix DePuy Synthes Companies), autogenous bone grafting, or free tissue transfer should be employed to help prevent nonunion (Figs. 23.4 and 23.5) [17, 18].

## Angle and Ramus

Because of the forces of mastication, angle fractures have the highest risk of post-surgical complications, including infection [14, 19, 20]. Management of third molars in mandibular angle fractures is a debatable subject and likely a contributing factor to the increased complication rate seen in these fractures [19, 21]. When the root is fractured, unsalvageable teeth due to caries or infection, unstable or loose teeth, and teeth preventing adequate fracture reduction are considerations for

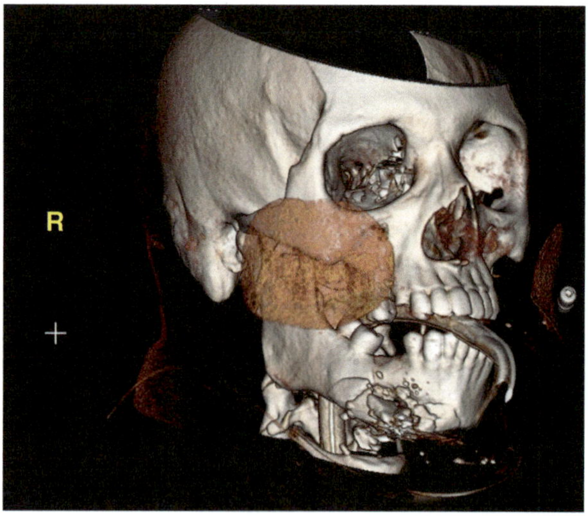


**Fig. 23.2** Mandible fracture after gunshot to the face with comminution and partial thickness continuity defect along the inferior border of the mandible

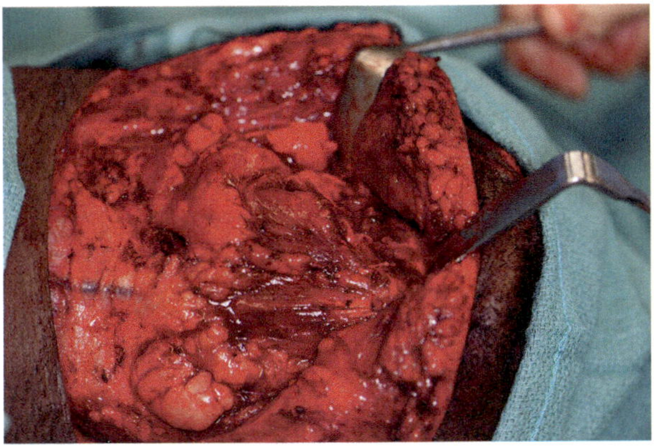

**Fig. 23.3** Mandibular body and parasymphysis exposed. Bone fragments have been removed, resulting in a partial thickness continuity defect along the inferior border of the mandible

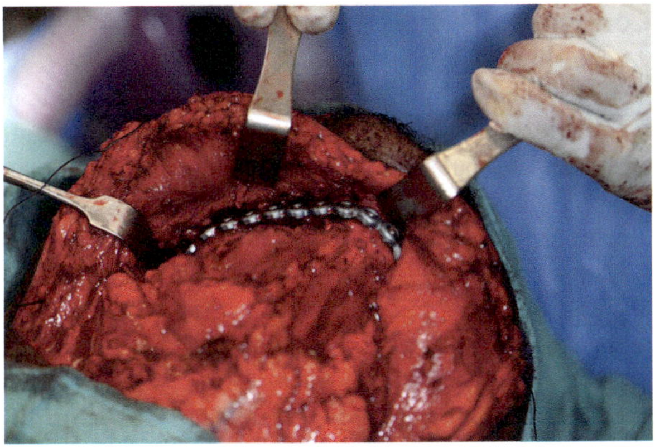

**Fig. 23.4** Fixation of fracture with 2.5 mm thick reconstruction plate. Three bicortical locking screws are present on each side of the partial thickness continuity defect

extraction [20, 21]. Treatment options for angle fractures include maxillomandibular fixation, two-miniplate fixation, three-dimensional square or rectangular-shaped miniplate fixation, and single miniplate fixation along the superior border of the mandible [19, 20, 22, 23]. In a prospective study examining the outcomes of angle fractures treated with either maxillomandibular fixation, single miniplate fixation, or two-miniplate fixation, it was found that the application of a single miniplate offered the shortest operative time with significantly fewer postoperative complications [19]. The advantages of the single miniplate technique along the oblique line of the mandible include decreased operative times, avoidance of transbuccal trocar placement, and avoidance of elevating the periosteum along the ramus and angle [19, 20]. However, there is some concern that the single superior miniplate provides inadequate fixation along the inferior mandibular border during functional loading, leading some surgeons to utilize either two miniplates or three-dimensional box plates [21, 24]. In a series of 88 patients with mandibular angle fractures treated with two-miniplate fixation using monocortical screws, the complication rate was minimal, and the infection rate was 2.9% [21].

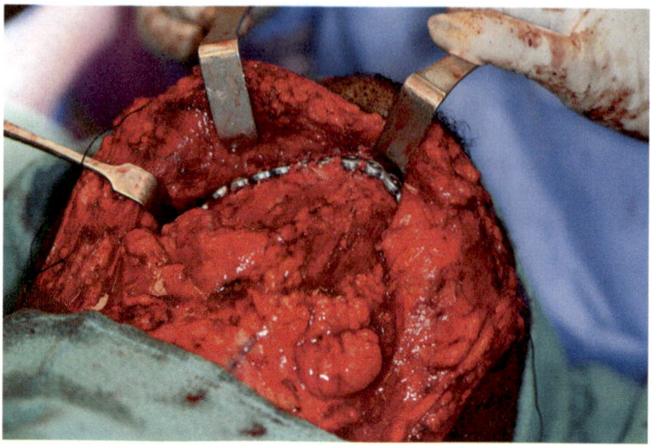

**Fig. 23.5** Partial thickness continuity defect reconstructed with cellular bone matrix (ViviGen® Cellular Bone Matrix DePuy Synthes Companies)

## Condylar

The management of condylar fractures varies significantly amongst institutions and surgeons. Over the past few decades, our understanding of the biomechanics of the temporomandibular joint and the biological adaptations that occur with the masticatory system after condylar fractures has significantly improved, allowing for better, albeit still controversial, treatment plans [25]. Management options for these fractures include closed treatment, open treatment, and endoscopic treatment options. Closed treatment options include a soft diet, jaw exercises, maxillomandibular fixation with elastics, and maxillomandibular fixation with wires. In the closed treatment of condylar process fractures, it is accepted that a degree of malunion will occur and that the patient will have a good outcome due to remodeling that occurs, allowing for a functional neoarticulation [25, 26]. Condylar fractures are the most common pediatric mandibular fracture, and closed treatment has been found to have good outcomes in these cases [27, 28]. Open approaches include the preauricular, retromandibular, and submandibular approaches, with the goal of placing at least one miniplate with two monocortical screws on each side of the fracture line. The endoscopic approach also has the same fixation goals as the open approach but utilizes a transoral approach with endoscopic assistance for visualization and typically requires a small facial incision for a transbuccal trochal that allows for screw placement [28–30]. The objectives of treatment include restoring premorbid occlusion, pain-free mouth opening with an interincisal distance of 40 mm, facial symmetry, sound temporomandibular joint function, and normal movement of the jaw in all directions [31]. The surgeon must, therefore, assess the characteristics of the condylar fracture and associated craniomaxillofacial injuries to develop an optimal treatment plan for that patient. In the 1980s, Zide and Kent proposed that displacement of the condyle into the middle cranial fossa, difficulty in obtaining occlusion with closed reduction, lateral displacement of the condyle, and presence of a foreign body in the condylar neck were absolute indications for open reduction internal fixation [31, 32]. However, since that time, the indications for open reduction internal fixation of condylar fractures have expanded, given the unfavorable outcomes in certain patients treated with closed approaches [29–31, 33]. Patients who can achieve good outcomes with closed treatment approaches include those with less than 2 mm of shortening of the height of the ramus and less than 10 degrees of deviation [30, 31]. Patients whose outcome would be improved with open or endoscopic reduction with internal fixation include those with more than 15 mm of shortening of the height of the ramus or more than 45 degrees of deviation [30, 31]. Patients with temporomandibular joint dislocation and associated midfacial or panfacial fractures also likely benefit from open reduction internal fixation [31]. In order for the patient to undergo successful internal fixation, there must be adequate bone in the segment proximal to the fracture line to allow for two screws to be placed. In cases where there is inadequate bone stock in the proximal segment for two screws, external fixation is an option [34]. For patients with 2–10 mm of shortening of the height of the mandible and 10–45 degrees of displacement, the optimal treatment option is less clear [30, 31].

## Preoperative Planning

Patients who present with acute mandibular fractures, particularly those involved in motor vehicle collisions, have commonly been involved in a high energy crashes and, therefore, should be evaluated according to advanced trauma life support protocols in order to identify and intervene on any acutely life-threatening injuries. A history regarding the mechanism of the injury should be inquired. Prior history of trauma, craniomaxillofacial surgery, bone diseases such as osteoporosis, and temporomandibular joint dysfunction should be elicited. Prior medical and psychiatric history should be obtained. Individuals with epilepsy may not be good candidates for postoperative maxillomandibular fixation. Current medications, prior surgeries, and allergies should be documented. Social history, such as alcohol intake and methamphetamine use, are also important preoperative considerations. After the trauma exam has been completed, tell-tale signs of craniomaxillofacial trauma are typically identified that lead to subspecialty consultation. A comprehensive head and neck examination should then be undertaken. Mobility of the midface and mandible should be assessed. The mandible should be palpated to identify any areas of tenderness and/or instability. The dentition and occlusal status should be assessed. Edentulous and partially dentulous mandibular fractures pose unique problems and typically need to be reconstructed with thicker plates in a load-bearing fashion [35]. In edentulous patients, the height of the mandible should be assessed, and if at least 20 mm in height can be treated with standard techniques [20]. It is in cases when the mandibular height is between 10 and 19 mm and particularly in cases where mandibular height is less than 10 mm that a load-bearing reconstruction and bone grafting needs to be considered [20]. Condylar fractures demonstrate premature occlusion ipsilateral to the fracture and an open bite contralateral to the fracture. Additionally, the mandible is noted to swing ipsilateral to the fracture when opening the mouth. In bilateral condylar fractures, an anterior open bite is seen with premature occlusion of the molars bilaterally. The gingival mucosa, the floor of mouth mucosa, and the remainder of the oral cavity mucosa should be carefully assessed. Mandibular fractures can commonly present with floor of mouth hematomas and gingival lacerations. Exposed bone should be noted. Sensation within the distribution of the mental nerve should be assessed to document this preoperatively. Bilateral mandibular body fractures can potentially lead to airway compromise and should be carefully assessed on physical exam. Computed tomography of the craniofacial skeleton with three-dimensional reconstruction allows for a precise evaluation of mandibular fractures and associated craniomaxillofacial injuries. Careful examination of the entire mandible on imaging studies is important given that multiple contralateral injuries are a frequent pattern of injury, with angle/contralateral body and symphyseal/contralateral condylar fractures being the most common combinations [36]. Double unilateral fractures are much less common; however, they pose a particular challenge in obtaining proper reduction given the floating nature of the segment of bone between the two fractures [36]. Preoperative and perioperative antibiotics are typically administered in mandible fractures, with the utility of postoperative antibiotics being less clear [20, 37].

## Instrument/Equipment

- Plates
- Screws
- Drill
- Drill bits
- Screwdrivers
- Drill guide
- Depth gauge
- Templates
- Plate benders
- Plate cutters
- Transbuccal instrumentation
- Bone holding forceps
- Fracture reduction forceps

## Surgical Technique

When open or endoscopic reduction with internal fixation is undertaken, there are a variety of approaches that can be utilized. Prior to internal fixation, arch bars are applied, and the patient is placed into premorbid occlusion. For symphyseal and parasymphyseal fractures, a transoral approach is most commonly employed utilizing a gingivobuccal sulcus incision located within the mobile gingiva approximately 10 mm from the junction of the mobile and attached gingiva to allow for closure. A transoral approach utilizing the gingivobuccal sulcus incision can also be utilized for mandibular body fractures with careful attention to preserving the mental nerve as it exits the mandible near the interspace of the premolars. For more posteriorly located mandibular body fractures, a small facial incision with a transbuccal trocar may be necessary to place the more posteriorly located screws in the proper trajectory.

The endoscopic approach has been shown to be an efficient and effective route to allow for the reduction and internal fixation of condylar process fractures while also obviating the need for large facial or neck incisions [29, 33]. Angulated screws and screwdrivers can avoid the need for any facial or neck incisions [29, 33]. A vertical incision is made following the anterior border of the ascending ramus erring this incision on the lingual surface of the ramus to facilitate soft tissue retraction laterally [29]. Subperiosteal dissection is then performed to widely expose the fracture [29]. The 30- and 70-degree endoscopes can then be placed into the optical cavity to assess the fracture [29, 30]. Reduction is performed, and this can be done by carving a silastic block that is cut to a vertical dimension of the overlap of the proximal and distal segments [29, 30, 33]. Once the fracture is reduced, a miniplate is then applied, and fixation is performed with either transbuccal trocar placement or with angulated screws and drills [29, 33].

The submandibular, retromandibular, and preauricular approaches are the open surgical techniques most commonly utilized when managing mandibular fractures. The preauricular approach affords excellent access to the condylar head and neck and is also useful in cases of medial condylar displacement [30, 31]. A preauricular incision is made extending from the superior pole of the helix to the inferior aspect of the tragus, and dissection is carried forth down through the superficial temporoparietal fascia and deep temporal fascia to the lateral aspect of the zygomatic arch [30]. Care must be taken to avoid injury to the superficial temporal vessels and the auriculotemporal nerve. The temporal branch of the facial nerve crosses the zygomatic arch between 8 and 35 mm anterior to the external auditory canal [31]. The superficial layer of the deep temporal fascial is contiguous with the periosteum of the zygomatic arch and can be elevated in the subperiosteal plane to protect the temporal branch of the facial nerve [30, 31]. Dissection then proceeds anteriorly to expose the articular eminence and the TMJ capsule, and dissection can proceed inferiorly to expose the condylar neck, although this soft tissue retraction does create the possibility of a traction injury to the facial nerve [31].

The submandibular approach affords excellent access to the mandibular body, angle, ramus, and condylar base fractures. An incision is made in a skin crease approximately 2 cm below the angle of the mandible. Subplatysmal flaps are then elevated, ensuring the superior elevation proceeds to the inferior border of the mandible. To protect the marginal mandibular nerve, it is either identified and protected, or the superficial layer of the deep cervical fascia can be elevated off the submandibular gland and retracted superiorly, thereby protecting the marginal mandibular nerve as it courses through this fascial layer [28, 30, 31]. The inferior border of the mandible is then exposed, the masseter is sharply divided, and subperiosteal dissection is performed widely, exposing the fracture.

The retromandibular approach affords excellent access to the ramus, condylar base, and condylar neck. There is limited access to medially displaced condylar segments [31]. An incision is made immediately posterior to the ramus, extending from just inferior to the lobule to the angle of the mandible. Dissection is carried forth down through the thin posterior extension of the platysma and the parotid capsule. Blunt dissection through the parotid is then performed parallel to the course of the facial nerve and with the utilization of a facial nerve monitor [30, 31]. Once the posterior aspect of the ramus is encountered, the masseter and periosteum are incised, and a subperiosteal dissection is performed, widely exposing the fracture [31]. An alternative to dissection through the parotid capsule is lifting the parotid tail from the sternocleidomastoid muscle to access the ramus or to identify the facial nerve using the standard parotidectomy technique [31].

## Postoperative Management

Although a clear benefit of postoperative antibiotics is lacking in the literature, it is a controversial topic and many surgeons do routinely prescribe postoperative antibiotics [20, 37]. Maintaining adequate oral hygiene postoperatively is important, and 0.1% chlorhexidine rinses can be prescribed for 7 days to help with this [20]. Maintaining patients in postoperative maxillomandibular fixation had been routine and is still routine at some centers for all mandibular fractures. However, in patients with noncomminuted fractures of the angle, body, parasymphysis, and symphysis, who undergo open reduction internal fixation, a period of postoperative maxillomandibular fixation carries the disadvantages of gingival trauma, patient discomfort, aspiration risk, and delayed temporomandibular joint mobility without any benefit of improved outcomes [38]. Nonetheless, in certain cases with comminuted fractures or concomitant midface fractures, postoperative maxillomandibular fixation with wires may be necessary. If the arch bars are left in place at the close of the case, this typically necessitates a return to the operating room for removal, depending on surgeon and patient preferences. Early mobilization decreases the risks of temporomandibular joint dysfunction and ankylosis, as well as improves the patient's quality of life. Maxillomandibular fixation with elastics and postoperative jaw exercises are an important component of postoperative treatment in many condylar fractures.

Patients should be carefully followed for signs of infection, malunion, or nonunion. Patients with multiple fractures and patients who use tobacco, alcohol, and drugs are at increased risk of postoperative infection and nonunion [26, 39]. Occlusion, maximal mouth opening, and facial symmetry should be assessed. The suture lines should be inspected for breakdown and plate exposure.

## References

1. Boole JR, Holtel M, Amoroso P, Yore M. 5196 mandible fractures among 4381 active duty army soldiers, 1980 to 1998. Laryngoscope. 2001;111(10):1691–6.

2. Chrcanovic BR, Abreu MHNG, Freire-Maia B, Souza LN. 1454 mandibular fractures: a 3-year study in a hospital in Belo Horizonte, Brazil. J Craniomaxillofac Surg. 2012;40(2):116–23.
3. Mukerji R, Mukerji G, McGurk M. Mandibular fractures: historical perspective. Br J Oral Maxillofac Surg. 2006;44(3):222–8.
4. Gahhos F, Ariyan S. Facial fractures: Hippocratic management. Head Neck Surg. 1984;6(6):1007–13.
5. Siegert R, Weerda H. Immobilization of fractures of the facial skeleton: past and present. Facial Plast Surg. 1990;7(3):137–51.
6. Romm S. Thomas Brian Gunning and his splint. Plast Reconstr Surg. 1986;78(2):252–8.
7. Buitrago-Téllez CH, Audigé L, Strong B, Gawelin P, Hirsch J, Ehrenfeld M, et al. A comprehensive classification of mandibular fractures: a preliminary agreement validation study. Int J Oral Maxillofac Surg. 2008;37(12):1080–8.
8. Cornelius C-P, Audigé L, Kunz C, Rudderman R, Buitrago-Téllez CH, Frodel J, et al. The comprehensive AOCMF classification system: mandible fractures—level 2 tutorial. Craniomaxillofacial Trauma Reconstr. 2014;7(Suppl 1):S015–30.
9. Neff A, Cornelius C-P, Rasse M, Torre DD, Audigé L. The comprehensive AOCMF classification system: condylar process fractures—level 3 tutorial. Craniomaxillofacial Trauma Reconstr. 2014;7(Suppl 1):S044–58.
10. Cornelius C-P, Audigé L, Kunz C, Rudderman R, Buitrago-Téllez CH, Frodel J, et al. The comprehensive AOCMF classification system: mandible fractures—level 3 tutorial. Craniomaxillofacial Trauma Reconstr. 2014;7(Suppl 1):S031–43.
11. Lee T, Sawhney R, Ducic Y. Miniplate fixation of fractures of the symphyseal and parasymphyseal regions of the mandible: a review of 218 patients. JAMA Facial Plast Surg. 2013;15(2):121–5.
12. Collins CP, Pirinjian-Leonard G, Tolas A, Alcalde R. A prospective randomized clinical trial comparing 2.0-mm locking plates to 2.0-mm standard plates in treatment of mandible fractures. J Oral Maxillofac Surg. 2004;62(11):1392–5.
13. Ellis E. Is lag screw fixation superior to plate fixation to treat fractures of the mandibular symphysis? J Oral Maxillofac Surg. 2012;70(4):875–82.
14. Cabrini Gabrielli MA, Real Gabrielli MF, Marcantonio E, Hochuli-Vieira E. Fixation of mandibular fractures with 2.0-mm miniplates: review of 191 cases. J Oral Maxillofac Surg. 2003;61(4):430–6.
15. Bouloux GF, Chen S, Threadgill JMC. Small and large titanium plates are equally effective for treating mandible fractures. J Oral Maxillofac Surg. 2012;70(7):1613–21.
16. Luhr HG, Reidick T, Merten HA. Results of treatment of fractures of the atrophic edentulous mandible by compression plating: a retrospective evaluation of 84 consecutive cases. J Oral Maxillofac Surg. 1996;54(3):250–4; discussion 254–255.
17. Shokri T, Misch E, Ducic Y, Sokoya M. Management of complex mandible fractures. Facial Plast Surg. 2019;35(6):602–6.
18. Zide MF, Ducic Y. Fibula microvascular free tissue reconstruction of the severely comminuted atrophic mandible fracture—case report. J Craniomaxillofac Surg. 2003;31(5):296–8.
19. Ellis E. A prospective study of 3 treatment methods for isolated fractures of the mandibular angle. J Oral Maxillofac Surg. 2010;68(11):2743–54.
20. Arosarena O, Ducic Y, Tollefson TT. Mandible fractures: discussion and debate. Facial Plast Surg Clin North Am. 2012;20(3):347–63.
21. Fox AJ, Kellman RM. Mandibular angle fractures: two-miniplate fixation and complications. Arch Facial Plast Surg. 2003;5(6):464–9.
22. Kalfarentzos EF, Deligianni D, Mitros G, Tyllianakis M. Biomechanical evaluation of plating techniques for fixing mandibular angle fractures: the introduction of a new 3D plate approach. Oral Maxillofac Surg. 2009;13(3):139–44.
23. Champy M, Loddé JP, Schmitt R, Jaeger JH, Muster D. Mandibular osteosynthesis by miniature screwed plates via a buccal approach. J Maxillofac Surg. 1978;6(1):14–21.

24. de Oliveira JCS, Moura LB, de Menezes JDS, Gabrielli MAC, Pereira Filho VA, Hochuli-Vieira E. Three-dimensional strut plate for the treatment of mandibular fractures: a systematic review. Int J Oral Maxillofac Surg. 2018;47(3):330–8.
25. Ellis E, Throckmorton GS. Treatment of mandibular condylar process fractures: biological considerations. J Oral Maxillofac Surg. 2005;63(1):115–34.
26. Reddy L, Lee D, Vincent A, Shokri T, Sokoya M, Ducic Y. Secondary management of mandible fractures. Facial Plast Surg. 2019;35(6):627–32.
27. Dahlström L, Kahnberg KE, Lindahl L. 15 years follow-up on condylar fractures. Int J Oral Maxillofac Surg. 1989;18(1):18–23.
28. Sawhney R, Brown R, Ducic Y. Condylar fractures. Otolaryngol Clin North Am. 2013;46(5):779–90.
29. Ducic Y. Endoscopic treatment of subcondylar fractures. Laryngoscope. 2008;118(7):1164–7.
30. Vincent AG, Ducic Y, Kellman R. Fractures of the mandibular condyle. Facial Plast Surg. 2019;35(6):623–6.
31. Cranford J, Kadakia S, Sawhney R, Ducic Y. Contemporary issues in the open management of subcondylar fractures of the mandible. Facial Plast Surg. 2016;32(4):424–30.
32. Zide MF, Kent JN. Indications for open reduction of mandibular condyle fractures. J Oral Maxillofac Surg. 1983;41(2):89–98.
33. Schön R, Schramm A, Gellrich N-C, Schmelzeisen R. Follow-up of condylar fractures of the mandible in 8 patients at 18 months after transoral endoscopic-assisted open treatment. J Oral Maxillofac Surg. 2003;61(1):49–54.
34. Kazi AA, Lee TS, Vincent A, Sokoya M, Sheen D, Ducic Y. The role of external fixation in trauma and reconstruction of the mandible in the age of rigid fixation. Facial Plast Surg. 2019;35(6):614–22.
35. Buchbinder D. Treatment of fractures of the edentulous mandible, 1943 to 1993: a review of the literature. J Oral Maxillofac Surg. 1993;51(11):1174–80.
36. Cillo JE, Ellis E. Treatment of patients with double unilateral fractures of the mandible. J Oral Maxillofac Surg. 2007;65(8):1461–9.
37. Abubaker AO, Rollert MK. Postoperative antibiotic prophylaxis in mandibular fractures: a preliminary randomized, double-blind, and placebo-controlled clinical study. J Oral Maxillofac Surg. 2001;59(12):1415–9.
38. Saman M, Kadakia S, Ducic Y. Postoperative maxillomandibular fixation after open reduction of mandible fractures. JAMA Facial Plast Surg. 2014;16(6):410–3.
39. Furr AM, Schweinfurth JM, May WL. Factors associated with long-term complications after repair of mandibular fractures. Laryngoscope. 2006;116(3):427–30.

# Midface Trauma Reconstruction

# 24

David A. Rengifo, Alexander P. Simko, and Raja Sawhney

## Introduction/History

The maxillofacial region is one of the most critical areas of the human body, providing anterior protection for the cranium, housing critical nerves and muscles related to function and cosmesis, and creating much of the contour and appearance of the face. The prominent position of the area leaves it vulnerable to injury, with the industrialization of society only increasing the number of midface fractures worldwide. Most commonly, injuries are the result of blunt trauma, with the leading cause being traffic accidents, followed by falls and interpersonal violence [1]. Primary prevention focuses on public policy, such as traffic laws and sports guidelines, but nonetheless, midfacial trauma remains an issue. The successful treatment of these patients requires extensive anatomical and functional knowledge of the region.

The fracture types that exist in the midface vary in severity and potential complications. The first widely developed classification system was published by Rene Le Fort in 1901 and is often still used today. Le Fort utilized traumatic forces to the midface of cadaver skulls to understand the transmission of force to various planes of the face and the resulting fractures. Reconstruction of the midface region was first successfully performed by Sir Harold Gillies, an Otolaryngologist often referred to as the "father of modern plastic surgery." He pioneered many novel techniques in the first half of the twentieth century that are still used today, such as the use of pedicled flaps. Developments in the mid and latter centuries include advances

D. A. Rengifo (✉) · R. Sawhney
Department of Otolaryngology-Head and Neck Surgery, University of Florida, Gainesville, FL, USA
e-mail: David.Rengifo@ent.ufl.edu

A. P. Simko
University of Florida School of Medicine, Gainesville, FL, USA
e-mail: ap.simko@ufl.edu



F. Sokoya, A. G. Vincent (eds.), *Manual of Head and Neck Reconstruction*,
https://doi.org/10.1007/978-3-031-65999-7_24

in internal fixation via suspension wires, as well as plates and screws in fracture treatment. Advancements in imaging grant better characterization of fractures, thereby allowing more precise preoperative planning. Computed tomography (CT) imaging is now the mainstay in facial fracture assessment. With a proper multidisciplinary team approach and thorough examination and planning, modern midface trauma reconstruction can often reestablish normal function and form.

## Anatomy

The midface contains several important structures and serves as a buffer between the external environment and the vital contents of the cranial skull (Fig. 24.1). Its frame allows for suitable protection of the brain by creating a cushion and transmitting forces via bony structures to reduce overall traumatic impact. Nahum studied the force necessary to generate midface fractures, concluding that these forces are relatively low in comparison to those necessary to create mandible and frontal sinus fractures [2].

The maxilla is composed of a central body that houses the pneumatized maxillary antrum, as well as the four processes:

1. Zygomatic
2. Frontal
3. Palatine

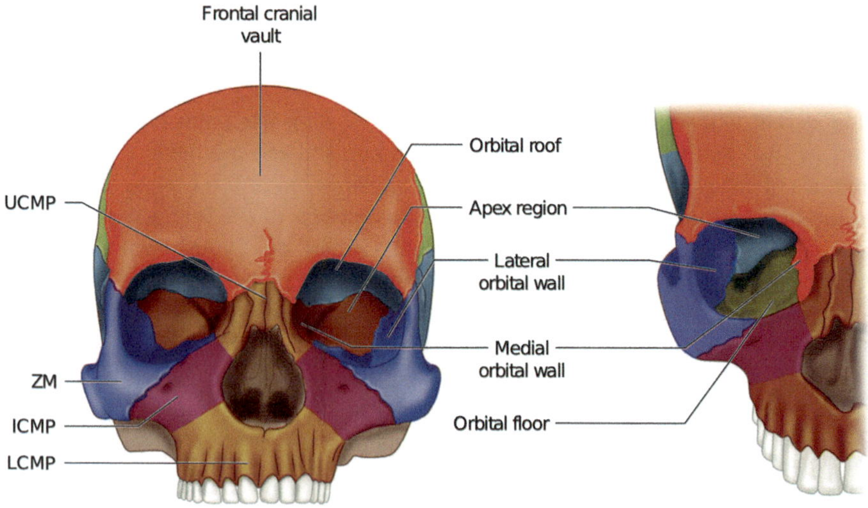


**Fig. 24.1** Skull Anatomy with a focus on the bones that are routinely fractured in maxillary trauma. LCMP, ICMP and UCMP refer to the AO CMF fracture classification charts of the skull base and cranial vault and be helpful in describing fracture location. *ZM* Zygomatic bone, *LCMP* Lower Central Midface Partition, *ICMP* Intermediate Central Midface Partition, *UCMP* Upper Central Midface Partition

4. Alveolar

The zygomatic bone is considered to have a central malar body and three distinct processes:

1. Temporal—Zygomatic arch is created by the articulation of this process to the temporal bone, which is responsible for the maintenance of the anterior projection of the malar eminence. The arch is also an attachment for the masseter muscle and the deep temporal fascia. The frontal branch of the facial nerve follows a course that is intimately associated with the anterior zygomatic arch. The temporomandibular joint and coronoid process are situated deep in the arch.
2. Orbital—Articulates with the orbital plate of the maxilla, forming the floor of the orbit. It is no surprise that nearly 40% of patient with zygoma fractures involving the orbital process have concomitant intraocular injury.
3. Maxillary—Inferior-medial articulation with the maxilla and forms part of the anterolateral wall of the maxillary antrum.

The malar body is the strongest portion of the zygoma. It also forms an important component of the lateral buttress. Traumatic disruption to the zygomatic complex and lateral buttress often creates an inferior-medial rotation of the zygomatic bone. This rotation is theorized to be the result of displacement by the masseter muscle [2].

It is imperative to understand the relationship between the maxilla, mandible, and skull base, with the knowledge of the facial buttresses (Fig. 24.2). There are four vertical buttresses, which act as supporting pillars for facial form and function. These buttresses represent the paths of a load of distribution for the powerful vertical forces of mastication. There are three paired buttresses:

1. Nasomaxillary (medial)—extending from the dentoalveolar arch near the canine region, along the pyriform aperture, and ends at the medial orbital rim and frontomaxillary suture.
2. Zygomaticomaxillary (lateral)—begins from the region of the maxillary first molar, running superiorly through the body of the zygoma, and ends at the lateral wall of the orbit and the frontozygomatic suture.
3. Pterygomaxillary (posterior)—begins at the maxillary tuberosity and extends through the pyramidal process of the palatine bone, medial plate of the pterygoid bone, and terminates at the basis of the sphenoid.
4. Additionally, there is a single midline vertical buttress termed the nasoseptum, which includes the crista galli, vomer, cartilaginous septum, and perpendicular plate of the ethmoid bone.

The alveolus, hard palate, infraorbital bar, and supraorbital bar make up the three horizontal buttresses. Of note, the alveolus is dependent upon the patient's dentition. Edentulousness predisposes the patient to a higher risk of traumatic disruption due to alveolar atrophy. Upon traumatic events, disruption of the vertical and horizontal buttresses leads to a release of the maxilla from its bony attachments. This

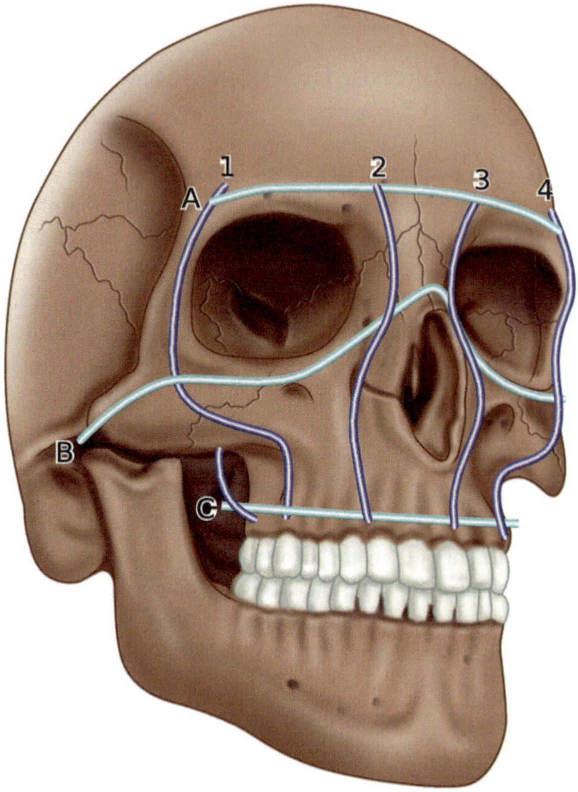


**Fig. 24.2** Vertical and Horizontal Buttress of the midface

disruption results in a pull of the maxilla in a posterior-inferior direction due to the forces of the medial and lateral pterygoid muscles, resulting in the commonly seen anterior open bite deformity.

Several components of the neurovascular supply to the midface are important to recognize and identify when planning for a safe surgical approach or to understand a patient's symptoms. The greater palatine artery and nerve emerge from the junction of the hard and soft palate and supply the mucosal and bone of the hard palate. Fractures of the orbital floor or anterior aspect of the maxilla may result in paresthesia to the anterior teeth due to injury of the anterior superior alveolar artery. Fractures of the posterior maxilla may result in molar paresthesia because of injury to the posterior superior alveolar artery and nerve. Trauma to the orbital floor may result in infraorbital nerve injury, which can present as numbness and pain in the entire ipsilateral cheek, ala of the nose, and upper lip.

## Classification

Le Fort's proposed classification system was published in 1901. His findings subsequently set the qualifications for different types of midface fractures, depending on severity [3].

Three patterns emerged from Le Fort's studies, termed Le Fort I, Le Fort II, and Le Fort III fractures (Fig. 24.3).

- Le Fort I
  - Clinical correlate of a floating maxilla
    - Horizontal fracture in the anterior maxilla that occurs above the palate and alveolus and includes the nasal septum.
    - Results in separation of the palate from the maxilla.
    - The fracture line passes along the nasal floor, pyriform aperture, canine fossa, and lateral maxillary wall. Occasionally involves the inferior aspect of pterygoid plates.
- Le Fort II
  - Characterized by a separation of the maxilla, nasal bones, and the nasal septum from the skull and lateral midface.

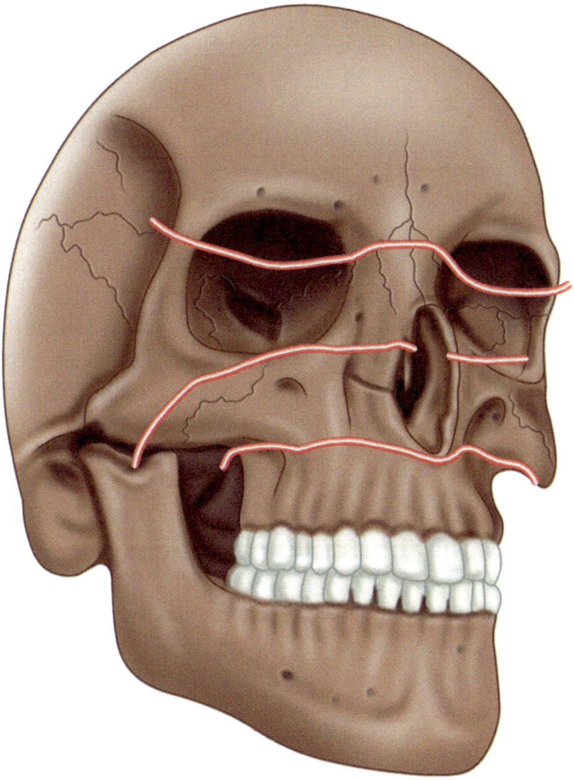

**Fig. 24.3** Le Fort fracture patterns

Fracture line follows the frontomaxillary suture, extending through the infraorbital margin to the zygomatic-alveolar crest.
Fracture line also courses around the maxillary tuberosity into the pterygoid process of the sphenoid bone and travels to the perpendicular plate of the palatine bone.

- Le Fort III
  - Results in craniofacial disjunction.
    Characterized by complete separation of the midface from the cranium.
    Fracture line follows the medial wall, floor, and the lateral wall of the orbit between the nasofrontal suture and the zygomatic-frontal suture.
    Fracture incorporates the zygomatic arches laterally and the ethmoid, lamina perpendicularis of the palatine bone, and pterygopalatine fossa medially.

This system is still widely used today, though only a minority of current maxillofacial fractures fit exactly with the initially described patterns. Le Fort acknowledged that his three fracture patterns often occurred in combination and often associated with several unclassified fractures. Thus, common nomenclature includes pure Le Fort fractures, as well as non-Le Fort fractures, such as palatal parasagittal, medial maxillary, and anterior maxillary fractures. The prevalence of non-Le Fort fractures may be due to the high forces that are more often involved in injuries in the modern world, as motor vehicles and industrial machinery have become commonplace. Le Fort's classification provides a solid foundation from which to organize a treatment plan; however, the surgeon must keep in mind that these classifications do not provide a full description of the degree of fracture displacement and comminution.

There are no standard classification systems for zygomatic complex fractures because of the impractical and inadequate quality of previously proposed classifications. The classification proposed by Jackson, however, is the more clinically relevant system that the authors of this chapter prefer. This classification encompasses four types of zygomatic fractures: (1) Nondisplaced that requires no surgical treatment, (2) Localized segmental fractures, requiring exposure and direct fixation, (3) Low velocity displaced tripod fractures, requiring simple elevation or direct exposure and rigid fixation, (4) High velocity comminuted tripod fractures, requiring wide surgical exposure and rigid fixation at multiple points [4].

## Indications and Contraindications

Surgical intervention and reconstruction may be necessary if there is a loss of function or obvious deformity. The absolute indication for surgical intervention of the midface is persistent diplopia and other vision changes that can be confirmed to be secondary to bony trauma. Secondary indications include malocclusion, trismus, airway concerns, and cosmetic deformities. Patients with significant medical co-morbidities and high surgical risk can also be offered observation and no treatment, in the case were major visual changes are not exhibited.

## Clinical Assessment

Prior to initiating any operative planning, it is imperative for the surgeon and their team to ensure surgical safety. This includes assessment of acute airway issues or other injuries sustained at the same time as facial injuries. It is not unusual for patients to suffer from traumatic brain injuries secondary to the same mechanism of injury that caused facial fractures. Secondary medical issues, especially those requiring long-term anticoagulation or those with a high propensity to cause poor healing, including tobacco abuse and diabetes, should be evaluated and treated appropriately.

Diagnosis and clinical assessment of midfacial trauma is mandatory to assure success in management despite the availability of radiographic studies. Assessment of neurologic function and cervical spine precede the evaluation of the fractures for operative intervention.

The examination should include the mechanism of injury, facial analysis to evaluate infraorbital ecchymosis or edema as well as changes in facial height and width, assessment of cerebrospinal fluid rhinorrhea, and evaluation of occlusal status. Occlusion tends to be dictated by fracture orientation. In the setting of transverse-style fractures of the midface, the clinical exam may reveal a retro-displaced maxilla, premature contact of the molars, and subsequent open bite deformities. Vertical fractures through the hard palate classically show crossbite on clinical exam. As part of the examination, palatal mobility should be assessed. This is performed by grasping the maxilla between the thumb and index finger and rocking the maxilla in a side-to-side and anterior-posterior direction.

The assessment of zygoma fractures involves the evaluation of malar projection, lateral canthus position, telecanthus and pseudo-telecanthus, tenderness along the frontozygomatic suture, trismus, lateral subconjunctival hemorrhage, paresthesia of midface and lip. Additionally, the elicitation of severe pain or decreased mobility when asking the patient to move their jaw in the direction away from the suspected side of trauma may key the surgeon to suspect severe displacement caused by a zygomaticomaxillary fracture due to impingement of the ipsilateral coronoid process.

Le Fort fractures of the midface can significantly affect the natural position of the patient's dentition, and therefore, foregoing repair of these fractures will interfere with mastication. Often, zygomatic fractures are reduced for cosmetic reasons;

however, these fractures may cause trismus and difficulty chewing due to impingement on the temporalis muscle. Additionally, zygomatic fractures may cause globe dysfunction and malposition, given the contribution of the zygoma to the bony orbit.

While this chapter does not include orbital reconstruction, ophthalmological examination is an absolute necessity prior to any operative intervention of the midface. The assessment of both the surgeon and ophthalmology will encompass the appropriate preoperative evaluation. Visual assessment should include measurement of orbital pressures as well as ruling out ocular and retinal injury by ophthalmology. Extraocular eye movements need to be assessed to define any concerns for entrapment and/or nerve injury.

## Preoperative Planning

The appropriate first step to achieve proper reconstruction consists of an in-depth evaluation of radiographical studies. 1.5–3 mm fine-cut CT scans are the standard for imaging evaluation of the midface. Imaging should extend from the cranial apex to the inferior edge of the mandible. This is important both for thorough assessment of the patient as well as setting up intraoperative navigation at the time of surgery. Assessment in all three radiographic planes should be performed. Added guidance can be gleaned from three-dimensional renderings of the CT scans which are becoming more widely available. These reconstructed CT images are excellent at examining the zygomatic complex, especially when there are comminuted fractures, which can disorientate when assessed in a single plane. The 3D renderings fall short when examining the orbit. Because of the thinness of the bone, there are often gaps in the image that can be mistaken for bone loss or fracture that are artifacts.

The order of reduction should also be planned during the imaging review. In the setting of multiple fractures, less distorted fractures should be addressed first to facilitate the reduction of the more severe fractures. Bilateral fractures should be addressed similarly, as the reduction of the less distorted side will facilitate the reconstruction of the more involved contralateral trauma.

## Instrument/Equipment Setup

To have success in midface reconstruction while decreasing the patient's risk under general anesthesia, the surgical team must make sure the appropriate instrumentation is available prior to surgery.

The room setup should ideally include the bed rotated 180° from anesthesia and the patient's imaging readily available. We have found surgical adjuncts such as the use of intraoperative endoscopy and navigation useful in many cases. The use of such instrumentation can require a unique setup as well as significant space within the operating room, which needs to be accounted for. Further, the use of intraoperative imaging, including CT scanners, has been invaluable, especially in complex cases. In many institutions, this modality is in high demand, and therefore, brought into the operating room when needed during a case. The placement of the OR table to expedite this process should be considered. Additionally, if preoperative planning of screws and plates has been performed, these diagrams should be in the room and available for the surgeon to evaluate during the entire procedure.

Nursing and scrub technicians should have the following available:

- Dilute betadine face prep.
- Local anesthetic.
- Items to protect the eye: lacrilube, corneal shield, erythromycin ophthalmic ointment.
- Peridex oral solution to adequately clean the oral cavity.
- Maxillo-mandibular fixation instruments of surgeon's choice.
- Trauma midface set that includes the following:
  - Oral retractor tray.
  - Rowe forceps.
  - McKesson bite block.
  - Army/Navy retractors.
  - Minnesota retractors.
  - Periosteal Elevator—(#9 Elevator).
  - Right angle retractor.
  - Drill and Irrigation—run at 20,000 rpms.
  - Carroll-Girard screw (*figure of Carroll Girard*).
  - Midface plates with associated screws.
  - Infraorbital instruments, which include Desmarres retractor, Jaeger lid plate retractor, as well as orbital floor plates.

## Surgical Approaches to the Midface

As with any facial trauma, care should be given to establishing and maintaining the airway. Most midface injuries do not result in malocclusion or require the need for mandibular-maxillary fixation (MMF); therefore, traditional oropharyngeal intubation is adequate. In cases where MMF may be necessary, transnasal intubation may be required. In these cases, assessment of any skull base injury is crucial. When airway instability is a major concern, the anesthesia and surgical teams must determine the best course of action. This may include fiberoptic transnasal intubation, transcutaneous submental intubation, or tracheostomy.

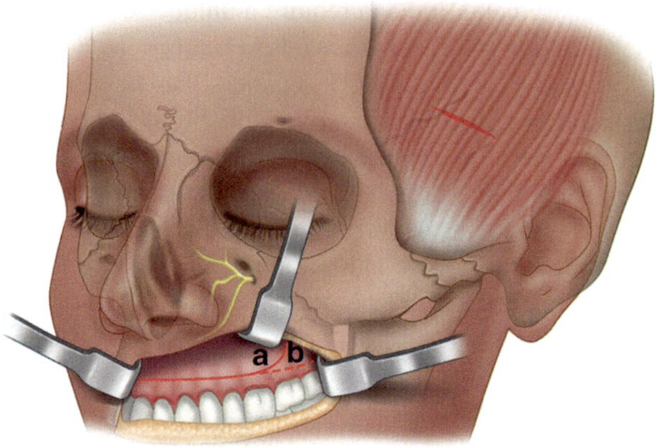


**Fig. 24.4** (**a**) maxillary vestibular approach. It can be extended (**b**) for greater lateral exposure. It is important to maintain at least a centimeter cuff of mucosa from the gingiva to assist with closure

All patients with midface fractures should receive prophylactic antibiotics since most of these fractures are considered to be open, and mucosal disruption is either caused by the injury or the surgical approaches. Often, intravenous steroids can aid in perioperative edema that is commonly encountered.

Prior to discussing the operative techniques addressing bony reconstruction, the surgeon must determine the appropriate incisions and approaches to the midface. When available, existing lacerations often provide the most direct approach to the bony skeleton.

The maxillary vestibular approach is the most common approach to the midface (Fig. 24.4). Local anesthetic/vasoconstrictor is injected submucosally, just above the mucogingival junction, to mitigate bleeding. After adequate time for vasoconstriction, the incision is made along the gingival mucosa, maintaining no more than a centimeter cuff of the mucosa. This provides enough tissue to close the incision at the completion of the case but does not limit exposure of inferior maxillary fractures or the ability to place reconstructive plates. The incision is carried down to the subperiosteal plane. From there, the soft tissue of the cheek is elevated in a subperiosteal plane. As dissection is carried superiorly, identification and protection of the infra-orbital nerve becomes important. Given that the nerve exists along the vertical mid-pupillary line, we routinely elevate the malar tissue by creating two pockets. One, aimed directly towards the most medial aspect of the infra-orbital rim which exposes the medial buttress. The other is along the most lateral aspect of the rim, which exposes the lateral buttress. Care is taken during elevation not to slip more than 1–2 mm superior to the rim edge to avoid injury of the globe. Once the elevator is slightly over the rim, the inferior aspect of the elevator is rotated superiorly, while the superior edge of the elevator remains fixed and acts as a fulcrum on the rim. When medial and lateral pockets are completely dissected in this fashion, most of the soft tissue between the pockets is also elevated, and the infraorbital nerve and foramen will come into view with minimal risk of injury. A right-angle clamp is

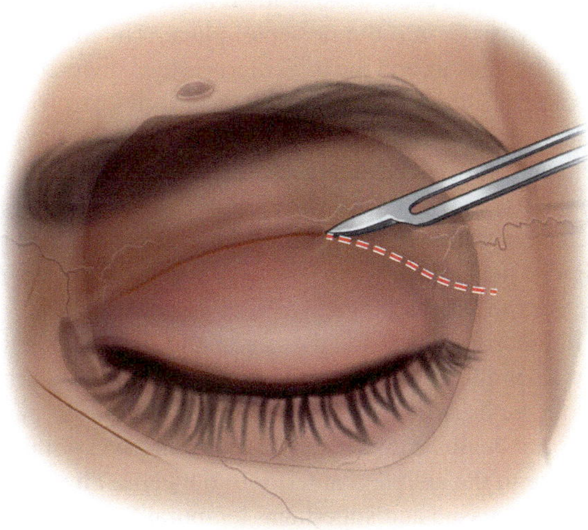

**Fig. 24.5** Lateral blepharoplasty incision. Placed within a natural skin rhytid, this incision can be used to expose the zygomatic-frontal suture line

then used to dissect the soft tissue sitting just superior to the infraorbital nerve. This will expose the mid portion of the infraorbital rim and, quite often, any infraorbital rim fractures. In our hands, this has allowed for assessment and, at times, plating of this fracture line without the need of a periorbital incision.

The transconjunctival approach is still useful when reduction and fixation of the orbital floor or infraorbital rim are required. This is our preference of surgical approaches to the region. The details of the approach, as well as other transcutaneous approaches to the orbit, are discussed in detail in the orbital trauma chapter.

The upper blepharoplasty incision (Fig. 24.5) is invaluable when assessing and treating zygomatico-frontal (ZF) fractures. It can also be used to evaluate the zygomatico-sphenoid (ZS) suture line within the orbit. The incision allows the surgeon to determine If the zygomatic complex has been elevated and rotated back into place appropriately. If the ZMC complex is under-elevated or under-rotated, an excess in overall orbital volume will remain, leading to postoperative enophthalmos and dystopia. These are two of the most common postoperative misalignments encountered, especially early in a surgeon's career. The upper blepharoplasty incision heals exceptionally well, so we have utilized this approach ever-increasingly. Prior to beginning the approach, the cornea can be protected with temporary tarsorrhaphy or corneal shields. The incision is designed in the lateral half of the upper lid in a curvilinear fashion and can be extended into the natural lateral lid rhytids, also known as the crow's foot. After this marking is completed, the planned incision can be injected with local anesthetic with vasoconstrictor. After adequate time has been given to local anesthesia with a vasoconstrictor, a 15-blade is used to incise the skin and subcutaneous tissue in a medial to lateral direction. Once the orbicularis oculi muscle is exposed, a slit should be made in the lateral aspect to allow the introduction of scissors into the preseptal plane. The dissection continues medially underneath the muscle, and the orbicularis is then divided, which leaves the orbital septum intact. The musculocutaneous flap is then sharply elevated in a medial-to-lateral fashion towards the superolateral rim to expose the periosteum. The periosteum is then sharply divided along the superolateral orbital rim. Periosteal elevators are used to expose the lateral rim and orbit. This allows for assessment of the ZF suture line and any fractures in the area. Dissection can then be carried into the orbit in the subperiosteal plane. As the dissection proceeds deeper into the orbit, the ZS suture line is exposed.

Indirect approaches to the zygomatic arch include the transoral (Keen) approach, as well as the temporal (Gillies) approach. These are useful when treating a pure zygomatic arch fracture without instability of the zygomatic complex. The Gillies approach begins with a 2-cm temporal incision within the hairline, designed 2.5 cm superior to the arch and anterior to the helix. Sharp dissection continues in the subcutaneous tissue and superficial temporal fascia and terminates at the deep portion of the deep temporal fascia. The deep temporal fascia is then incised, and a sharp elevator is introduced deep to the temporalis fascia and moved in the windshield wiper motion until it sits medial to the zygomatic arch. Dissection under the superficial layer of the deep temporalis fascial avoids injury to the frontal branch of the facial nerve. An elevator of choice can then be introduced for the reduction of the fracture. The surgeon should not use the squamous portion of the temporal bone as a fulcrum.

The Keen approach begins by design of a 2-cm lateral maxillary vestibular incision and the mucosa is incised with electrocautery or a scalpel blade. The elevator of choice is then introduced and advanced towards the medial aspect of the zygomatic arch fracture that needs reduction. We have found that in the majority of cases, a Keen approach enables adequate reduction without leaving a scar on the skin or risking injury to the temporal branch of the facial nerve. In rare cases, the limited leverage obtained by the keen approach is not enough to reduce the fracture. In such cases, the Gilles approach may be necessary. In both of these indirect approaches, palpation will confirm the appropriate reduction. We have found the use of intraoperative imaging beneficial in confirming reduction.

The coronal approach is rarely used in the setting of midface reconstruction unless there are severe fractures of the zygomatic arch or trauma is in conjunction with panfacial fractures. In these cases, this approach is used to treat the zygomatic arch or the ZF suture line via a direct approach. The incision should be designed to sit several centimeters posterior to the hairline . Care should be given to the regression of the natural hairline with time, which may lead to exposure of a once-hidden scar. The incision is extended inferiorly, either pre- or postauricular, to expose the zygomatic arch. Hair preparation and design of incision (zigzag, bow, wave pattern) should be performed per the surgeon's preference. Local anesthetic with vasoconstrictor is then injected into the subgaleal plane, and after the appropriate time for effect is allowed, the initial incision is made with a scalpel or electrocautery. We routinely utilize bipolar cautery for hemostasis of the skin edge of the coronal flap.

Studies have shown possible alopecia with the use of hemostatic clips. After hemostasis, the incision is carried down to the supraperiosteal plane. We routinely elevate a pericranial flap as part of our dissection. If not utilized during the case, the pericranial flap can be sutured back in place for future use. We often raise the coronal flap and pericranial flap as a single unit after making the lateral and inferior cuts of the pericranial flap. The combo flap is then raised from posterior to anterior in the subperiosteal plane as dissection is carried anteriorly until the superior orbital rims are encountered. Care should be taken to protect the supraorbital and supratrochlear neurovascular units. Dissection can be carried anteriorly along the midline down over the root of the nose. The superior aspects of the orbits can also be entered with this approach if the supraorbital complex enters the area through a foramen; a chisel and blunt dissection may be required to free them from the foramen and elevate the soft tissue unit of the coronal flap.

After carrying the incision down to the supraperiosteal plane, the surgeon should begin the lateral component of the coronal flap just superficial to the temporalis fascia and continue towards the level of the zygomatic arch. Soft tissue elevation proceeds anteriorly and inferiorly along this plane until the superficial temporal fat pad is seen through the superficial layer of the deep temporal fascia. The fascia is transected at a 45-degree angle (in the same direction that the temporal branch of the facial nerve runs) to enter the fat pad. The dissection is carried antero-inferiorly to the arch by staying immediately deep to the superficial layer of the temporalis fascia. Staying in this plane will protect the temporal branch of the facial nerve. Care is given to limit trauma to the fat pad itself, thereby limiting post-operative temporal hallowing, which is caused by devascularization of the fat pad. If the reconstruction necessitates the maximum midface exposure, the lateral subperiosteal dissection can be continued from the lateral orbital rim downward over the body of the zygoma. This exposure allows for direct reduction of the lateral half of the orbital floor. The exposure necessary to reach the upper midface, medial orbital wall, infratemporal fossa, temporomandibular joint, and mandibular condyle/ramus is covered in other chapters of this text.

## Site-Specific Surgical Techniques

1. *Isolated ZMC*
2. *Le Fort I*
3. *Le Fort II*

### Zygomaticomaxillary Complex Fractures

While there are always multiple fractures with any zygomatic complex fractures, a significant portion does not require multiple approaches. Often, depending on the mechanism of injury, the force applied to the complex causes it to rotate medially, posteriorly, and inferiorly without vertical separation of the ZF suture line or significant disruption of the orbital floor. Often, this can be determined preoperatively through imaging and physical exam. In simple, straightforward injuries, the appropriate reduction can often be achieved by simply disimpacting the complex and reducing it by rotating the zygomatic complex anteriorly and laterally through a transoral approach. In many cases, once the complex is reduced, it will not fall back to its injury position. We routinely utilize an elevator for reduction. After elevation of the soft tissue envelope through a vestibular incision, the elevator is passed through the comminuted bone of the anterior maxillary sinus into the sinus itself. The elevator edge is then placed against the most anterior lateral edge of the maxillary sinus. Then, either lifting the elevator or cantilevering it off the nonfractured portion of the maxilla, the ZMC complex can be rotated back into place. In these cases, often, a single reconstructive plate placed along the ZM suture line is enough to fixate the fracture.

After reduction and fixation, it is important to confirm that the ZF suture line is still in correct alignment/reduction. This can be assessed by digital palpation along the lateral orbital rim. If uncertain, then intraoperative imaging or direct assessment of the suture line through a lateral blepharoplasty incision is warranted. The other area that must be assessed is the orbital floor. It is possible that during the reduction of the ZMC complex, the orbital floor fracture has shifted and is now of a significant size that requires treatment or shift, causing the inferior rectus muscle of the orbit to become entrapped. We have found that it is possible to assess the quality of the orbital floor after reduction by placing an elevator within the maxillary sinus along the orbital floor and then gently pushing on the globe. The surgeon can feel if there is significant displacement of orbital contents. Similarly, an angled endoscope can be passed into the sinus for direct observation of the floor. Once again, if there is any doubt, imaging or direct surgical assessment and treatment may be performed. Finally, a forced duction test should be performed at the conclusion of any ZMC case to rule out entrapment of the inferior rectus muscle.

In cases that are more complex with significant disruption of the ZMC complex, a single transoral approach will not suffice. These cases typically require multiple approaches, including lateral upper blepharoplasty to assess the ZF and ZS suture lines and a transconjunctival approach to examine and treat the orbital floor and rim. We have found in complex cases, it is best to utilize multiple approaches early in the surgery to identify fractures, assess their reduction, and, when needed, fixate. When reducing the ZMC in multiple vectors at the same time, it is not uncommon to correctly reduce and fixate one fracture line while misaligning the other.

Once the soft tissue is elevated and the fractures are exposed, the surgeon needs to determine the best manner in which to reduce the fracture. As with simple ZMC fractures, reduction with periosteal elevator or bone hook, may be enough to reduce the complex and hold it place. In other cases, the amount of malar deformity is too substantial, or adequate torque to reduce the fracture cannot be generated by the use of an elevator or hook. In such cases, a Carroll-Girard screw can be used. The instrument can either be placed transcutaneous through a small stab incision through the overlying skin or the soft tissue can be elevated and the instrument placed through the trans vestibular incision. When utilizing a Carroll-Girard screw, it is important to place it in an area of adequate bone stock so that it does not become dislodged when manipulating the malar complex. Once placed, this instrument cannot be removed and replaced multiple times. A disadvantage of the Carroll-Girard screw is that its overall size and placement can often make it difficult to observe the skeleton directly behind the instrument. This can also make the placement of screws and plates markedly more difficult. To circumvent these drawbacks, we often utilize the placement of a longer midface or mandible recon screw in the same location as we would normally place the Carroll-Girard. The midface screw is not completely tightened, with a significant portion of the screw left exposed above the bone edge. A clamp or hemostat can then be used to grab onto the screw, and the new construct can be manipulated like the Carroll-Girard. The hemostat can also be removed or replaced depending on necessity.

It is not unusual in complex cases to find that the fractures remain mobile after reduction, making it difficult to maintain ZMC reduction in all directions while plating. As each fracture line is fixated, the amount of mobility in the other directions decreases, thereby making each subsequent reduction easier to hold in place. Unfortunately, it is quite easy to plate one fracture in appropriate reduction, only to find that the other fracture lines have shifted out of correct reduction, and that the plate that was placed, will not allow the rest of the complex to be reduced accurately. Therefore, the order of fixation that that the surgeon chooses has its own benefits and limitations. While each surgeon has an order that they prefer to fixate fractures, we find that with a mobile ZMC, we routinely fixate the ZF fracture first. By doing this, we have corrected the vertical height of the midface. Fixation of the ZF suture line first still allows manipulation of the ZMC in some directions. The medial portion of the complex can be rotated in the superior-inferior direction as well as in the anterior-posterior direction. This limited mobility lets us rotate the ZMC complex and reset the zygomatico-sphenoid (ZS) suture line correctly, thereby correcting the orbital volume. We do not find that the ZS suture line routinely needs fixation, though some surgeons prefer to place a small plate there. With the persistent mobility allowed by ZF fixation, we can also correctly reduce the infraorbital (IO) rim, which is the fracture line we fixate second. Finally, after confirming that the ZF, ZS, and IO lines are reduced correctly, we fixate the zygomatic maxillary (ZM) suture line. Of all the fracture lines, it is the easiest to access and plate. Also, slight malposition of the ZM has a limited impact on malar projection and overall appearance. We rarely find that the zygomatic arch (ZA) requires plating unless there is a significant palpable step-off noted on palpation. After fixation of the ZF, IO and ZM fractures, we then treat the orbital floor fracture if necessary. Occasionally, when there is significant comminution of the infraorbital rim along with an orbital floor fracture, we will next place an orbital floor plate that extends over the rim to treat both the floor and IO areas simultaneously.

## Le Fort I Fractures

Le Fort I fracture treatment aims to restore normal occlusion and vertical height to the midface. Treatment begins by confirming occlusion. If there is no malocclusion, then the patient is placed in maxilla-mandibular fixation (MMF) prior to performing a vestibular incision. This is done so that the reduction of the midface fractures does not alter the patient's occlusion. When the patient does not easily go back into occlusion, reduction of the maxilla may be required. Often, this can be done with a simple periosteal elevator after exposure of the fracture lines. In cases where greater traumatic forces were applied to the maxilla, Rowe disimpaction forceps may be required to mobilize the maxilla prior to MMF utilization. After occlusion is reestablished with MMF and the fractures are exposed, stabilization is required. While all four vertical buttresses can be fixated, a minimum of two are required so that the maxilla does not shift or rotate when the patient chews. When placing midface plates, at least two screws must be placed on either side of the fracture line. L- or T-shaped plates are very useful in this area because they allow the placement of enough screws along the inferior aspect of the fracture while simultaneously avoiding the tooth roots. If there is bone loss within the vertical buttress, bone grafts should be used. Bridging gaps with plate fixation alone may lead to an alteration of the achieved occlusion or plate exposure. Generally, if bone grafting is not required and when reduction is rigid, the surgeon may elect to discontinue MMF at the end of the case.

## Le Fort II Fractures

Le Fort II fracture reconstruction begins with the sequence as a Le Fort I fracture; however, the surgeon may need to expose the orbital rim and floor. The rim may be repaired with low-profile miniplates, and bone loss can be addressed via bone grafting to avoid cosmetic deformities. The reconstruction of the orbital floor is further explained in the orbital trauma chapter of this text. In cases where there are bilateral midface fractures, we once again address occlusion first. From there, treatment begins on the side of the face that is less comminuted and, therefore, easier to correctly reduce and fixate fracture. As variables become reestablished, they can be used to help confirm the correct reduction on the more comminuted side. Minimizing the number of variables gives the best chance of a successful outcome.

## Pan Facial Fractures

Determining the order of reduction and fixation varies greatly from case to case in pan facial fractures. There is no definitive order of reconstruction. At best, general guidelines can be given. Function is the main concern, and therefore, reestablishing occlusion when possible is paramount. From there, the literature describes various directional reconstructions, such as a bottom-to-top or inside-to-out reconstruction, for example. As with bilateral midface fractures, after establishing occlusion, we start with the areas of least comminution and move on to progressively more complex areas. Experience also teaches us to monitor for common mistakes such as over-widening of the lateral face. This can be caused by something as seemingly innocuous as overly curving the zygomatic arches, which, despite their name, are mostly a straight structure in the anterior-posterior direction. Beyond just falling back on previous experience, the use of modern technology has made these exceptionally tough cases easier. Liberal utilization of intraoperative navigation and imaging allows the surgical team to assess their work in real time and adjust quickly. Ever increasing ease of use and application of surgical planning software with patient specific hardware is quickly taking the guesswork out of these cases and optimizing outcomes.

## Pediatric Midface Fracture Management

Midface fractures in the pediatric population, while uncommon, are often the result of blunt trauma from sports injuries, falls, transportation incidents, and assault and tend to occur in the older pediatric population. The pediatric facial bones have more elasticity and cartilage framework when compared to the adult facial skeleton. Also, late aeration of the maxillary sinus, along with unerupted teeth in younger children, act as buttresses and limit displaced fracture occurrence. The majority of ZMC fractures occur with limited displacement and are best treated with observation and a soft diet. Fractures of the zygomatic complex with significant displacement, comminution or diplopia should be treated with open reduction and internal fixation. Maxillary fractures with malocclusion are often best managed with a short course of MMF with elastics for no longer than 1–2 weeks. If the ZMC is significantly displaced, fixation with miniplates should be performed. Great care should be taken to avoid placing screws into the undescended tooth buds. There continues to be a lack of consensus regarding internal fixation plate management because of the controversial risk of halting facial growth. Some surgeons will elect to remove plates around 3–6 months after fixation, while others do not believe permanent plates significantly impact facial growth. Unfortunately, there is no significant evidence to sway the decision towards a standard of care. Literature does suggest for consideration of plate removal in the setting of highly complex and involved facial fractures, younger patients, and the presence of facial deformity. Absorbable plates are another option; however, there is no significant evidence to prove their superiority over non-absorbable plating. There is also a learning curve to their correct placement; therefore, they have not become the standard of care. Overall, a thorough discussion with the parents or guardians should include the potential risks and benefits of surgical management, absorbable and nonabsorbable plates, as well as temporary and permanent plating.

## Complications

Complications of midface trauma may result from sequelae of injury, delayed therapy, infection, and improper surgical technique. It is important to keep in mind that the severity of injury and incidence of complications have a direct relationship. Severely comminuted fractures may often exhibit associated bone loss, which further complicates appropriate fixation. The vast vascular supply of the midface aids in decreased risk of nonunion and infection, and the feared complication of osteomyelitis is thankfully rarely encountered due to this vascularity.

While nasal bone fractures are covered in more detail in other chapters of this text, it should be noted that they are the most common fractures of the midface. Minimal displacement of the nasal bones and septum may result in epistaxis, septal hematoma, cosmetic deformity, and nasal obstruction. Proper initial management and subsequent septo-rhinoplasty are important to address these risks. Postoperatively, residual deformities and continual nasal obstruction are the most common complications. Sufficient time to heal after initial repair is important to keep in mind, even with suboptimal results. This time allows edema and inflammation, making for a proper facial analysis to consider revision.

A full review of orbital fractures and associated complications is beyond the scope of this chapter; however, it is important to briefly cover the basics of these complications. When orbital fractures are included in ZMC injury, symptoms may include periorbital bruising, swelling, diplopia, enophthalmos, and hypoesthesia of the inferior orbital (V2) nerve. Entrapment of the inferior rectus can also limit extraocular movement, while traumatic palsy of CN III can present in a similar or more severe fashion. Oculocardiac reflex is the one true emergency complication of orbital fractures and should be addressed in a timely fashion. Postoperative complications include inferior orbital nerve paresthesia, as well as diplopia and enophthalmos due to malposition of the reconstructed zygoma. Persistent diplopia may, unfortunately, be a relatively common complication, with literature noting up to 7% incidence postoperatively. Long-term enophthalmos may be due to perioperative edema and orbital fat atrophy.

Complications of ZMC fractures can include loss of facial lateral projection, trismus due to impingement of depressed zygomatic arch on the coronoid process or direct compression of the temporalis by the zygomatic arch. As discussed previously, several orbital complications may present as sequelae of ZMC injury. Common complication from improperly repaired ZMC fractures include facial asymmetry, poor aesthetics, and cheek ptosis. The subciliary approach can lead to persistent lower lid edema. Likewise, ectropion may also present as a complication of the transconjunctival approach. Daily massage of the area postoperatively may result in the spontaneous resolution of these complications.

Le Fort I fractures result in mobile palatomaxillary segment, mucosal lacerations and palatal ecchymosis. Le Fort II fractures often result in infraorbital nerve paresthesia, with these patients exhibiting reduced sensitivity in the frontal teeth, upper lip, cheeks, and skin of the lateral nose. Le Fort III fractures may exhibit epistaxis, massive swelling of oral mucosa and orbit, cerebrospinal fluid rhinorrhea. All Le

Fort fractures may additionally present in malocclusion after reconstruction despite the surgeon's best attempts. This may be caused by early mobilization and subsequent malunion. This complication may be addressed by orthognathic reconstruction at a later time.

## References

1. Motamedi MH, Dadgar E, Ebrahimi A, Shirani G, Haghighat A, Jamalpour MR. Pattern of maxillofacial fractures: a 5-year analysis of 8,818 patients. J Trauma Acute Care Surg. 2014;77(4):630–4. https://doi.org/10.1097/TA.0000000000000369. PMID: 25250606.
2. Nahum AM. The biomechanics of maxillofacial trauma. Clin Plast Surg. 1975;2:59.
3. Le Fort R. Etude expérimentale sur les fractures de la mâchoire inférieure. I, II, III. Rev Chir Paris. 1901;23:208.
4. Jackson IT. Classification and treatment of orbitozygomatic and orbitoethmoid fractures. The place of bone grafting and plate fixation. Clin Plast Surg. 1989;16(1):77–91. PMID: 2647349.

# Frontal Sinus Reconstruction

# 25

Laura Petrauskas, Eli Gordin, and David Chan

## Introduction

Disruption of the frontal sinus is usually the result of oncologic ablative surgery, blunt or penetrating trauma, and chronic infection [1, 2]. Frontal sinus fractures account for 5–15% of facial fractures. Approximately two-thirds of frontal sinus fractures involve both the anterior and posterior table, while isolated anterior table fractures occur in one-third of cases, and isolated posterior table fractures are the least common (7–11%) [3]. The frontal sinuses may function as a "crumple zone" for protection of the cranial vault [4, 5]. Neoplasms affecting the frontal sinus are rare, with osteomas being the most common, and are present in up to 3% of all CT scans [6]. While inverted papillomas are benign and usually originate from the lateral nasal wall, they can rarely present in the frontal sinus and carry a 5–15% risk of malignant transformation. Malignant neoplasms of the frontal sinus are rare and only account for 2% of all sinonasal malignancies [7].

Frontal sinus injury, whether iatrogenic or traumatic, can lead to significant morbidity and mortality if not properly diagnosed and repaired. Obstruction of the frontal sinus outflow tract impairs mucociliary flow, leading to mucocele formation in up to 33% of anterior table fractures and 60% of combined anterior/posterior table fractures. Depressed anterior table fractures may lead to cosmetic deformity of the forehead, while posterior table fractures may result in cerebrospinal fluid leak and

L. Petrauskas · D. Chan (✉)
Section of Otolaryngology—Head and Neck Surgery, University of Chicago, Chicago, IL, USA
e-mail: Laura.petrauskas@vumc.org

E. Gordin
Department of Otolaryngology—Head and Neck Surgery, UT Southwestern Medical Center, Dallas, TX, USA
e-mail: Eli.Gordin@UTSouthwestern.edu



F. Sokoya, A. G. Vincent (eds.), *Manual of Head and Neck Reconstruction*,
https://doi.org/10.1007/978-3-031-65999-7_25

intracranial infection (e.g. meningitis, extra or intradural abscess, osteomyelitis) [2, 3].

Therefore, the goals of frontal sinus reconstruction, regardless of cause, are to (1) create a safe sinus by reopening or eliminating the frontal sinus drainage system, (2) separate the sterile intracranial compartment from the contaminated sinonasal space, (3) create a watertight dural seal if there is a CSF leak, (4) provide an acceptable cosmetic outcome, and (5) minimize long-term complications. Failure to properly address the frontal sinus may result in chronic sinusitis, forehead deformity, mucocele, mucopyocele, meningitis, or brain abscess [8].

## Anatomy

The frontal sinus is absent at birth; by 2 years, the anterior ethmoid cells invade the frontal bone and continue to develop to adult size by the age of 15 [9]. The frontal sinuses usually take the shape of a pyramid. The borders of the frontal sinus are as follows: anteriorly, the frontal sinus is bounded by the nasofrontal suture line and extends to below the frontal protuberance. Laterally, it extends to the angular prominence of the frontal bones. Inferiorly, it forms the roof of the orbit. The superior border of the frontal sinus is the frontal bone [10]. The anterior table (2–12 mm) is usually significantly thicker than the posterior (0.1–4 mm), which protects the anterior cranial fossa [4]. The shape of the frontal sinus is variable and, in some cases, may be unilateral (10%), rudimentary (5%), or absent (4%) [11]. The frontal sinus outflow tract is traditionally described as an hourglass shape with the infundibulum superiorly. The ostium is usually the narrowest portion (3–4 mm), leading to the inferior frontal recess [4]. The boundaries of the frontal recess include the middle turbinate (medially), lamina papyracea (laterally), posterior wall of agger nasi (anteriorly), and the ethmoid bulla (posteriorly) [12]. The frontal sinus drainage pathway is dependent on the location of the attachment of the uncinate process. Most commonly, the uncinate process attaches to the skull base, and the frontal sinus drains into the ethmoid infundibulum. When the uncinate attaches to the lamina, the frontal sinus drains into the middle meatus [13].

The frontal bone is one of the strongest of the facial bones, tolerating forces up to 800–1600 lbs [14]. Thus, injury is most commonly caused by high velocity impacts such as motor vehicle accidents, assaults, industrial accidents, and sports injuries [15]. Frontal injuries are often associated with other facial fractures (65%) [16], ophthalmologic and intracranial injuries. Long-term sequelae include mucocele, chronic sinusitis, and mucopyocele [17].

## Evaluation and Management

Evaluation of frontal sinus defects is usually performed by physical exam and imaging. The anterior table, posterior table, and frontal sinus outflow tracts should be carefully assessed to determine the extent of injury, anticipate sequelae, and plan surgery. Soft tissue injures should be noted, as well as lacerations that may accommodate sufficient surgical exposure. The presence of CSF rhinorrhea should also be noted, as this will influence the extent of repair. CT imaging is essential. Axial images are useful to evaluate displacement of the anterior and posterior tables, while coronal and sagittal images are useful for assessing the frontal sinus outflow tract.

## Anterior Table

Anterior table fractures account for 18–27% of frontal sinus fractures. If the outflow tract and posterior table are not affected, an isolated anterior table fracture represents a purely cosmetic issue, and observation can be considered depending on the degree of deformity [4]. Unfortunately, there is no consensus regarding indications for anterior table repair, as this depends on what is considered acceptable between the surgeon and the patient. Small, depressed fractures of 4 mm or less may heal without significant cosmetic deformity once scarring and bone remodeling occur [18, 19].Multiple approaches to the frontal sinus are available. The coronal approach offers the best exposure but carries some morbidity, including scalp paresthesia, alopecia, scarring, and facial nerve injury. This approach is best reserved for severe depressions, severely comminuted fractures, the need to obliterate or cranialize the frontal sinus, or in cases where a craniotomy is needed to address neurologic injuries.

Less invasive approaches include the upper eyelid incision, suprabrow approach, endoscopic brow, and transnasal endoscopic approach [20–23]. The endoscopic approach is unique in that it can address both depressed anterior table fractures, CSF leaks, and the frontal sinus outflow tract in well-selected patients [3, 24].

## Posterior Table

Fractures of the posterior table can be associated with intracranial injuries or dural tears, which predispose the patient to intracranial infections, mucoceles, and CSF leaks. Historically, cranialization was the recommended treatment for significantly displaced posterior table fractures (greater than one table width or 2 mm) or persistent CSF leaks. However, Choi et al. showed that even displaced, comminuted posterior table fractures can be managed without cranialization, regardless of the presence of CSF leak, in their 10-year, retrospective review of 59 patients [25]. Furthermore, for persistent CSF leaks, an endoscopic approach can be attempted prior to committing to an open procedure. Complication rates after cranialization or obliteration range from 10 to 17%, including headache, wound infection, persistent CSF leak, mucocele formation, intracranial infection, and cosmetic deformity [26]. Therefore, it may be prudent to observe mild to moderate posterior table fractures prior to surgical intervention. In cases with persistent CSF leak, persistent obstruction of the frontal outflow tract, significant posterior table disruption or comminution, or intracranial injury requiring neurosurgical intervention, surgery should not be delayed, and the patient will likely need cranialization.

## Frontal Sinus Outflow Tract

The frontal sinus outflow tract is necessary for mucociliary clearance to prevent mucocele formation. In traumatic injuries, if the frontal sinus is to be preserved, the outflow tract must be intact and patent [3]. Indeed, Rodriguez et al. [27] and Chen et al. [28] both identified the importance of nasal-frontal duct function as key to sinus preservation. These authors advocate for obliteration or cranialization in cases where the nasofrontal ducts are compromised. Obliteration can be used in cases where the posterior table is unscathed, but frontal outflow compromise is identified. Cranialization is generally utilized when the posterior table is significantly damaged. Both procedures involve plugging the frontal outflow tract and carry a complication rate of 10–17%.

To prevent mucocele formation, all frontal sinus mucosa must be completely removed, which can be difficult [26]. This has been corroborated by several other authors who found expectant management to be reasonable [3, 29, 30]. On the other hand, Rodriguez et al. showed that patients with frontal sinus outflow tract obstruction had a higher incidence of complications with observation, as compared to obliteration or cranialization, in their study of 857 patients [27].

There has been a recent trend towards more conservative management of frontal sinus fractures. In 2002, Smith et al. demonstrated good results with observation, followed by staged endoscopic frontal sinusotomy when indicated. This is applied to patients with anterior table fractures with extension into the frontal recess [29]. In a small study by Jafari et al., resolution of frontal recess obstruction on interval imaging was noted in 87% of patients with observation alone [30].

Although observation and endoscopic treatment of the frontal sinus outflow tract have gained popularity over the last couple of decades, open approaches are still indicated for severe cases, particularly in those necessitating neurosurgical intervention for intracranial injuries.

## Role of Cranialization

Cranialization of the frontal sinus was first described by Donald and Bernstein in 1978 to prevent complications associated with frontal sinus trauma, such as meningitis and intracranial abscess [31]. Cranialization involves the removal of the posterior table (either bilateral or unilateral), thorough removal of all remaining frontal sinus mucosa, and obliteration of the outflow tract, thereby allowing the frontal lobe to expand to the outer table of the frontal sinus.

Traditionally, cranialization was advocated in cases in which either the posterior table was displaced greater than one table width or when frontal outflow tract obstruction was identified [32]. Cranialization, however, still carries a risk of secondary mucocele formation even decades after the initial injury.

Similar to the management of the frontal outflow tract, advances in endoscopic sinus surgery and improved intraoperative navigation have allowed surgeons to employ endoscopic techniques to repair traumatic CSF leaks. Grayson et al. demonstrated success in repairing both anterior and posterior table fractures with or without CSF leaks in carefully selected patients [3]. However, the authors note that patients requiring a craniotomy are not ideal candidates for an endoscopic procedure and will likely need cranialization. They also echo the utility of endoscopic techniques in managing the frontal outflow tract. A 10-year review of 59 patients by Choi et al. showed that even in cases with significant comminuted fracture patterns and a high rate of CSF leak, only a single patient required cranialization [25]. Recently, Miller et al. describe their preliminary result of open repair with frontal sinus preservation [33]. In their series of 23 patients who required major open surgical intervention due to trauma or tumor resection, the frontal sinuses were preserved, and an allograft and pericranial flap was used to "compartmentalize" the extracranial and intracranial contents. This allowed the repair of any dural defects and CSF leaks while maintaining the function of the frontal sinus as long as the outflow tract was intact. The authors note that having an intact pericranium is vital to the success of this technique and if not available, then traditional obliteration or cranialization should be employed.

Despite the trend towards endoscopic and conservative management, there is still a place for the open approach with cranialization, as Dedhia et al. noted in their review of patients with severely depressed and comminuted posterior table fractures with refractory CSF leak [8]. Additionally, Chegini et al. reported a lower complication rate in patients treated with cranialization compared to patients who would have otherwise been cranialized but were observed due to comorbidities [34].

While cranialization now plays a more limited role in the contemporary management of frontal sinus fractures, in our current practice, the open approach with or without cranialization is appropriate for severely displaced and/or comminuted fractures that require rigid fixation, management of refractory CSF leak, and the need for craniotomy to simultaneously address neurosurgical issues. Frontal sinus obliteration for severely compromised frontal sinus outflow is more controversial.

The use of obliteration, cranialization, or endoscopic management of frontal sinus fractures will vary among institutions and clearly depends on the surgeon's training and comfort with endoscopic sinus surgery. Decision-making should be multidisciplinary and involve input from the facial trauma surgeon, neurosurgeon, and endoscopic sinus surgeon when available. Patient factors should be considered as well, such as the patient's reliability and ability or desire to follow-up frequently when observation is an option. Considering the time-course by which mucocele develops, which is on the order of years to decades, most studies are limited by a lack of long-term follow-up. The patient needs to be educated regarding signs and symptoms of complications, regardless of the technique employed.

## Reconstructive Options for Frontal Sinus Defects

There are a variety of options for reconstructing the frontal sinus depending on the pathology and needs. Isolated anterior table contour deformities can be corrected with internal fixation but larger defects may require contouring with bone grafts, titanium mesh, or other alloplastic materials. Vascularized flaps and nonvascularized grafts have also been used for obliteration of the sinus cavity, and in the most extreme cases, free tissue transfer is an option as well.

## Grafts

### Autologous Bone Grafts

Autologous bone grafts can be used to reconstruct anterior table defects but have also been used to obliterate the frontal sinus outflow tracts [35–38]. The most common donor sites of bone grafts include the iliac crest and calvarium [37, 38]. Dova et al. reported good results with using calvarial bone grafts for reconstruction of the frontal sinus, given its proximity to the frontal region, natural aesthetic outcome, and minimal donor site morbidity [39]. Calvarial bone grafts also demonstrate better graft survival than other grafts and can be used in contaminated spaces such as the paranasal sinuses [40, 41]. Calvarial bone grafts are typically harvested from the temporoparietal region for curved grafts, but straighter grafts can be harvested from the occipitoparietal region. Graft size should be no longer than 6 cm or wider than 2 cm as there is a higher risk of fracture [42]. Compared to the common method of using autologous abdominal fat to obliterate the frontal sinus outflow tract [43], bone is more reliably monitored on CT scans, as fat can be mistaken for mucoceles or infection [4]. In addition, over time, some of the fat graft atrophies and is replaced with fibrous tissue, whereas bone grafts have new bone formation [44]. Other advantages of using autologous bone grafts include resistance to infections, re-ossification, and high biocompatibility [45]. Disadvantages include donor site morbidity, the requirement of an open approach, variable resorption, and difficulty in contouring [46].

## Alloplastic Implants

### Titanium Mesh

Titanium mesh is an alternative option for alloplastic reconstruction of the anterior table (Fig. 25.1a and b). It has been described for reconstruction of the mandible [47], zygomatic arch [48], orbit [49], and cranium [35]. Advantages of titanium mesh include its strength and malleability that make it ideal for contour and stability [50, 51]. Studies examining both gross and histologic soft tissue response show good compatibility with soft tissue, with tissue incorporation and resurfacing by

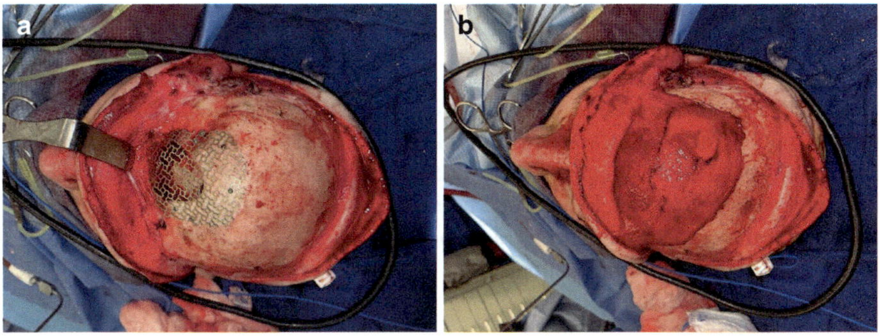


**Fig. 25.1** Titanium mesh. After the removal of a frontal sinus osteoma, the anterior table was reconstructed with a titanium mesh (**a**) and then covered with a pericranial flap (**b**)

indigenous cells, even when exposed to sinuses or mucosa of nasopharyngeal and oral regions [52]. In addition, titanium mesh does not produce significant artifacts on CT or MRI when compared to other metals [53]. Titanium mesh is useful for severely comminuted fractures, where small depressed fragments can be brought into reduction by drilling a hole and inserting a nonlocking screw, bringing the fragment up to the mesh from the sinus [35]. Disadvantages include risk of infection, headache, and mesh exposure [54, 55]. Lakhani et al. demonstrated a 17% (2/12) incidence of mild infection that resolved with antibiotics and 1/12 patients who had persistent headaches [50]. Similarly, the most common complication of titanium mesh cranioplasty was infection in a retrospective study by Mukherjee, looking at 174 patients (8.6% infection rate) [56].

## Medpor (Porous Polyethylene)

Porous polyethylene or Medpor is a biomaterial used for facial contour. The main benefit of porous polyethylene is that the pore sizes allow fibrous tissue ingrowth, as opposed to smooth implants that become encapsulated as a part of the body's foreign body response [57]. Medpor is often used as an onlay to recontour a persistent deformity after primary repair. Strong described an endoscopic technique for placement of a Medpor implant with the advantage of: not needing to manipulate the bone fragments, can be done in delayed fashion, reduces donor site morbidity, and can be done as an outpatient [58]. Porous polyethylene has the advantage of being quickly available and low cost ($260–$460). In addition, patient-specific implants can be constructed from postinjury computed tomography scans but require more time and cost ($3500–$4500) [59]. The advantages of using porous polyethylene are that the material is easy to handle, insert, and remove and has been used for facial contour for many years. In addition, the endoscopic approach results in less scarring and morbidity relative to the coronal incision. Studies have shown that once implants are in place, they may be palpable but demonstrate no deformity, movement, or displacement [59].

## PEEK (Polyether-Ether Ketone)

Polyether-Ether Ketone is a polyaromatic semicrystalline thermoplastic polymer that is ideal for use in reconstructive procedures. It has been used in a multitude of subspecialties, including trauma, orthopedics, neurosurgery, and craniofacial reconstruction [60, 61]. Specifically, Suresh et al. performed reconstruction using PEEK implants with sinus contact and found no instances of sinusitis or implant rejection, suggesting they may be ideal for craniofacial reconstruction in the paranasal sinus region [62]. It has good biocompatibility, with strength similar to bone, and structural stability at high temperatures allowing it to be sterilized [60, 61, 63]. PEEK is also nonimmunogenic, causing no clinically significant inflammation in in-vivo and in-vitro studies, and is radiolucent on imaging [64, 65]. In addition, studies suggest that chemical modifications of PEEK can enhance osseointegration [66]. However, a review of literature suggests that larger scale, and further studies may need to be performed to better understand the osseointegration properties of PEEK [67]. Another advantage includes the ability to create 3D customized models based on CT scans, which decreases intraoperative time and also donor site morbidity compared to other methods [68, 69]. However, it is not possible to use PEEK implants immediately for emergency situations; static implants may not be ideal for growing pediatric patients, implants do not become revascularized, and may be costly for patients [70].

## Hydroxyapatite Cement

Hydroxyapatite is a calcium phosphate compound and is one of the primary mineral components of bone. Hydroxyapatite cement (HAC) is a compound that hardens via isothermic chemical reaction to form a paste in-vivo; thus, there is no surrounding thermal injury, and it has been used to repair bony defects in craniofacial reconstruction [71, 72]. It is also used in otologic surgeries for temporal bone reconstruction, cranioplasty for translabyrinthine approaches, and for jugular bulb dehiscence [73–75]. Histologic studies have shown good biocompatibility of HAC with minimal inflammation, osseointegration, and osteo conversion, leading to decreased risk of extrusion [76, 77]. HAC benefits from ease of application and ability to contour well especially when compared to preformed hydroxyapatite ceramic [71]. The most common complications were edema (10%), tenderness (6%), sinusitis (4%), and surgical site infections (3%) [76]. Risk factors associated with increased risk of infection or implant removal include placing the implant underneath the bicoronal incision, postoperative radiation, secondary pediatric craniofacial reconstruction, or exposure to the sinus mucosa [78–81]. Data, however, is limited by mixtures of pediatric and adult populations, small sample sizes, and varied pathologies ,including trauma, neoplasms, and congenital defects.

## Methyl Methacrylate

Methyl methacrylate (MMA) is an acrylic-based resin. MMA has good tension and compression stress resistance, is inert, and is relatively cheap compared to other materials [82]. This material is often used for cranioplasties and in a variety of other medical procedures [83]. Its use is ideal for partial thickness or contour deformities, as monomeric MMA functions as a liquid that fills defects and then can be molded once hardened. In addition, for partial thickness defects, the dura remains protected from thermal reactions [84].

Disadvantages of MMA include the formation of a capsule [72] and exothermic reaction while hardening, which can result in injury to surrounding tissues [85]. It is a static implant that will not grow over time which may make it not an ideal choice for children [86]. There is no osseointegration, making it easy to remove if necessary; however, it increases susceptibility to infection [86]. MMA has been shown to have a high risk of infection and is not recommended when exposed to sinus tissues [87] An older but comprehensive study looking at the use of MMA showed a 0% infection rate in patients undergoing isolated cranioplasty. However, if patients also had cranial vault reconstruction or reconstruction of the orbital wall or nose had an infection rate of 23% [88]. This is confirmed by other studies that have also shown an increased risk of infection when the implant is exposed to the paranasal sinuses [82, 89]. The exothermic reaction and higher risk of infection, when exposed to sinus mucosa, suggest that MMA may not be ideal for the repair of frontal sinus fractures.

## Vascularized Flaps for Frontal Sinus Reconstruction

### Pericranial Flap

The pericranial flap has been a versatile workhorse in frontal sinus reconstruction and has been widely used for CSF leak repair, obliteration of the frontal sinus, separation of the anterior cranial fossa from the sinonasal cavity, and repair of skin and facial skeletal defects (Fig. 25.2) [90–93]. By bringing in well-vascularized tissue, wound healing potential is improved, as well as the delivery of antibiotics to sites of infection. The vascularity of the pericranial flap is supplied anteriorly by the supratrochlear and supraorbital vessels, laterally by the superficial temporal vessels, and posteriorly from the occipital and greater auricular vessels. This rich network of vascular supply allows the flap to be based anteriorly or laterally to fill various defects of the anterior and lateral skull base [92]. The pericranial flap is the deepest layer of the scalp (skin, subcutaneous tissue, galea aponeurotica, subgaleal loose areolar tissue, and periosteum). The pericranial flap is typically harvested via a coronal approach, although endoscopic techniques have been described [94, 95].

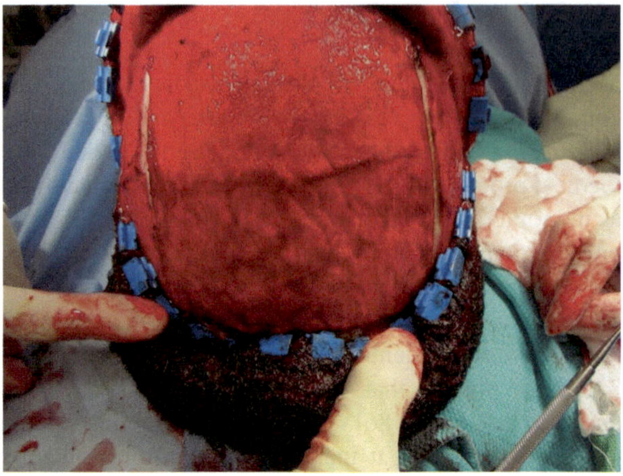

**Fig. 25.2** Pericranial flap. An extended-length pericranial flap can be harvested by elevating the posterior scalp flap as far as possible to expose the pericranium prior to making the cuts

## Other Locoregional Flaps for Frontal Sinus Reconstruction

Alternative local flaps used for frontal sinus and anterior skull base reconstruction have been used when the pericranial flap is not available or insufficient. Smith et al. described their use of the temporalis muscle flap for reconstruction of the anterior and middle cranial fossa. In their series of 35 patients, there were no flap failures, one transient CSF leak, and three hardware exposures. Donor site complications were also noted with their use of hydroxyapatite for reconstructing the donor site deformity and the need for secondary procedures [96]. Other authors have also described the use of temporalis muscle flaps for frontal sinus obliteration or anterior skull base reconstruction as an alternative when the pericranium is no longer available [97–99]. The paramedian forehead flap, while most notably used for nasal reconstruction, has also been used for anterior skull base reconstruction when typical options are no longer available (e.g. pericranial flap, nasoseptal flap) [100]. In a preclinical study, the temporoparietal fascia flap was evaluated by Ferrari et al. as another option for anterior skull base defects by passing the flap through a side door [101].

## Free Tissue Transfer in Reconstruction of the Frontal Sinus

Free tissue transfer offers advantages in tissue bulk to fill dead space and improve healing potential [2]. Various types of free flaps have been used in this situation, including muscle flaps, musculocutaneous, fasciocutaneous, and osteocutaneous flaps (Fig. 25.3a–c). Rodriguez et al. showed in their series of seven patients with a recurrent frontal sinus infection that elimination of the frontal plate with simultaneous obliteration and reconstruction of the frontal bone with a fibula-free flap helped resolve the infection [102]. Shimbo et al. used a de-epilethialized latissimus dorsi musculocutaneous free flap for the treatment of chronic frontal osteomyelitis.

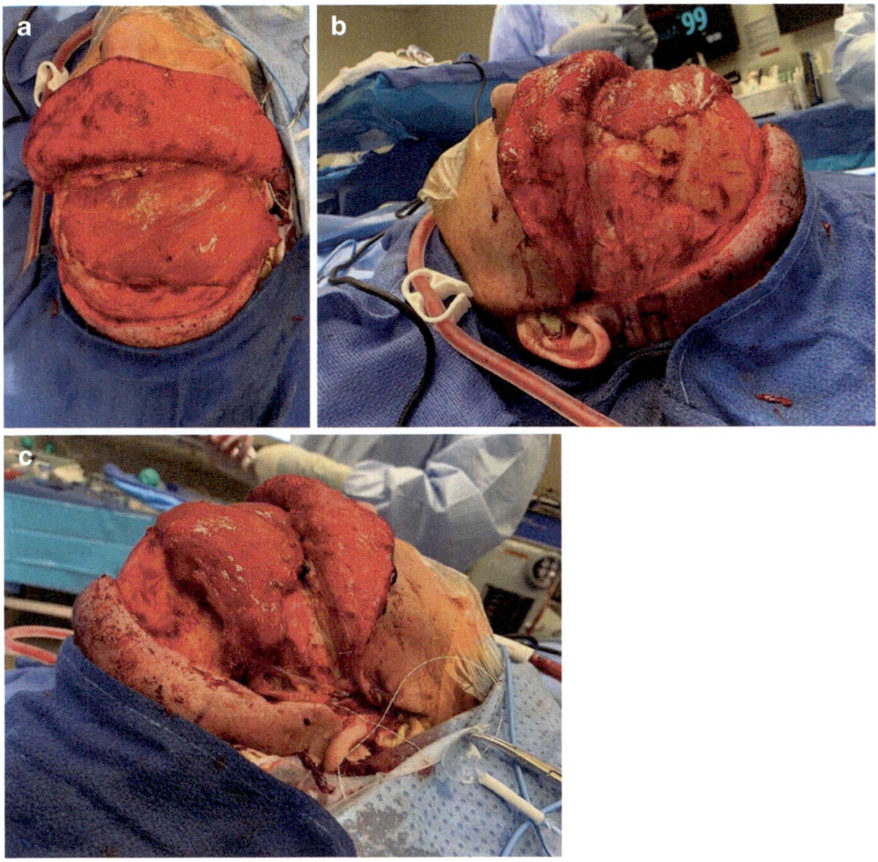


**Fig. 25.3** Serratus free tissue transfer. Serratus free flap was used to reconstruct the anterior skull base after a failed pericranial flap due to a delayed infection (**a** and **b**). The vascular pedicle was anastomosed to the superficial temporal vessels (**c**)

Musculocutaneous flaps seem to perform better than fasciocutaneous flaps for controlling infections. The advantage of their technique was that they were able to reconstruct a larger frontal bone deformity with the de-epitheliazed skin paddle than what can be achieved by an osteocutaneous fibula-free flap. One downside that they noted was that over time, the muscle atrophies and some patients will develop a concavity that may require a secondary cranioplasty [103].

## Surgical Technique for Open Approach to Frontal Sinus

Typically, a bicoronal approach is employed for full exposure of the frontal bone, which can be extended down to the nasal bones and lateral orbital rims; however, if a convenient laceration is available, it can be used as an alternative. The incision is made about 1–1.5 cm posterior to the hairline. A common mistake is designing the incision directly over the vertex, necessitating additional elevation. The superficial temporal vessels should preserved if the flap is to be based laterally, especially the posterior branch.

A subgaleal flap is elevated first, taking care to leave a thick pericranial layer. The pericranial flap is elevated separately, especially in cases where cranialization, obliteration, or skull base repair is planned. Even in cases of severe frontal sinus and calvarial fracture, the pericranial flap may still be viable. A unilateral blood supply from the supratrochlear/supraorbital bundle is sufficient to perfuse a pericranial flap spanning the entire width between temporal lines.

It is useful to harvest an extended pericranial flap, whereby the posterior scalp is elevated, and a pericranial flap is developed, starting near the occiput. The flap is then bluntly elevated with a periosteal elevator down to the supraorbital rims. The supraorbital neurovascular bundle is visualized, and if more mobility is needed, osteotomies can free the neurovascular bundle from its canal. The flap is then covered with a moist gauze to prevent desiccation while the rest of the surgical repair is being addressed.

In cases where the pericranium has been resected or the vascular supply has been disrupted bilaterally, another flap option may be necessary. A laterally based pericranial flap can be utilized, though it will provide less length than an extended, anteriorly based flap. The superficial temporoparietal fascia flap represents another local option.

Once exposure is complete, we consider our reconstructive needs and options based on the injury. If only the anterior table needs to be addressed and the frontal sinus outflow tract is patent, then open reduction internal fixation is performed. If there is no usable bone available for fixation, reconstruction of the anterior table can be accomplished with alloplastic materials (titanium, medpor, and PEEK), bone grafts, or free flaps. We prefer a simple reconstruction with titanium mesh in these situations. Soft tissue defects may necessitate local scalp flaps or free tissue transfer.

Obliteration or cranialization is accomplished by removing all frontal sinus mucosa with an elevator. Care must be taken to fully explore all the nooks and crannies of the frontal sinus to ensure all mucosa is removed all the way down to the frontal sinus outflow tracts. Once the mucosa has been removed, the bony surfaces are either drilled with a diamond burr or cauterized to remove any possible mucosal remnants. The outflow tract is then plugged with either free muscle grafts taken from the temporalis muscle or bone wax. Obliteration of the frontal sinus can then be accomplished by filling it with a pericranial flap, fat graft, or free tissue transfer, depending on the reconstructive needs. Our preference is for a vascularized pericranial flap; however, many surgeons prefer a fat graft.

Cranialization requires the removal of the posterior table. Typically, this may be performed by the neurosurgical team while they are repairing any dural defects. Anterior skull base reconstruction, which is addressed in another chapter, is also accomplished at this time by creating a barrier between the cranial and sinonasal compartments. This is typically done by placing vascularized tissue beneath the dura, such as a pericranial flap.

## Conclusion

Management of injuries to the frontal sinus has evolved significantly over the past couple of decades. Improved understanding of the frontal sinus outflow tract and modern endoscopic techniques have relegated traditional open approaches to only the most severe cases that already require craniotomy. It is, however, still important for the reconstructive surgeon to be familiar and facile with open techniques and concepts to prevent further morbidity and sequela for patients needing more invasive treatment.

## References

1. Rimmer RA, Duffy AN, Knops AM, Rabinowitz MR, Koszewski IJ, Rosen MR, Ortlip T, Heffelfinger RN, Garcia HG, Evans JJ, Nyquist GG, Curry JM. The role of free tissue transfer in the management of chronic frontal sinus osteomyelitis. Laryngoscope. 2019;129:1497–504.
2. Soto E, Ovaitt AK, Clark AR, Tindal RR, Chiasson KF, Aryanpour Z, Ananthasekar S, Grant JH, Myers RP. Reconstructive management of gunshot wounds to the frontal sinus: an urban trauma center's perspective. Ann Plast Surg. 2021;86:S550.
3. Grayson JW, Jeyarajan H, Illing EA, Cho DY, Riley KO, Woodworth BA. Changing the surgical dogma in frontal sinus trauma: transnasal endoscopic repair. Int Forum Allergy Rhinol. 2017;7:441–9.
4. Arnold MA, Tatum SA. Frontal sinus fractures: evolving clinical considerations and surgical approaches. Craniomaxillofac Trauma Reconstr. 2019;12:85–94.
5. Donath A, Sindwani R. Frontal sinus cranialization using the pericranial flap: an added layer of protection. Laryngoscope. 2006;116:1585–8.
6. Harvey RJ, Sheahan PO, Schlosser RJ. Surgical management of benign sinonasal masses. Otolaryngol Clin North Am. 2009;42:353–75.
7. Vázquez A, Baredes S, Setzen M, Eloy JA. Overview of frontal sinus pathology and management. Otolaryngol Clin North Am. 2016;49:899–910.
8. Dedhia RD, Morisada MV, Tollefson TT, Strong EB. Contemporary management of frontal sinus fractures. Curr Opin Otolaryngol Head Neck Surg. 2019;27:253–60.
9. Strong EB. Frontal sinus fractures: current concepts. Craniomaxillofac Trauma Reconstr. 2009;2:161–75.
10. Al-Bar MH, Lieberman SM, Casiano RR. In: Kountakis SE, Senior BA, Draf W, editors. The frontal sinus. Springer; 2016. p. 573.
11. Strong EB. In: Johnson J, editor. Bailey's head and neck surgery—Otolaryngology. Lippincott Williams & Wilkins; 2014. pp. 1255–1271.
12. Walden MJ. In: Flint PW, Haughey BH, Robbins KT, Thomas JR, Niparko JK, Lund VJ, Lesperance MM, editors. Cummings otolaryngology—Head and neck surgery E-book. Elsevier Health Sciences; 2015. pp. 658–677.
13. Daniels DL, Mafee MF, Smith MM, Smith TL, Naidich TP, Brown WD, Bolger WE, Mark LP, Ulmer JL, Hacein-Bey L, Strottmann JM. The frontal sinus drainage pathway and related structures. AJNR Am J Neuroradiol. 2003;24:1618–27.
14. Pappachan B, Alexander M. Biomechanics of cranio-maxillofacial trauma. J Maxillofac Oral Surg. 2012;11:224–30.
15. Strong EB, Pahlavan N, Saito D. Frontal sinus fractures: a 28-year retrospective review. Otolaryngol Head Neck Surg. 2006;135:774–9.
16. Wallis A, Donald PJ. Frontal sinus fractures: a review of 72 cases. Laryngoscope. 1988;98:593–8.

17. Metzinger SE, Metzinger RC. Complications of frontal sinus fractures. Craniomaxillofac Trauma Reconstr. 2009;2:27–34.
18. Kim DW, Yoon ES, Lee BI, Dhong ES, Park SH. Fracture depth and delayed contour deformity in frontal sinus anterior wall fracture. J Craniofac Surg. 2012;23:991–4.
19. Patel SA, Berens AM, Devarajan K, Whipple ME, Moe KS. Evaluation of a minimally disruptive treatment protocol for frontal sinus fractures. JAMA Facial Plast Surg. 2017;19:225–31.
20. Alinasab B, Fridman-Bengtsson O, Sunnergren O, Stjärne P. The supratarsal approach for correction of anterior frontal bone fractures. J Craniofac Surg. 2018;29:1906–9.
21. Kinzinger M, Steele TO, Chin O, Strong EB. Degree of frontal bone exposure via upper blepharoplasty incision: considerations for frontal sinus fracture. Otolaryngol Head Neck Surg. 2019;160:468–71.
22. Fattahi T, Salman S. An aesthetic approach in the repair of anterior frontal sinus fractures. Int J Oral Maxillofac Surg. 2016;45:1104–7.
23. Strong EB, Buchalter GM, Moulthrop TH. Endoscopic repair of isolated anterior table frontal sinus fractures. Arch Facial Plast Surg. 2003;5:514–21.
24. Steiger JD, Chiu AG, Francis DO, Palmer JN. Endoscopic-assisted reduction of anterior table frontal sinus fractures. Laryngoscope. 2006;116:1978–81.
25. Choi M, Li Y, Shapiro SA, Havlik RJ, Flores RL. A 10-year review of frontal sinus fractures. Plast Reconstr Surg. 2012;130:399–406.
26. Adelson RT, Wei C, Palmer JN. Frontal sinus fractures. In: Atlas of endoscopic and sinonasal skull base surgery. Philadelphia: Elsevier; 2013. p. 337–56.
27. Rodriguez ED, Stanwix MG, Nam AJ, St Hilaire H, Simmons OP, Christy MR, Grant MP, Manson PN. Twenty-six-year experience treating frontal sinus fractures: a novel algorithm based on anatomical fracture pattern and failure of conventional techniques. Plast Reconstr Surg. 2008;122:1850–66.
28. Chen KT, Chen CT, Mardini S, Tsay PK, Chen YR. Frontal sinus fractures: a treatment algorithm and assessment of outcomes based on 78 clinical cases. Plast Reconstr Surg. 2006;118:457–68.
29. Smith TL, Han JK, Loehrl TA, Rhee JS. Endoscopic management of the frontal recess in frontal sinus fractures: a shift in the paradigm. Laryngoscope. 2002;112:784–90.
30. Jafari A, Nuyen BA, Salinas CR, Smith AM, DeConde AS. Spontaneous ventilation of the frontal sinus after fractures involving the frontal recess. Am J Otolaryngol. 2015;36:837–42.
31. Donald PJ, Bernstein L. Compound frontal sinus injuries with intracranial penetration. Laryngoscope. 1978;88:225–32.
32. Morse JC, Chandra RK. Is there still a role for cranialization in modern sinus surgery. Curr Opin Otolaryngol Head Neck Surg. 2021;29:53–8.
33. Miller C, Weisbrod L, Beahm D, Chamoun R. Compartmentalization: an open technique for frontal sinus repair and preservation-description of technique and early case series. J Neurol Surg B Skull Base. 2021;82:189–95.
34. Chegini S, Gallighan N, Mcleod N, Corkill R, Bojanic S, Griffiths S, Dhariwal D. Outcomes of treatment of fractures of the frontal sinus: review from a tertiary multispecialty craniofacial trauma service. Br J Oral Maxillofac Surg. 2016;54:801–5.
35. Abu-Ghname A, Banuelos J, Oliver JD, Vyas K, Daniels D, Sharaf B. Outcomes and complications of pediatric cranioplasty: a systematic review. Plast Reconstr Surg. 2019;144:433e–43e.
36. Muderris T, Bercin S, Sevil E, Kiris M. Management of frontal sinus fracture: reconstruction of the sinus with iliac bone graft. J Craniofac Surg. 2013;24:e194–5.
37. Shumrick KA, Smith CP. The use of cancellous bone for frontal sinus obliteration and reconstruction of frontal bony defects. Arch Otolaryngol Head Neck Surg. 1994;120:1003–9.
38. Vironneau P, Coste A, Prulière-Escabasse V. Frontal sinus obliteration with autologous calvarial bone graft: indications and results. Eur Arch Otorrinolaringol. 2014;271:2957–62.
39. Dova S, Karkos PD, Constantinidis J. Reconstruction of frontal defects with calvarial grafts. Rhinology. 2018;56:297–302.

40. Elisevich K, Bite U. En block forehead reconstruction with split-thickness cranial bone. Surg Neurol. 1991;35:384–8.
41. Goodrich JT, Argamaso R, Hall CD. Split-thickness bone grafts in complex craniofacial reconstructions. Pediatr Neurosurg. 1992;18:195–201.
42. Frodel JL, Marentette LJ, Quatela VC, Weinstein GS. Calvarial bone graft harvest. Techniques, considerations, and morbidity. Arch Otolaryngol Head Neck Surg. 1993;119:17–23.
43. Eledeissi A, Ahmed M, Helmy E. Frontal sinus obliteration utilizing autogenous abdominal fat graft. Open Access Maced J Med Sci. 2018;6:1462–7.
44. Owens M, Klotch DW. Use of bone for obliteration of the nasofrontal duct with the osteoplastic flap: a cat model. Laryngoscope. 1993;103:883–9.
45. Rodríguez IZ, Uceda MI, Lobato RD, Aniceto GS. Postraumatic frontal sinus obliteration with calvarial bone dust and demineralized bone matrix: a long term prospective study and literature review. Int J Oral Maxillofac Surg. 2013;42:71–6.
46. Delaney SW. Treatment strategies for frontal sinus anterior table fractures and contour deformities. J Plast Reconstr Aesthet Surg. 2016;69:1037–45.
47. Dai J, Shen G, Yuan H, Zhang W, Shen S, Shi J. Titanium mesh shaping and fixation for the treatment of comminuted mandibular fractures. J Oral Maxillofac Surg. 2016;74:337.e1–337.e11.
48. Mahmoud SM, Liao HT, Chen CT. Aesthetic and functional outcome of zygomatic fractures fixation comparison with resorbable versus titanium plates. Ann Plast Surg. 2016;76(Suppl 1):S85–90.
49. Nowinski D, Messo E, Hedlund A. Treatment of orbital fractures: evaluation of surgical techniques and materials for reconstruction. J Craniofac Surg. 2010;21:1033–7.
50. Lakhani RS, Shibuya TY, Mathog RH, Marks SC, Burgio DL, Yoo GH. Titanium mesh repair of the severely comminuted frontal sinus fracture. Arch Otolaryngol Head Neck Surg. 2001;127:665–9.
51. Chattopadhyay C. Reconstruction of acquired frontal bone defects using titanium mesh implants: a retrospective study. J Maxillofac Oral Surg. 2019;18:34–9.
52. Schubert W, Gear AJL, Lee C, Hilger PA, Haus E, Migliori MR, Mann DA, Benjamin CI. Incorporation of titanium mesh in orbital and midface reconstruction. Plast Reconstr Surg. 2002;110:1022–30.
53. Sullivan PK, Smith JF, Rozzelle AA. Cranio-orbital reconstruction: safety and image quality of metallic implants on CT and MRI scanning. Plast Reconstr Surg. 1994;94:589–96.
54. Maqbool T, Binhammer A, Binhammer P, Antonyshyn OM. Risk factors for titanium mesh implant exposure following cranioplasty. J Craniofac Surg. 2018;29:1181–6.
55. Gundeslioglu OA, Ince B. Exposed titanium mesh and dura persisting for 8 years after cranioplasty. J Craniofac Surg. 2013;24:655–6.
56. Mukherjee S, Thakur B, Haq I, Hettige S, Martin AJ. Complications of titanium cranioplasty—a retrospective analysis of 174 patients. Acta Neurochir (Wien). 2014;156:989–98; discussion 998.
57. Yaremchuk MJ. Facial skeletal reconstruction using porous polyethylene implants. Plast Reconstr Surg. 2003;111:1818–27.
58. Strong EB. Endoscopic repair of anterior table frontal sinus fractures. Facial Plast Surg. 2009;25:43–8.
59. Kim KK, Mueller R, Huang F, Strong BE. Endoscopic repair of anterior table: frontal sinus fractures with a Medpor implant. Otolaryngol Head Neck Surg. 2007;136:568–72.
60. Kurtz SM, Devine JN. PEEK biomaterials in trauma, orthopedic, and spinal implants. Biomaterials. 2007;28:4845–69.
61. Panayotov IV, Orti V, Cuisinier F, Yachouh J. Polyetheretherketone (PEEK) for medical applications. J Mater Sci Mater Med. 2016;27:118.
62. Suresh V, Anolik R, Powers D. The utility of polyether-ether-ketone implants adjacent to sinus cavities after craniofacial trauma. J Oral Maxillofac Surg. 2018;76:2361–9.
63. Camarini ET, Tomeh JK, Dias RR, da Silva EJ. Reconstruction of frontal bone using specific implant polyether-ether-ketone. J Craniofac Surg. 2011;22:2205–7.

64. Nieminen T, Kallela I, Wuolijoki E, Kainulainen H, Hiidenheimo I, Rantala I. Amorphous and crystalline polyetheretherketone: mechanical properties and tissue reactions during a 3-year follow-up. J Biomed Mater Res A. 2008;84:377–83.
65. Rudman K, Hoekzema C, Rhee J. Computer-assisted innovations in craniofacial surgery. Facial Plast Surg. 2011;27:358–65.
66. Zhao Y, Wong HM, Wang W, Li P, Xu Z, Chong EY, Yan CH, Yeung KW, Chu PK. Cytocompatibility, osseointegration, and bioactivity of three-dimensional porous and nanostructured network on polyetheretherketone. Biomaterials. 2013;34:9264–77.
67. AlOtaibi N, Naudi K, Conway D, Ayoub A. The current state of PEEK implant osseointegration and future perspectives: a systematic review. Eur Cell Mater. 2020;40:1–20.
68. Gerbino G, Zavattero E, Zenga F, Bianchi FA, Garzino-Demo P, Berrone S. Primary and secondary reconstruction of complex craniofacial defects using polyetheretherketone custom-made implants. J Craniomaxillofac Surg. 2015;43:1356–63.
69. Wang W, Namin A, Shokri T, Ducic Y. Customized orbit and frontal bone implants. Facial Plast Surg. 2020;36:711–4.
70. Manrique OJ, Lalezarzadeh F, Dayan E, Shin J, Buchbinder D, Smith M. Craniofacial reconstruction using patient-specific implants polyether ether ketone with computer-assisted planning. J Craniofac Surg. 2015;26:663–6.
71. Costantino PD, Friedman CD, Jones K, Chow LC, Pelzer HJ, Sisson GA. Hydroxyapatite cement. I. Basic chemistry and histologic properties. Arch Otolaryngol Head Neck Surg. 1991;117:379–84.
72. Lee DW, Kim JY, Lew DH. Use of rapidly hardening hydroxyapatite cement for facial contouring surgery. J Craniofac Surg. 2010;21:1084–8.
73. DeHart AN, Shaia WT, Coelho DH. Hydroxyapatite cement resurfacing the dehiscent jugular bulb: novel treatment for pulsatile tinnitus. Laryngoscope. 2018;128:1186–90.
74. Kveton JF, Coelho DH. Hydroxyapatite cement in temporal bone surgery: a 10 year experience. Laryngoscope. 2004;114:33–7.
75. Volsky PG, Hillman TA, Stromberg KJ, Buchinsky FJ, Chen DA, Jackson NM, Arriaga MA. Hydroxyapatite cement cranioplasty following translabyrinthine approach: long-term study of 369 cases. Laryngoscope. 2017;127:2120–5.
76. Friedman CD, Costantino PD, Synderman CH, Chow LC, Takagi S. Reconstruction of the frontal sinus and frontofacial skeleton with hydroxyapatite cement. Arch Facial Plast Surg. 2000;2:124–9.
77. Kokoska MS, Friedman CD, Castellano RD, Costantino PD. Experimental facial augmentation with hydroxyapatite cement. Arch Facial Plast Surg. 2004;6:290–4.
78. Verret DJ, Ducic Y, Oxford L, Smith J. Hydroxyapatite cement in craniofacial reconstruction. Otolaryngol Head Neck Surg. 2005;133:897–9.
79. Wong RK, Gandolfi BM, St-Hilaire H, Wise MW, Moses M. Complications of hydroxyapatite bone cement in secondary pediatric craniofacial reconstruction. J Craniofac Surg. 2011;22:247–51.
80. David L, Argenta L, Fisher D. Hydroxyapatite cement in pediatric craniofacial reconstruction. J Craniofac Surg. 2005;16:129–33.
81. Singh KA, Burstein FD, Williams JK. Use of hydroxyapatite cement in pediatric craniofacial reconstructive surgery: strategies for avoiding complications. J Craniofac Surg. 2010;21:1130–5.
82. Marchac D, Greensmith A. Long-term experience with methylmethacrylate cranioplasty in craniofacial surgery. J Plast Reconstr Aesthet Surg. 2008;61:744–52; discussion 753.
83. Reddy S, Khalifian S, Flores JM, Bellamy J, Manson PN, Rodriguez ED, Dorafshar AH. Clinical outcomes in cranioplasty. Plast Reconstr Surg. 2014;133:864–73.
84. Cavalieri-Pereira L, Assis A, Olate S, Asprino L, de Moraes M. Surgical treatment of frontal sinus fracture sequelae with methyl methacrylate prosthesis. Int J Burns Trauma. 2013;3:225–31.
85. Dunne NJ, Orr JF. Curing characteristics of acrylic bone cement. J Mater Sci Mater Med. 2002;13:17–22.

86. Cho YR, Gosain AK. Biomaterials in craniofacial reconstruction. Clin Plast Surg. 2004;31:377–85, v.
87. Blum KS, Schneider SJ, Rosenthal AD. Methyl methacrylate cranioplasty in children: long-term results. Pediatr Neurosurg. 1997;26:33–5.
88. Manson PN, Crawley WA, Hoopes JE. Frontal cranioplasty: risk factors and choice of cranial vault reconstructive material. Plast Reconstr Surg. 1986;77:888–904.
89. Greene AK, Warren SM, McCarthy JG. Onlay frontal cranioplasty using wire reinforced methyl methacrylate. J Craniomaxillofac Surg. 2008;36:138–42.
90. Ducic Y, Stone TL. Frontal sinus obliteration using a laterally based pedicled pericranial flap. Laryngoscope. 1999;109:541–5.
91. Noone MC, Osguthorpe JD, Patel S. Pericranial flap for closure of paramedian anterior skull base defects. Otolaryngol Head Neck Surg. 2002;127:494–500.
92. Smith JE, Ducic Y. The versatile extended pericranial flap for closure of skull base defects. Otolaryngol Head Neck Surg. 2004;130:704–11.
93. Thaller SR, Donald P. The use of pericranial flaps in frontal sinus fractures. Ann Plast Surg. 1994;32:284–7.
94. Chakravarthi S, Gonen L, Monroy-Sosa A, Khalili S, Kassam A. Endoscopic endonasal reconstructive methods to the anterior skull base. Semin Plast Surg. 2017;31:203–13.
95. García-Fernández A. Single-port approach to endoscopic pericranial scalp flap for anterior cranial fossa closure. Laryngoscope. 2017;127:2721–4.
96. Smith JE, Ducic Y, Adelson RT. Temporalis muscle flap for reconstruction of skull base defects. Head Neck. 2010;32:199.
97. Gagliardi F, Bailo M, Spina A, Boari N, Donofrio CA, Piloni M, Gragnaniello C, Caputy AJ, Mortini P. Bilateral temporal myofascial flap for the reconstruction of frontal sinus defects. World Neurosurg. 2017;107:477–81.
98. Kwon SG, Kim YO, Rah DK. Anterior cranial base reconstruction with a reverse temporalis muscle flap and calvarial bone graft. Arch Plast Surg. 2012;39:345–51.
99. Mohammed-Ali RI, Robbins AE, Hussain O, Fitzgerald A, Carroll T, Smith AT, Yousefpour A. Six-year retrospective study of reconstructive options for defects of the skull base after resection of tumour. Br J Oral Maxillofac Surg. 2013;51:719–24.
100. Bresler AY, Mir G, Grube J, Hegazin M, Liu JK, Eloy JA, Paskhover B. Endoscopic paramedian forehead flap reconstruction of the anterior skull base for recalcitrant cerebrospinal fluid leaks: minimally invasive adaptation of ancient flap. World Neurosurg. 2019;130:37–41.
101. Ferrari M, Vural A, Schreiber A, Mattavelli D, Gualtieri T, Taboni S, Bertazzoni G, Rampinelli V, Tomasoni M, Buffoli B, Doglietto F, Rodella LF, Deganello A, Nicolai P. Side-door temporoparietal fascia flap: a novel strategy for anterior skull base reconstruction. World Neurosurg. 2019;126:e360–70.
102. Rodriguez ED, Stanwix MG, Nam AJ, St Hilaire H, Simmons OP, Manson PN. Definitive treatment of persistent frontal sinus infections: elimination of dead space and sinonasal communication. Plast Reconstr Surg. 2009;123:957–67.
103. Shimbo K, Okuhara Y, Yokota K. Dual purpose of de-epithelialized latissimus dorsi musculocutaneous flap for treatment of chronic frontal sinusitis and frontal bone defect. J Craniofac Surg. 2021;32:1122–5.

# Orbital Trauma Reconstruction

# 26

Derek Sheen and Eli Gordin

## Intro/History

Orbital injuries usually occur from blunt force, causing a transfer of energy throughout the orbit, displacing the globe into the surrounding bony walls [1]. Specifically, motor vehicle accidents, falls, and assaults account for most of these injuries and occur more commonly in 20- to 30-year-old males [2–4]. In pediatric patients, falls and sports-related injuries are more prevalent [5]. Protective factors in children include the proportionally larger cranium and reduced aeration of the paranasal sinuses, decreasing the dead space into which orbital contents can potentially extrude [4]. With age, increased bony resorption weakens surrounding areas, leading to higher fracture rates. The most commonly injured orbital walls are regions composed of very thin bone, with studies that support variable rates between the medial orbital wall versus the floor [1, 2, 4, 6, 7]. The orbital roof is involved much more rarely, usually secondary to very high energy impacts and multisystem injuries, with an incidence of about 1–9% of all orbital wall fractures [8].

Because of the mechanism of injury, a high proportion of fractures are complex and involve surrounding facial bones, including the nasal, maxillary, and zygomatic bones [1] as well as the ethmoid and maxillary sinuses. When high velocity forces are involved, other multisystem trauma may take priority in terms of acute management. Regardless, significant damage to the surrounding structures of the eye can lead to devastating consequences to function and cosmesis, significantly affecting a patient's quality of life.

Two main theories explain how fractures occur. In the "hydraulic" theory, a sudden increase in intraorbital pressure fractures the weakest points of the thin orbital

D. Sheen · E. Gordin (✉)
Department of Otolaryngology Head and Neck Surgery, University of Texas Southwestern Medical Center, Dallas, TX, USA
e-mail: Derek.sheen@utsouthwestern.edu; Eli.Gordin@UTSouthwestern.edu



F. Sokoya, A. G. Vincent (eds.), *Manual of Head and Neck Reconstruction*,
https://doi.org/10.1007/978-3-031-65999-7_26

bone, while the globe is usually spared [6, 7]. This is due to the direct transmission of pressure from the globe to the surrounding tissues [2]. Presumably, this is a natural protective mechanism of human evolution, sparing the globe from rupturing during rapid increases in pressure. The other "buckling" or "bone conduction" theory explains a transfer of kinetic energy along the facial skeleton from direct force, causing fracture without displacement of orbital contents [2, 5–7].

The contemporary management of orbital fractures has evolved with advancements in both evidence-based practice and technology, including imaging, intraoperative navigation, and implant designs.

## Anatomy

In general, the orbit comprises a pyramidal shaped cavity, housing the globe in its center. It is surrounded by extraocular muscles, and all interconnected through a network of orbital fibers, fat, and muscular fascia. There are four rectus muscles as well as the superior and inferior obliques. The connective tissue and fat serve to preserve orbital volume, as well as reduce the pressure exerted by the extraocular muscles [3]. The seven bones of the orbit include the frontal, zygomatic, maxillary, palatine, lacrimal, ethmoidal, and sphenoid [3]. Orbital fractures can occur in isolation, but it is crucial to understand that certain unique fracture patterns can also be present. These include the zygomaticomaxillary complex, Le Fort II, and naso-orbito-ethmoid complex fractures [9]. These specific fractures are discussed in other chapters, while this chapter discusses isolated orbital trauma.

The orbital walls contribute to one horizontal and two paired, vertical structural buttresses, which support the facial skeleton. The horizontal midfacial buttress runs from the squamous temporal bone through the zygomatic arch along the inferior orbital rim (including the orbital floor), ending at the nasofrontal junction medially [9]. The fronto-zygomatic-maxillary buttresses are positioned laterally, extending vertically from the frontal bone, through the zygomaticofrontal suture, and down to the maxillary molars. They include the lateral orbital rim [9]. The medial maxillary buttresses run vertically, from the anterior nasal spine, along the piriform aperture, up to the nasofrontal area and include the medial orbital wall [9].

The lateral orbital wall is formed by the zygomatic bone, with additional support provided by the temporalis muscle [10]. Superiorly, the frontal bone creates the orbital roof. The apex represents the deepest portion within the orbit, where the sphenoid bone forms the posterior wall. The superior orbital fissure and optic canal lie in this region. The optic canal contains the optic nerve and ophthalmic artery. The superior orbital fissure contains cranial nerves III, IV, and VI, as well as the lacrimal, frontal, and nasociliary nerves from cranial nerve V. Cranial nerve V also gives off the infraorbital and zygomatic nerves, which travel through the inferior orbital fissure, along with the infraorbital vessels, and the inferior ophthalmic vein.

The maxillary and lacrimal bones together form the lacrimal fossa and contribute to the medial orbital wall, along with the lamina papyracea of the ethmoid bone [3]. Medially, within the lacrimal fossa, the lacrimal sack receives drainage from the superior and inferior lacrimal puncta located on the medial lid margins. The sack drains into the lacrimal duct, which empties into the inferior meatus, inferior and about 1 cm posterior to the head of the inferior turbinate [11]. Just medially, adjacent to the orbit lie the ethmoid sinuses, which are a pneumatized system of usually 8–15 separate bony partitions [11]. The inferior orbital rim and most of the orbital floor are formed by the maxillary bone and are positioned just superior to the maxillary sinus.

The orbital floor and medial walls are most susceptible to fracture. The medial wall is composed of the thin, fragile lamina papyracea. The orbital floor lacks support as it lies above the aerated maxillary sinus. Additionally, the infraorbital canal may represent an area of structural weakness. Certain authors have noticed a relationship between ethnicity and a tendency towards certain fractures. Afro-Caribbean patients were found to have thicker orbital floors and fewer ethmoid bony partitions, leading to higher rates of medial orbital wall fractures; on the other hand, Asians (both Eastern and Indian) and Caucasians had higher rates of orbital floor fractures [2]. It is also possible that variation in reported rates of fracture patterns is related to a discrepancy in symptoms, depending on the location of injury. For example, orbital floor fractures may cause entrapment of extraocular muscles, whereas medial orbital fractures typically do not and thus lack symptoms [2].

There is some variability in the vascular orbital anatomy. Variations have been reported where the ophthalmic artery branches off the middle meningeal artery and enters the orbit through the superior orbital fissure [12, 13]. From the ophthalmic artery, branches of the ethmoidal artery enter through the medial orbit into the ethmoid sinuses. The relationship is described as the rule of 24-12-6 mm, representing the distances between the anterior lacrimal crest and the anterior ethmoid artery, between the anterior ethmoid artery to the posterior ethmoid artery, and between the posterior ethmoid artery back to the optic canal, respectively [14]. In regards to the blood supply adjacent to the orbit, the anterior ethmoid artery supplies a portion of the lateral nasal wall [11]. Other relevant vessels that may be damaged include the infraorbital artery (a branch of the maxillary artery) as well as its paired vein which runs in the infraorbital groove adjacent to the infraorbital nerve [14]. Given the close relationship of these delicate structures, presurgical imaging is recommended to ascertain anatomical variations [14].

The majority of issues that arise from orbital wall fractures involve the displacement of orbital contents into the adjacent sinuses. Diplopia may result from muscular entrapment by bony fragments, displacement of the globe, edema, or nerve injury. Infraorbital nerve damage and enophthalmos are also common. In rare instances, orbital infection can develop in high-risk patients [15].

## Indications/Contraindications

Careful selection of surgical versus nonsurgical candidates is crucial. The severity of symptoms may not always correlate with significant anatomical deformity. Both surgical intervention and observation may result in long-term deficits of globe position and function. In general, indications for surgery include (1) limitation of extraocular movement, specifically noted on forced duction testing, which suggests a mechanical cause rather than motor nerve injury, (2) evidence of muscle entrapment on imaging, (3) enophthalmos >2 mm when compared to the contralateral side with persistent diplopia, and (4) orbital defects larger than 2 cm squared or representing greater than 50% of the orbital floor area [2, 16, 17].

Greenstick fractures are more common in children because of their increased bone elasticity, leading to muscle entrapment and incarceration, which may elicit a life-threatening oculocardiac reflex [18]. Symptoms may be limited to restricted eye movement or just catching or pausing during eye movement. Other symptoms include nausea, vomiting, and even bradycardia because of the oculocardiac reflex.

The oculocardiac reflex involves stretch receptors in the afferent limb of the ciliary ganglion through the V1 branch of cranial nerve V and efferent stimulation originating from the Vagus nerve. This manifests as the development of marked bradycardia and hypotension, and sometimes asystole secondary to orbital injuries [19]. Patients at risk for this phenomenon include younger age (due to increased vagal tone), hypercarbia or hypoxemia, patients under light anesthesia, or the use of high-dose narcotics because of a suppressed sympathetic response and increased vagal tone [19]. The role of surgery is to remove the stimulus by relieving any impingement on the orbital soft tissues. Prior to surgery, vagolytic medications can be administered under close cardiopulmonary monitoring.

Any life-threatening injuries clearly take priority over the management of isolated orbital fractures. However, in certain instances, an ophthalmologic emergency may be present. Urgent operative management is only necessary in certain circumstances, such as soft tissue entrapment, which may lead to irreversible tissue necrosis, or if there is hemodynamic instability triggered by the oculocardiac reflex, as mentioned earlier. Other injuries to the orbit that require urgent management include a ruptured globe, retinal tears and detachment, vitreous hemorrhage, hyphemia, extraocular muscle injury, foreign body causing orbital impingement, and traumatic optic neuropathy [10, 20]. Traumatic optic neuropathy is reported in about 3% of isolated orbital fractures [5, 21]. Damage to the optic nerve can be identified by testing for red color perception, asking the patient to assess the hue and color intensity, one eye at a time. Concern should be raised if the same color is perceived differently from one eye to the other [10].

Studies have shown that specific symptoms other than visual acuity may be more reliable to indicate the presence of a serious injury. These include having at least one of the following: sudden onset blurred vision, severe pain and pressure, diplopia, photophobia, nausea, floaters, photopsias, scotomas, dizziness, or intense tearing [20]. Significant hemorrhage and soft tissue edema can lead to the rapid development of orbital compartment syndrome, leading to ophthalmic infarction and permanent vision loss within about 90 min [10].

In patients with preexisting monocular vision who sustain orbital wall fractures, surgery to the only seeing eye represents an increased risk. Typical surgical indications may not apply. For example, globe malposition will not cause diplopia in the monocular patient. Attention should be paid to other aspects of cosmetic or functional outcomes, as previously mentioned.

## Preop Planning/Workup

Patients who have sustained an orbital fracture typically present to the emergency room and have about a 29% chance of concurrent ocular injury [5]. As with any examination, a careful history and physical must be taken. A focused physical examination should include all components of the trauma assessment along with a thorough eye exam including "vision, eye pressure, ocular motility, pupil exam, visual field, slit lamp ocular exam, retinal exam, and external exam," as well as an assessment for the presence of foreign bodies [5]. Palpation is used to determine areas of bony step-off, tenderness, and the presence of crepitus [10].

Any eye that cannot close needs to be addressed immediately with lubrication or moisture chamber placement to prevent keratosis and corneal damage. Because of the potential complexity of injuries, all patients with orbital fractures should be evaluated for possible global injuries. Red flag symptoms include 360 degrees of the subconjunctival hemorrhage, a misshapen pupil, and a flat anterior chamber [5]. The authors uniformly request preoperative ophthalmologic consultation and believe surgical management should be undertaken by the facial trauma surgeon only after ophthalmologic clearance.

All patients should be placed on sinus precautions, including no nose blowing, no straining, sneezing with mouth open, and no aggressive sniffing. The sudden introduction of air may become entrapped by ball valving of the orbital fat, raising intraocular pressure and causing vascular and visual compromise from compartment syndrome [10]. Furthermore, sinus precautions are recommended to prevent additional bacterial contamination and infection.

While tonometry is the most reliable indicator of intraocular pressure, a quick examination of orbital pressure can be done by simply pressing against the orbits with the eyelids closed to compare both sides as well as manually opening the eyelids. High intraocular pressure prevents the lids from opening easily [10]. With any suspicion of orbital compartment syndrome, emergent decompression must be performed [10]. Typically, this involves a lateral canthotomy and cantholysis. Needle aspiration of orbital emphysema may be helpful. Failure to relieve pressure on the optic nerve may lead to optic neuropathy and irreversible blindness.

When patients are discharged for outpatient follow-up, they should be given clear emergency room precautions necessitating return, such as a sudden change in pain and swelling or the development of fever or chills. Evidence is lacking to support the use of prophylactic or postoperative antibiotics to prevent orbital infections. Clinical judgement should be used to determine which patients are high risk and may benefit from prophylactic antibiotics, namely, those with concurrent upper respiratory infections, immunocompromised patients, or long-term steroid users [15, 22]. Antibiotics should protect against orbital cellulitis of sinus origin, covering *Staphylococcus aureus*, *Streptococcus pneumoniae*, *Streptococcus pyogenes*, anaerobic organisms, and in children under 5 years, *Haemophilus influenzae* [15, 23]. On the other hand, intraoperative antibiotics are well supported to reduce the incidence of postoperative infections [5, 24].

The initial treatment algorithm also involves the reduction of inflammation and edema and the treatment or prevention of infection. Intravenous corticosteroids should be administered preoperatively to help reduce edema and allow a more accurate assessment of globe position [10]. However, there is no clear literature recommendation on the specific dosage or type of corticosteroid.

A fine-cut CT scan is recommended when there is concern for orbital trauma. This is due to the limitations of physical diagnosis and for operative planning should a fracture be identified. Fractures along the orbital roof and floor are best visualized with coronal and sagittal images, as well as extraocular muscle involvement. Axial images are helpful for visualizing medial and lateral wall fractures [10].

There is debate regarding the timing of orbital repair in the absence of indications for urgent surgery. If surgery is delayed, it may be easiest to operate within 1–2 weeks of the inciting trauma, after inflammation has subsided but prior to fibrosis setting in [1, 3, 5, 10, 25]. In cases of muscle entrapment, operative intervention within the first few days may provide the best chance of preventing permanent motility restriction, especially in older individuals [4, 5].

It is the authors' opinion that the ideal timing of nonurgent orbital repair is multifactorial. In the absence of entrapment or the oculocardiac reflex, the decision of when to proceed with surgery will depend on surgeon availability, operating room time, prioritization of other injuries, and patient preference. Unfortunately, while many isolated orbital fractures may not warrant admission, outpatient follow-up may not be possible for patients who lack insurance. Admission and urgent repair may be ideal for these patients. Orbital repair can be performed in the acute setting, though it may be somewhat more challenging in the presence of significant edema. The authors prefer to operate around 5–7 days after injury. In cases where surgery is planned within the acute setting, we administer 8 mg of dexamethasone every 8 hours and maintain head-of-bed elevation to mitigate edema.

## Instruments/Setup

Orbital fracture repair is performed under general anesthesia. The patient is positioned supine on the operating room table with the head positioned away from the anesthesia machine. A Mayo table is positioned over the patient's chest. A Bovie electrocautery is used with a Colorado tip on a setting of 13–15 watts. A bipolar cautery is also ready. The key instrumentation includes Desmarres lid retractors, a metal Jaeger lid plate, a #9 periosteal elevator, a Freer elevator, small coated malleable retractors, and a plating system.

Several materials may be used to repair the orbital defect [4]. These range from autologous bone grafts (such as calvarium, iliac, or anterior maxillary wall), to cartilage grafts (septum or auricular), to absorbable materials such as polydioxanone sheets, to alloplastics, such as silastic, porous polyethylene, or titanium. Titanium implants may be formed by hand by cutting and bending mesh or preformed, 3-dimensional implants. These are readily available as titanium mesh or as titanium mesh coated with porous polyethylene.

Coated titanium implants are theoretically less prone to adhesion formation between the inferior rectus muscle and the plate. The drawback of coated titanium is that it may be more prone to infection and may be more difficult to remove. There is no definitive, evidence-based recommendation. The authors generally use preformed titanium orbital implants coated in porous polyethylene for the orbital floor. The authors do not usually operate on isolated medial wall fractures. Though, in these situations, porous polyethylene or PDS sheeting is preferred. It is cut and bent to fit the defect. Autologous grafts may present less cost than an alloplastic implant; however, they increase operative time and carry some donor site morbidity.

Difficult fractures may benefit from the use of surgical navigation, endoscopic visualization, or intraoperative imaging modalities. Navigation can be used to assess the position of the posterior portion of a plate if visualization is difficult because of the posterior extent of a fracture in the region of the orbital apex. It can also be used to verify bony landmarks in an extensive facial fracture where there is little stable bone. Endoscopy can also prove useful. An endoscope may be passed through the incision or through a window made in the anterior wall of the maxillary sinus through a sub-labial approach. A trans-antral endoscopic approach into the maxillary sinus may be utilized as well. Some surgeons find this helpful to identify the posterior fracture ledge or to verify plate positioning.

While the authors rarely use navigation or endoscopic visualization, the intraoperative CT scanner has proven useful at our institution. This is not frequently employed, but in an extensive fracture where visualizing the posterior extent of the defect is difficult or where the entire inferior and medial walls are heavily comminuted, and accurate anatomic positioning of the implant is made difficult due to a lack of visual reference, a scan can be of use to assure proper placement. Rather than obtain postop imaging, we prefer to scan select patients in the operating room so that the plate can be easily repositioned if need be.

## Surgical Technique/Pearls (Treatment)

The main surgical goals are to restore function and form. Any entrapped or extruded orbital contents must be reduced, followed by restoration of the surrounding orbital walls. Displaced fractures of the orbital rim must also be reduced to restore cosmesis and eyelid function.

For the most part, studies evaluating the surgical outcomes of orbital surgery focus on comparison to the contralateral eye; however, in many instances, orbits may not be symmetric in their three-dimensional structure and form [26].

As mentioned previously, intraoperative antibiotics and steroids are recommended. Once the patient is under general anesthesia, forced duction testing is performed to assess any restriction in the ocular range of motion.

Approaches to the orbital floor include the transconjunctival and transcutaneous approaches. While transcutaneous incisions have largely fallen out of favor, these include the subciliary, subtarsal, and orbital rim approaches. In general, these external approaches carry higher rates of ectropion and retraction compared to the transconjunctival approach [4, 5, 10, 27–29]. The subtarsal approach is used more frequently compared to the orbital rim approach, as it positions scars in natural skin creases, particularly in the elderly [5, 29]. If present, lacerations can be used, especially to access the lateral and superior orbital rims.

The transconjunctival approach is most commonly used and can be combined with a lateral canthotomy and cantholysis to maximize exposure in larger, complex fractures. This approach can be performed with either the preseptal or postseptal techniques [10]. The preseptal approach involves a conjunctival incision just inferior to the inferior tarsal plate. To assist, a traction suture is placed in the inferior lid margin, and the lower lid is everted over a Desmarres retractor. The dissection then bluntly follows the superficial surface of the orbital septum down to the inferior orbital rim. A traction stitch can then be placed through the conjunctival flap and clamped to the forehead to protect the cornea. Some surgeons prefer this approach because the septum helps to retain some orbital fat, improving visualization.

The retro-septal approach is usually employed by the authors and may be a simpler and safer technique [27]. The Desmarres is used to retract the lower lid and is held by the assistant. The Jaeger lid plate is used to retract the globe.

A corneal shield is not routinely used by the authors. The tip of the Jaeger lid plate is directed just posterior to the orbital rim and applies posterior and inferior retraction. A #9 periosteal elevator is used in the other hand, and a hand-over-hand technique is used to sweep the orbital fat posteriorly away from the orbital rim. Once there is very little soft tissue overlying the orbital rim, the Jaeger lid plate is held firmly against the orbital floor. The periosteal elevator is exchanged for the Bovie, and an incision is made through the fornix of the lower lid down to the inferior orbital rim.

At this point, the postseptal and preseptal approaches are identical. Once the rim is exposed, the periosteal elevator is used to elevate the periorbita over the orbital floor. The orbital floor fracture is usually encountered medial to the infraorbital nerve. Once the fracture is identified, the elevator is used to reduce the orbital contents back into the orbit and out of the sinus. Depending on the time from injury, this can sometimes require some degree of force because of fibrosis. Pushing the orbital floor fragments into the sinus and removing them can aid in visualization, as this allows any blood to drain into the sinus rather than immediately collecting in the operative bed. It also allows the surgeon to gain a sense of the size of the orbit and the location of the orbital apex (Fig. 26.1).

The medial orbital floor and the medial orbital wall are more easily dissected than the lateral border of the fracture. This is because of the infraorbital neurovascular bundle. Vascular tributaries should be carefully cauterized with bipolar so as to prevent orbital hematoma upon emergence from anesthesia. The nerve is dissected away from the orbital contents when necessary.

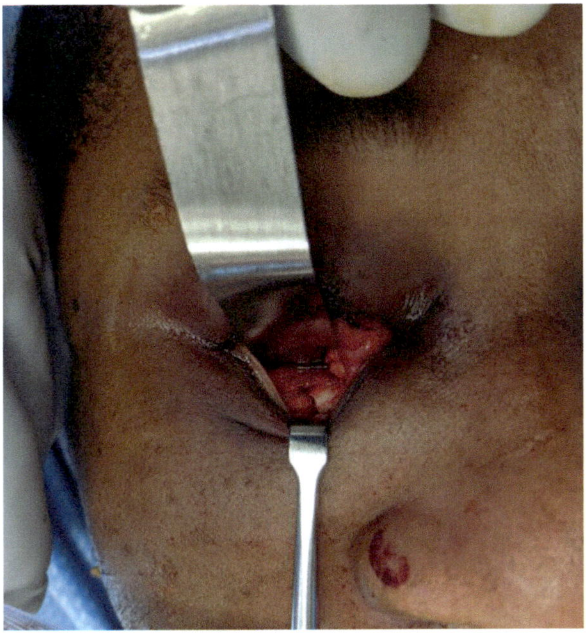

**Fig. 26.1** Exposure of an inferior orbital rim fracture through a trans-conjunctival approach. Reduction has already been performed

The authors usually use a lateral canthotomy and cantholysis to improve visualization unless the fracture is small. This incision is connected to the transconjunctival incision. If additional exposure is needed medially, the inferior oblique can be detached from the inferior orbital rim. A prolene suture can be used to mark the muscle, and it can be reattached at the end of the case. Not all surgeons feel the need to reattach the inferior oblique [30].

When the orbital rim is fractured, it is advisable to repair it prior to proceeding with orbital floor repair (Fig. 26.2).

Similarly, when the orbital floor is fractured in the context of a zygomaticomaxillary fracture, the zygoma should be reduced and plated prior to addressing the orbital floor. This is because the orbital shape may be altered by the reduction of the main zygomatico-maxillary fragment. Furthermore, fixating the rim provides stable bone anteriorly, which is necessary for floor repair.

In cases where there is significant medial orbital involvement or when an isolated medial orbital wall fracture is treated, a trans-caruncular incision is made. A malleable retracts the globe laterally and an incision is made through the conjunctiva through the semilunar fold, ensuring that the dissection is posterior to the lacrimal system. Tenotomy scissors are used to dissect the posterior lacrimal crest, where the periosteum is then incised. The trans-caruncular incision can be used in conjunction with the trans-conjunctival incision of the lower lid and can be connected if need be.

Again, less commonly, a transcutaneous incision can be made to maximize exposure over the medial canthus region, which can potentially injure the medial canthal tendon, lacrimal system, and supratrochlear nerve [16]. Similar to orbital floor

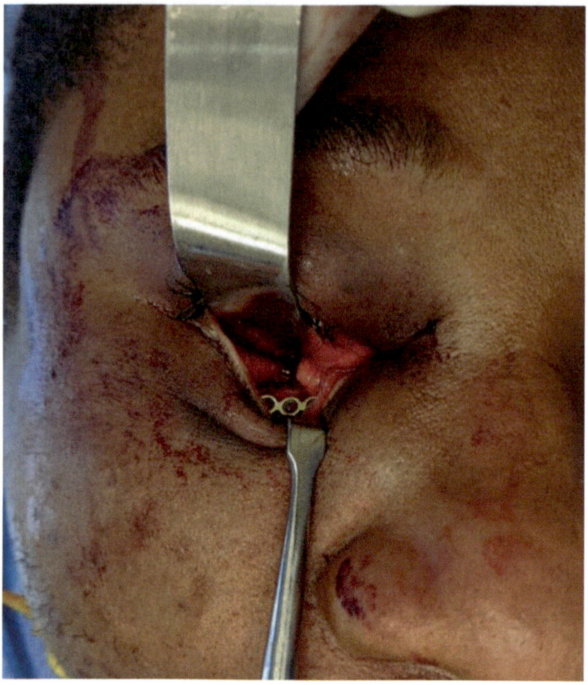

**Fig. 26.2** Fixation of the inferior orbital rim prior to placement of the floor implant

fractures, the endoscopic, endonasal surgical approach can be used but is less favored due to its limited visualization [5].

Exposure of the lateral orbital rim can be gained either through a lateral canthotomy or through an upper blepharoplasty incision or brow incision [5]. Exposure of the superior orbit can also be obtained through an upper blepharoplasty incision or a brow incision. Often, superior orbital trauma necessitates a bicoronal approach because of additional craniofacial injuries. Significant superior orbital trauma with skull base violation should prompt neurosurgical participation.

Fractures can also be repaired through endoscopic transantral or endonasal approaches [10, 18, 29]. Other authors have described using urinary bladder catheter inflation to treat orbital floor fractures with full resolution of diplopia. The overall benefit of endoscopic approaches is a less invasive option to free entrapped soft tissue and restore normal ocular movements with reduced recovery time and complication rates, with the downfall of decreased visualization and potentially inadequate exposure [18, 31].

While autografts were historically employed for orbital wall reconstruction, advancements in biomaterial engineering have led to the common use of alloplasts today [5]. Porous polyethylene is a material that has good biocompatibility; however may be difficult to remove, is expensive, and lacks radiopacity, making visualization on imaging challenging. Titanium orbital mesh is also commonly used because of its availability, biocompatibility, low risk of infection, and rigidity [32, 33]. Titanium implants are available as mesh or in various two-dimensional and three-dimensional configurations specific to orbital use. Molding to achieve proper alignment may be difficult and holes within the mesh make future removal challenging due to tissue ingrowth. As mentioned earlier, titanium coated in porous polyethylene is the authors' usual choice.

Increased precision may be possible with individualized, custom-designed implants (Fig. 26.3).

These are made using selective laser melting or 3D printing and may reduce revision rates [33, 34]. Additionally, operative time is reduced when individualized implants are premade [33]. However, custom implants carry a high cost [33] and may require 1–2 weeks to manufacture, delaying surgery. Custom implants should be considered when surgery is not urgent, especially in complex cases, such as revisions (Fig. 26.4).

The implant should be placed beneath the periorbita, ensuring that no orbital contents are entrapped beneath it. Ideally, it should overlap stable bone circumferentially. We usually fixate with one 4 mm self-drilling screw. After successful implant placement, forced duction testing is critical, the wound is irrigated, and Valsalva is performed. If lateral canthotomy was performed, the lateral canthus is resuspended. In older patients, tightening the lid may be beneficial to prevent ectropion.

## Postop Management

Postop imaging is another area of controversy. As mentioned earlier, the authors utilize intraoperative CT imaging in complex cases where there is doubt or difficulty in implant placement. True postoperative imaging after emergence from anesthesia is only employed when there is a concern for malposition based on patient symptoms. Of note, intraoperative CT scanning only added about 14.5 minutes per

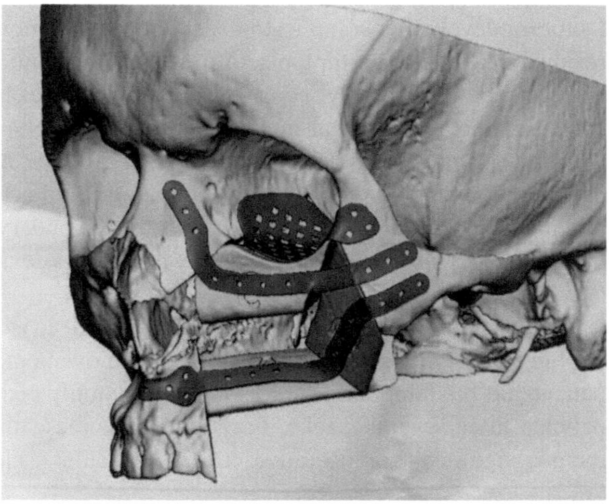

**Fig. 26.3** Customized orbital implant designed through virtual surgical planning. This implant was designed in the context of an oncologic resection and reconstruction. However, the technique is similar to custom implants for traumatic applications

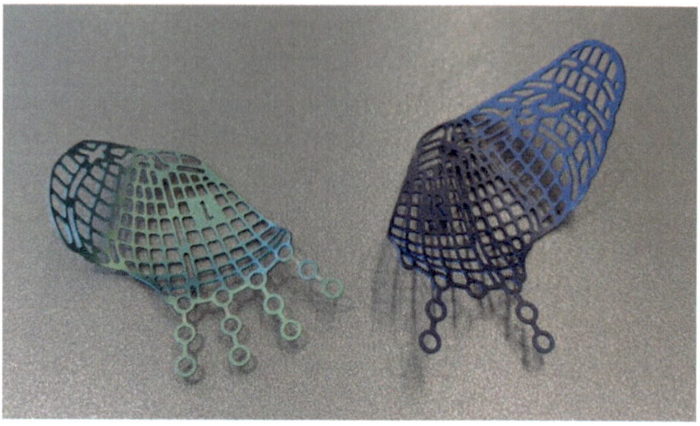

**Fig. 26.4** Three-dimensional stock implants are available and easily trimmed to fit most traumatic orbital floor defects

case, with intraoperative revisions arising in up to 24% of complex procedures [5, 35]. Our philosophy is that if the surgeon plans to obtain a post-operative scan to determine the need for revision, it is most efficient to accomplish this in the operating room.

Once in the recovery unit, a postoperative physical exam should be performed early to assess for visual acuity. It is imperative to assess corneal protection in cases of early postoperative edema or chemosis preventing proper eye closure [10]. Specific discharge instructions should be given to monitor for early warning signs of retrobulbar hemorrhage formation, such as sudden worsening pain, edema, or vision loss. Appropriate pain control should be paired with adjuncts to reduce edema, such as ice packs, elevating the head of the bed, and using ophthalmologic lubricants as needed. Avoidance of straining and heaving lifting, as well as sinus precautions listed earlier, should be recommended for 2–4 weeks after surgery. The first follow-up visit should occur 1 week following surgery, with interval visits thereafter. Throughout the follow-up course, postoperative photographs should be taken for documentation.

Complications can be categorized into early versus late regarding functional and aesthetic outcomes, with some overlap. Studies have shown that older age is a risk factor for developing complications, as patients are more predisposed to developing residual postoperative diplopia. As previously mentioned, early ophthalmologic emergencies significantly increase complication rates because of either early unresolved edema making an accurate assessment of alignment difficult, or delayed surgical intervention with entrapment [1, 10, 25]. The most common postoperative complications include diplopia, enophthalmos, and ectropion. The most important complication to identify is optic neuropathy secondary to a hematoma, edema, or direct compression from an implant. It is rare but devastating, and vision loss can occur between 0 and 0.4% of cases [5].

Once edema resolves in the subacute period, it is important to check for any ongoing or new limitations in extraocular movement. It is important to counsel patients on the temporary diplopia that commonly occurs, which resolves in most patients after several weeks. Factors that increase the risk of residual diplopia include significant preoperative edema, muscular ischemia or inflammation, and improper graft/implant placement, causing impingement. These can occur in 8–42% of cases [5, 10, 36]. Some factors beyond the surgeon's control include preoperative alterations of the orbital connective tissue, which leads to long-term tethering and restrictions of extraocular muscles, as well as intrinsic fibrosis, which may occur during the normal healing process, despite proper surgical reduction [5, 36]. Additionally, extraocular muscle or nerve damage suffered during trauma is a common cause of sustained diplopia [1, 4, 5, 25]. This is an important concept to counsel patients on preoperatively.

Ectropion occurs due to scar contracture, shortening of the anterior lamella of the eyelid, and loss of muscle tone [37]. Early enophthalmos is commonly due to failure to restore orbital volume with implant positioning or improper fracture reduction. This risk is greater in patients who have more than one orbital wall fractured [10].

Enophthalmos occurs at a frequency of about 7–27%, with the most likely cause being the expansion of the orbital cavity after displacement [5, 17, 38]. Even after ideal implant placement, it may occur due to loss of orbital volume from fat atrophy or necrosis, fibrosis of the retrobulbar tissues causing tethering of the globe, or loss of ligamentous support [6, 38]. Enophthalmos can be addressed with implant replacement or augmentation at around 3 months after surgery [5].

Patient counseling should also include V1 or V2 distribution hypoesthesia, dysesthesia, and numbness. This is more prevalent in the orbital roof or orbital floor and zygomatic complex fractures involving the supraorbital or supratrochlear and infraorbital nerves, respectively [39]. Infraorbital nerve dysfunction can be reduced by performing rigid fixation to the infraorbital rim to decompress the infraorbital canal [40]. While there is no recognized treatment, certain antiepileptic medications such as topiramate have shown some benefit in recovery of neuropathic symptoms when given early [39].

In conclusion, orbital reconstruction is evolving with newer biomaterials and techniques to improve surgical precision, reduce operative time, and decrease cost. Enhanced preoperative planning, intraoperative navigation, and customized implants are all increasing the predictability of surgical outcomes. More research is needed to clearly define gold standards for the optimal timing of repair, detailed dosing of perioperative steroids, ideal selection of implant materials, and precise evaluation of intraoperative and postoperative bony reduction and implant placement. With all these advancements, promising developments in individualized medicine can ultimately enhance patient outcomes.

**Acknowledgments** University of Texas Southwestern Medical Center, Department of Otolaryngology, Head and Neck Surgery, Parkland Health and Hospital System.

## References

1. Converse JM, Smith B, Obear MF, Wood-Smith D. Orbital blowout fractures: a ten-year survey. Plast Reconstr Surg. 1967;39(1):20–36. https://doi.org/10.1097/00006534-196701000-00002.

2. de Silva DJ, Rose GE. Orbital blowout fractures and race. Ophthalmology. 2011;118(8):1677–80. https://doi.org/10.1016/j.ophtha.2011.05.001.
3. Koenen L, Waseem M. Orbital floor fracture. In: StatPearls. StatPearls Publishing; 2021. http://www.ncbi.nlm.nih.gov/books/NBK534825/.
4. Shin JW, Lim JS, Yoo G, Byeon JH. An analysis of pure blowout fractures and associated ocular symptoms. J Craniofac Surg. 2013;24(3):703–7. https://doi.org/10.1097/SCS.0b013e31829026ca.
5. Boyette JR, Pemberton JD, Bonilla-Velez J. Management of orbital fractures: challenges and solutions. Clin Ophthalmol. 2015;9:2127–37. https://doi.org/10.2147/OPTH.S80463.
6. Chang EW, Manolidis S. Orbital floor fracture management. Facial Plast Surg. 2005;21(03):207–13. https://doi.org/10.1055/s-2005-922861.
7. Rhee JS, Kilde J, Yoganadan N, Pintar F. Orbital blowout fractures: experimental evidence for the pure hydraulic theory. Arch Facial Plast Surg. 2002;4(2):98–101. https://doi.org/10.1001/archfaci.4.2.98.
8. Haug RH, Van Sickels JE, Jenkins WS. Demographics and treatment options for orbital roof fractures. Oral Surg Oral Med Oral Pathol Oral Radiol Endod. 2002;93(3):238–46. https://doi.org/10.1067/moe.2002.120975.
9. Hopper RA, Salemy S, Sze RW. Diagnosis of midface fractures with CT: what the surgeon needs to know. Radiographics. 2006;26(3):783–93. https://doi.org/10.1148/rg.263045710.
10. Roth FS, Koshy JC, Goldberg JS, Soparkar CNS. Pearls of orbital trauma management. Semin Plast Surg. 2010;24(4):398–410. https://doi.org/10.1055/s-0030-1269769.
11. Jones N. The nose and paranasal sinuses physiology and anatomy. Adv Drug Deliv Rev. 2001;51(1):5–19. https://doi.org/10.1016/S0169-409X(01)00172-7.
12. Bertelli E, Regoli M, Bracco S. An update on the variations of the orbital blood supply and hemodynamic. Surg Radiol Anat. 2017;39(5):485–96. https://doi.org/10.1007/s00276-016-1776-9.
13. Hayreh SS. Orbital vascular anatomy. Eye. 2006;20(10):1130–44. https://doi.org/10.1038/sj.eye.6702377.
14. Felding UA, Karnov K, Clemmensen A, Thomsen C, Darvann TA, von Buchwald C, Tranum-Jensen J. An applied anatomical study of the ethmoidal arteries: computed tomographic and direct measurements in human cadavers. J Craniofac Surg. 2018;29(1):212–6. https://doi.org/10.1097/SCS.0000000000004157.
15. Reiss B, Rajjoub L, Mansour T, Chen T, Mumtaz A. Antibiotic prophylaxis in orbital fractures. Open Ophthalmol J. 2017;11:11–6. https://doi.org/10.2174/1874364101711010011.
16. Bonsembiante A, Valente L, Ciorba A, Galiè M, Pelucchi S. Transnasal endoscopic approach for the treatment of medial orbital wall fractures. Ann Maxillofac Surg. 2019;9(2):411–4. https://doi.org/10.4103/ams.ams_173_19.
17. Clauser L, Galiè M, Pagliaro F, Tieghi R. Posttraumatic enophthalmos: etiology, principles of reconstruction, and correction. J Craniofac Surg. 2008;19(2):351–9. https://doi.org/10.1097/SCS.0b013e3180534361.
18. Park I-H, Lee H-M, Yanagi K. Endoscopic transantral and transnasal repair of orbital floor fracture with the ballooning technique, and classification and characterization of orbital floor fractures. Am J Rhinol Allergy. 2015;29(6):445–8. https://doi.org/10.2500/ajra.2015.29.4222.
19. Pham CM, Couch SM. Oculocardiac reflex elicited by orbital floor fracture and inferior globe displacement. Am J Ophthalmol Case Rep. 2017;6:4–6. https://doi.org/10.1016/j.ajoc.2017.01.004.
20. Ho TQ, Jupiter D, Tsai JH, Czerwinski M. The incidence of ocular injuries in isolated orbital fractures. Ann Plast Surg. 2017;78(1):59–61. https://doi.org/10.1097/SAP.0000000000000748.
21. He D, Blomquist PH, Ellis E. Association between ocular injuries and internal orbital fractures. J Oral Maxillofac Surg. 2007;65(4):713–20. https://doi.org/10.1016/j.joms.2006.09.006.
22. Mundinger GS, Borsuk DE, Okhah Z, Christy MR, Bojovic B, Dorafshar AH, Rodriguez ED. Antibiotics and facial fractures: evidence-based recommendations compared with experience-based practice. Craniomaxillofac Trauma Reconstr. 2015;8(1):64–78. https://doi.org/10.1055/s-0034-1378187.

23. Shuttleworth GN, David DB, Potts MJ, Bell CN, Guest PG. Orbital trauma: do not blow your nose. BMJ. 1999;318(7190):1054–5.
24. Chole RA, Yee J. Antibiotic prophylaxis for facial fractures. A prospective, randomized clinical trial. Arch Otolaryngol Head Neck Surg. 1987;113(10):1055–7. https://doi.org/10.1001/archotol.1987.01860100033016.
25. Hossal BM, Beatty RL. Diplopia and enophthalmos after surgical repair of blowout fracture. Orbit. 2002;21(1):27–33. https://doi.org/10.1076/orbi.21.1.27.2598.
26. Felding UNA. Blowout fractures—Clinic, imaging and applied anatomy of the orbit. Dan Med J. 2018;65(3):B5459.
27. Barcic S, Blumer M, Essig H, Schumann P, Wiedemeier DB, Rücker M, Gander T. Comparison of preseptal and retroseptal transconjunctival approaches in patients with isolated fractures of the orbital floor. J Craniomaxillofac Surg. 2018;46(3):388–90. https://doi.org/10.1016/j.jcms.2017.12.013.
28. Korchia D, Braccini F, Paris J, Thomassin J. Transconjunctival approach in lower eyelid blepharoplasty. Can J Plast Surg. 2003;11(3):166–70.
29. Ridgway EB, Chen C, Colakoglu S, Gautam S, Lee BT. The incidence of lower eyelid malposition after facial fracture repair: a retrospective study and meta-analysis comparing subtarsal, subciliary, and transconjunctival incisions. Plast Reconstr Surg. 2009;124(5):1578–86. https://doi.org/10.1097/PRS.0b013e3181babb3d.
30. Rodriguez J, Galan R, Forteza G, Mateos M, Mommsen J, Bouso OV, Piera V. Extended transcaruncular approach using detachment and repositioning of the inferior oblique muscle for the traumatic repair of the medial orbital wall. Craniomaxillofac Trauma Reconstr. 2009;2(1):35–40. https://doi.org/10.1055/s-0029-1202598.
31. Otori N, Haruna S, Moriyama H. Endoscopic endonasal or transmaxillary repair of orbital floor fracture: a study of 88 patients treated in our department. Acta Otolaryngol. 2003;123(6):718–23. https://doi.org/10.1080/00016480310000584a.
32. Chattopadhyay C, Dev V, Pilania D, Harsh A. Reconstruction of orbital floor fractures with titanium micromesh: our experience. J Maxillofac Oral Surg. 2022;21:369. https://doi.org/10.1007/s12663-020-01407-x.
33. Zimmerer RM, Ellis E, Aniceto GS, Schramm A, Wagner MEH, Grant MP, Cornelius C-P, Strong EB, Rana M, Chye LT, Calle AR, Wilde F, Perez D, Tavassol F, Bittermann G, Mahoney NR, Alamillos MR, Bašić J, Dittmann J, et al. A prospective multicenter study to compare the precision of posttraumatic internal orbital reconstruction with standard preformed and individualized orbital implants. J Craniofac Surg. 2016;44(9):1485–97. https://doi.org/10.1016/j.jcms.2016.07.014.
34. Tavassol F, Gellrich NC. [Competence and communication in the implementation of computer-assisted surgical planning]. Der Chirurg; Zeitschrift Fur Alle Gebiete Der Operativen Medizen. 2021;92(3), 194–199. https://doi.org/10.1007/s00104-020-01348-8.
35. Shaye DA, Tollefson TT, Strong EB. Use of intraoperative computed tomography for maxillofacial reconstructive surgery. JAMA Facial Plast Surg. 2015;17(2):113–9. https://doi.org/10.1001/jamafacial.2014.1343.
36. Balaji SM. Residual diplopia in treated orbital bone fractures. Ann Maxillofac Surg. 2013;3(1):40–5. https://doi.org/10.4103/2231-0746.110078.
37. Kesselring AG, Promes P, Strabbing EM, van der Wal KGH, Koudstaal MJ. Lower eyelid malposition following orbital fracture surgery: a retrospective analysis based on 198 surgeries. Craniomaxillofac Trauma Reconstr. 2016;9(2):109–12. https://doi.org/10.1055/s-0035-1567813.
38. Chen C-T, Huang F, Chen Y-R. Management of posttraumatic enophthalmos. Chang Gung Med J. 2006;29(3):251–61.
39. Lone PA, Singh RK, Pal US. Treatment of traumatic infra orbital nerve paresthesia. Natl J Maxillofac Surg. 2012;3(2):218–9. https://doi.org/10.4103/0975-5950.111390.
40. Westermark A, Jensen J, Sindet-Pedersen S. Zygomatic fractures and infraorbital nerve disturbances. Miniplate osteosynthesis vs. other treatment modalities. Oral Surg Oral Diagn. 1992;3:27–30.

# Part VIII

# Skull Base Reconstruction

# Endoscopic Skull Base Reconstruction

27

Britney Scott, Collin Smith, Luka Bahra, Ricardo L. Carrau, and Sameep P. Kadakia

## Introduction

Advancements in transnasal endoscopic surgery of the skull base have allowed for safe and effective management of both benign and malignant lesions of the skull base. With the help of technological advances, improvements in surgical techniques, and the use of multidisciplinary teams, endoscopic surgery of the skull base has seen rapid development over the last several decades [1]. Beginning with purely pituitary and sellar approaches, surgical resection has expanded to include suprasellar lesions, as well as a myriad of lesions extending from the cribriform plate to C2 and laterally out to the infratemporal fossa and petrous apex [2]. With the development of expanded ablative techniques, the surgeon is often left with large skull base defects that require reconstruction to separate the cranial cavity from the sinonasal cavity and obliterate the remaining dead space. Today, endoscopic reconstruction using local and regional vascularized grafts has allowed for successful reconstruction of the skull base with a reduction in postoperative complications such as CSF leaks and meningitis. This chapter is intended to review the key principles of

B. Scott · C. Smith
Department of Otolaryngology—Head and Neck Surgery, Kettering Health, Kettering, OH, USA

L. Bahra
College of Osteopathic Medicine, Rocky Vista University, Englewood, CO, USA
e-mail: luka.bahra@rvu.edu

R. L. Carrau
Department of Otolaryngology—Head and Neck Surgery, The Ohio State University Wexner Medical Center, Columbus, OH, USA

S. P. Kadakia (✉)
Department of Plastic and Reconstructive Surgery, Wright State University Boonshoft College of Medicine, Dayton, OH, USA


F. Sokoya, A. G. Vincent (eds.), *Manual of Head and Neck Reconstruction*,
https://doi.org/10.1007/978-3-031-65999-7_27

endoscopic skull base reconstruction as well as describe endoscopic surgical reconstructive techniques using local and regional vascularized flaps. The primary goal is to provide a framework to help guide selection for skull base reconstruction and to allow for successful outcomes while minimizing morbidity to the patient.

## Endoscopic Anatomy of the Skull Base

An understanding of skull base anatomy is critical to the success of both its resection and reconstruction. Historically, certain anatomical areas were thought to only be accessible via an open transcranial and/or external approach. Over time, expanded endonasal approaches (EEA) developed, leading to advancements in techniques, allowing for safe and reliable surgical resection and reconstruction with limited need for open approaches. By providing a minimally invasive option, the surgeon has the opportunity for safe surgical resection and reconstruction, minimizing the tissue disruption, brain retraction, and neurovascular manipulation that come along with many open approaches [3]. Using a rod-lens endoscope, the surgeon has access and high-quality visualization of several distinct anatomic regions of the skull base, allowing for a safe and successful endoscopic skull base surgery. These areas include the anterior cranial fossa, sella/suprasellar regions, clivus/posterior cranial fossa, cavernous sinus, and the petrous apex. The anatomy of these regions is briefly reviewed below.

### Endoscopic Anatomy of the Anterior Cranial Fossa

Transnasal endoscopic access to the anterior skull base allows the resection of a variety of anterior skull base tumors. A purely endoscopic anterior skull base resection is ideal for malignancies confined to the area between the orbits and benign lesions of the anterior cranial fossa. Larger tumors require the use of endoscopic-assisted approaches in combination with external craniofacial approaches. Important anatomical landmarks include the frontal recess anteriorly, the planum sphenoidale posteriorly, and the lamina papyracea laterally. To expose the anterior skull base bilaterally, removal of the middle turbinate, anterior and posterior ethmoid air cells, and the superior part of the nasal septum are required until a rectangular area of the cranial base is exposed limited by the lamina papyracea laterally, the planum sphenoidale posteriorly, and the frontal recess anteriorly [4]. Superiorly in the midline is the cribiform plate, along with the small olfactory nerves extending from the olfactory bulb. Key vascular structures in this region include the anterior and posterior ethmoid arteries, which can be identified and isolated along the ethmoid roof. Removing the bone of the anterior skull base between the orbits exposes the dura and, if needed, the intracranial contents.

## Endoscopic Anatomy of the Sella/Suprasellar Region

The sellar and suprasellar regions encompass the midline portion of the middle cranial fossa. The sella is housed within the sphenoid bone that contains the pituitary gland and is covered superiorly in a thin dural layer known as the diaphragma sellae. The anterior boundary is made up of a portion of the sphenoid bone known as the tuberculum sellae and posteriorly by the bony dorsum sellae. Endoscopic surgical access to these areas is achieved through the transsphenoidal approach. This approach requires wide removal of the anterior face of the sphenoid sinus along with any intersinus septa. Once removed, exposure of the posterior and lateral walls of the sphenoid sinus allows identification of the rostrum and floor of the sella, most commonly within the midline central portion of the posterior wall but can vary depending on the degree of pneumatization (i.e., sellar, presellar, and conchal) within the sphenoid sinuses [5]. Superior to the sellar floor lies the planum sphenoidale, and inferiorly lies the superior portion of the clivus. Within the lateral walls, the bony protuberances of the optic nerves superiorly, and inferiorly the intracavernous portion of the internal carotid arteries. Between these two projections is the optico-carotid recess [6]. The removal of the upper half of the sella, tuberculum sellae, and the posterior portion of the planum sphenoidale offers the possibility of exploring the suprasellar region [5]. This region contains key neurovascular structures, including the pituitary stalk, the optic chiasm, the medial portion of bilateral optic nerves, along with the anterior cerebral artery.

## Endoscopic Anatomy of the Clivus and Posterior Cranial Fossa

When viewing the posterior wall of the sphenoid sinus, immediately below the sellar floor lies the anterior surface of the clivus. From an endoscopic view, the clivus is located along the inferior portion of the sphenoid sinus and represents the posterior cranial fossa. The bony landmark acts to separate the nasopharynx from the posterior cranial fossa. Extending inferiorly, the clivus transitions into the craniocervical junction. Endoscopic access to the clivus is achieved via the removal of the inferior portion of the sphenoid sinus down to the sphenoid-vomer junction. The junction, including the sphenoid rostrum and vomer, is removed. This is carried out laterally until the vidian nerves are identified at the floor of the sphenoid sinus. Once identified, the vidian nerves represent the lateral and inferior limit of the bony resection and serve as useful landmarks to prevent injury to the intrapetrous portion of the carotid artery [7]. Further access to the craniocervical junction is achieved by the downward extension of the dissection from the clivus. When the clival bone is fully removed, the dura covering the posterior cranial fossa is exposed and can be opened to allow access to key structures such as the basilar artery, brain stem, and upper cranial nerves.

## Endoscopic Anatomy of the Cavernous Sinus

The cavernous sinuses are paired structures located lateral to the sella turcica bilaterally. They form the parasellar region and extend from the superior orbital fissure anteriorly to the petrous part of the temporal bone posteriorly [8]. Housed within these venous sinuses are a number of important neurovascular structures, including the intracavernous portion of the internal carotid artery and cranial nerves III, IV, V1, V2, and VI. Endoscopic access to this region can be achieved through a transsphenoidal route with wide removal of the anterior face of the sphenoid sinus. This exposure is then extended to include removal of the bony coverings of the lateral wall of the sphenoid sinus and carotid protuberances. Key structures helping to guide dissection in this area are the paraclival and intracavernous portions of the internal carotid artery, V2, and the vidian canal [9].

## Endoscopic Anatomy of the Petrous Apex

The petrous apex forms a portion of the medial temporal bone and is the area housed between the inner ear laterally, the floor of the middle fossa superiorly, the posterior cranial fossa posteriorly, and the clivus medially. Anatomically, this area is a pyramidal shape and develops with a variable degree of pneumatization. The orientation of the petrous apex lies in an oblique plane with the apex positioned anteromedially and its base located posterolaterally [10]. It is divided into an anterior and posterior portion by the internal auditory canal. Key anatomical landmarks to endoscopic surgery of the petrous apex include the petrous carotid canal, Dorello's canal housing the abducens nerve, Meckel's cave contains the trigeminal ganglion and is associated with the vidian canal, and vidian artery (quadrangular space). Endoscopic access to this area involves expert techniques and anatomical knowledge of these key landmarks.

# Indications and Contraindications

The minimal access nature of endoscopic endonasal approaches to the skull base provides inherent advantages over open approaches. Although technically different, the fundamentals are universal, including surgical access that delivers maximal visualization of the lesion, tumor resection occurs in accordance with oncological principles, and conservation of key neurovascular elements [11]. The surgeon must be aware of the indications and contraindications, advantages and disadvantages of each approach, and the degree of tumor involvement with surrounding anatomical structures. If the most direct path to the lesion is impeded by critical neurovascular components and significant manipulation of these components is required, other surgical approaches should be considered in the surgical decision-making [12].

Both benign and malignant pathologies can warrant the need for resection and reconstruction of the skull base, and their extent depends on the nature and spread of the tumor. Nonhematopoietic malignancies usually mandate a surgical resection if complete tumor extirpation can be achieved with satisfactory morbidity [13]. Benign lesions that often necessitate these practices include pituitary adenoma, craniopharyngioma, meningocele or encephalocele, arachnoid cyst, chordoma, schwannoma, inverted papilloma, osteoma, and fibro-ossifying lesions with skull base involvement. It should be noted that with regards to craniopharyngiomas, a nuanced surgical approach that considers the origin, lesion morphology (i.e., cystic vs. solid), as well as pituitary function is required for successful treatment. Additionally, the treatment planning is dependent on the craniopharyngioma subtype. In recent literature, craniopharyngiomas of the papillary type have been shown to have a strong response to BRAF (e.g., vemurafenib, dabrafenib) and MEK inhibitors (e.g., trametinib, selumetinib) in the neoadjuvant setting. Contrarily, surgical intervention remains the primary indication in the adamantinomatous subtype as drugs targeting the WNT/CTNNB1 pathway remain largely in the in-vitro phase [14]. Malignant lesions that warrant surgical resection include sinonasal malignancies such as esthesioneuroblastoma, adenocarcinoma, sinonasal undifferentiated carcinoma, and neuroendocrine carcinoma, as well as intracranial lesions such as anaplastic meningioma, chondrosarcoma, and malignant schwannoma [15].

Typically, the primary objective of skull base reconstruction is to prevent postoperative complications such as CSF leak and subsequent meningitis or pneumocephalus via separation of the intra- and extracranial spaces. Secondary objectives include reconstructive efforts to promote efficient healing, protect neurovascular elements, and reduce postoperative morbidity [16]. To determine if reconstruction is indicated, the surgeon first determines the extent of the defect and the presence of the CSF leak. Second, the character of the leak is described—absent, low flow, or high flow. In the absence of a CSF leak or intracranial opening, reconstruction is typically not indicated. However, the repair and technique are at the acumen of the surgeon. The surgeon may choose to repair with a simple epidural or subdural synthetic graft (with packing and sealant) that can be further augmented with a free mucosal graft or a similar autograft [17]. The CSF leak classification system and the algorithm for flap selection will be described in detail.

It is important to note that factors that increase the likelihood of postoperative CSF leak indicate the use of vascularized flaps. These include the pathologies previously described, as well as Cushing disease (reduced healing from hypercortisolemia) and morbid obesity (increased intracranial pressure). In the case of extradural defects, especially those previously irradiated or that will undergo radiation therapy, vascularized flaps have shown better reliability and resilience when compared to nonvascularized flaps. In this case, the primary objective would be to provide coverage of the defect with enhanced healing [17, 18].

Tumor extirpation is dependent on its extent, aggressiveness, and involvement of critical structures. Generally speaking, anatomic contraindications to skull base surgery are lesion involvement of the brainstem, specific areas of the cerebrum, superior sagittal sinus, both internal carotid arteries, both cavernous sinuses, and vital bridging veins. Purely endoscopic approaches are contraindicated when the tumor demonstrates extensive invasion of the nasal bones, lacrimal apparatus or structures of the orbit, lateral recesses or anterior walls of the maxillary sinus, or dura overlying the roof of the orbit [12]. Other contraindications that are dependent on the nature of the lesion include spread to distant locations. It should be noted that even in cases with distant metastatic disease, it is appropriate to surgically decompress neuroanatomical structures to preserve neurological function [19].

## Preoperative Planning

Preoperative planning in endoscopic skull base reconstruction is of the utmost importance in optimizing postoperative outcomes. As with most reconstructive surgeries, a thorough evaluation of past medical history and preexisting risk factors should be assessed. This includes identifying risk factors such as obesity, diabetes mellitus, cardiovascular disease and atherosclerosis, use of anticoagulation, hematologic malignancies such as leukemias or lymphomas, as well as overall functional and nutritional status. A thorough social history should also be reviewed, including smoking and alcohol consumption, as well as any nonprescription supplements being used. Any prior nasal surgeries should also be reviewed, including prior septorhinoplasty or sphenopalatine artery ligation, as well as any prior internal maxillary artery embolization procedures, as this may influence the reconstructive options that are available. All these factors play a role in predicting success in reconstructive surgery as they heavily impact the reconstructive options available to the surgeon as well as the wound healing process.

In a recent retrospective study looking at patients who underwent endoscopic endonasal approach for resection of intradural skull base tumors the risk factors identified to increase the risk of postoperative CSF leak was BMI >25 and tumors located in the posterior fossa. Sex and use of perioperative lumbar drain did not affect CSF leak rates [20].

Additionally, any endoscopic skull base surgery is best executed as part of a multidisciplinary team, often composed of a neurosurgeon and an otolaryngologist. Transparency and open communication between the respective disciplines are imperative to a successful surgery. This includes discussing preoperative imaging and pathology to gain insight into the characteristics of the anticipated skull base defect that will need to be repaired. The size and location of the defect, the potential need for dural repair, the presence of a CSF leak, plans for a lumbar drain, as well as the need for adjuvant postop treatment such as radiation to the newly reconstructed wound bed should also be communicated amongst disciplines preoperatively if possible, but certainly intra and postoperatively as appropriate.

The use of lumbar spinal drains remains controversial. Many studies show that the use of lumbar drains does not decrease postoperative CSF leak rates and can increase the risk of postoperative meningitis [20, 21]. While others have shown the use of a short-term lumbar drain following endoscopic skull base surgery demonstrated CSF leak rates of 8.2% compared to 21.2% in patients who did not receive a lumbar drain [22]. Nonetheless, a graded approach to skull base reconstruction denoting the severity of the CSF leak has proven beneficial in identifying the necessary components needed to increase the success of the repair [21]. This grading system and steps to repair will be outlined in further detail in the surgical technique section.

## Instruments and Equipment

Endoscopic skull base reconstruction requires a broad skill set as well as a wide range of instruments. A standard anterior skull base reconstruction will require an endoscopic sinus tray with a variety of angled scopes and a septorhinoplasty tray. Instruments of particular interest in these procedures include Kerrison rongeurs, a sickle knife, microdebrider, Freer, suction Freer or Cottle dissectors, a septal scissor, a 15-blade scalpel, a curved beaver blade, and a Takahashi forceps. An endoscopic, high-speed, diamond-bit drill may also be needed to refine the bony defect. An ultrasonic aspirator can also be helpful in removing additional bone if needed based on the operating surgeon's preference. An extended Colorado or insulated needle-tip electrocautery has also been proven useful in these procedures. The fine tip can be slightly bent with forceps and used to make mucosal incisions endoscopically within the nose. This technique provides a good balance between sharp dissection and hemostasis, minimizing the need for repetitive suctioning within the nasal cavity. Suction cautery and/or endoscopic bipolar forceps are also excellent supportive instruments in the event that profuse intraoperative bleeding is encountered.

Aside from instrumentation, endoscopic skull base reconstruction also utilizes a variety of synthetic materials that should be on hand for skull base repair. Commonly used materials include collagen matrix and sealants, although some surgeons prefer to avoid sealants because of the cost and potentially questionable efficacy. Stereotactic CT or MRI navigation can also be quite helpful for the reconstructive surgeon with respect to intraoperative orientation.

## Surgical Technique: Endoscopic Skull Base Reconstruction

This section will outline the basics of skull base defect assessment and grading of CSF leaks, as well as a stepwise approach to the planning and harvesting of vascularized pedicled flaps that are commonly used in endoscopic skull base reconstruction.

### Assessment and Severity of CSF Leak

When technically executing skull base reconstruction, as with any reconstructive case, it is important to have a good working knowledge of the reconstructive options that are available and to have multiple options that can be reliably pursued in the event that the defect evolves and certain reconstructive options become contraindicated or less feasible. As mentioned in the previous section, the major characteristics of a skull base defect that will need to be accounted for are the location and size of the defect as well as the presence and severity of a CSF leak. The classification system and repair protocol for intraoperative CSF leaks were initially described by Esposito et al. in 2007; it has since been updated following the adoption of endoscopic techniques and introduction of the pedicled nasoseptal flap. In the updated system outlined by Conger et al., it is recommended that CSF leaks be graded 0–3 with a stepwisereconstructive protocol for the respective grades. The following algorithm for grading CSF leaks is adapted from Conger et al. and provides a good framework for assessing skull base defects. However, the authors understand that variations in assessing skull base defects will exist on a case-by-case basis as well as between surgeons and institutions.

**Grade 0**

Grade 0 is the absence of a CSF leak, as confirmed by the intraoperative Valsalva maneuver. This defect calls for an intrasellar fat graft in the setting of large sellar dead space, collagen sponge on-lay, repositioning of sphenoid sinus mucosa, if available, over sella and collagen, followed by a second layer of collagen sponge over mucosa and posterior sphenoid. Finally, a layer of fibrin sealant is applied.

**Grade 1**

Grade 1 is defined by a small "weeping" CSF leak, confirmed by intraoperative valsalva with small diaphragmatic or dural defect. Repair of this defect entails an intrasellar fat graft in the setting of large sellar dead space and collagen sponge on-lay, much like a grade 0. However, unlike grade 0, it is recommended that a bone or synthetic buttress (intrasellar, extradural) be placed if it is safe to do so. Repositioning of sphenoid mucosa over the sellar defect and buttress, followed by a second layer of collagen sponge, then fibrin sealant. If it is not possible to bolster the defect with bone within the sella then a unilateral or bilateral merocel nasal packing is recommended and left in place for 5 days.

**Grade 2**

Grade 2 is classified as a moderate CSF leak with obvious dural defect. This repair calls for an intrasellar fat graft in the setting of large sellar dead space, collagen sponge on-lay, placement of intrasellar buttress using bone or other rigid synthetic material, and repositioning of the sphenoid sinus mucosa over the defect with the placement of additional fat within the sphenoid. A second layer of collagen sponge over the fat graft and fibrin sealant is then placed. In the scenario where an intrasellar rigid buttress cannot be placed, a unilateral or bilateral merocel nasal packing is positioned and left in place for 5 days.

**Grade 3**

Grade 3 is defined as a large CSF leak that is usually the result of an extended transsphenoidal approach (transplanum or transclival). This repair calls for intrasellar, suprasellar, or clival fat graft, collagen sponge on-lay, bone or synthetic buttress wedged within the bony defect, a pedicled nasoseptal or other vascularized mucosal flap, as well as additional fat bolstering over the flap. Finally, a second layer of collagen sponge is applied with fibrin sealant, and bilateral merocel nasal packing is placed on opposing the flap to the skull base.

Of note, all repairs necessitate a multilayer technique, but not all CSF leaks require a pedicled vascularized flap for successful repair as the postoperative CSF leak rates for grades 0, 1, 2, and 3 were 0%, 1.9%, 3.1%, and 4.8%, respectively [22]. Nonetheless, it is important to note that these recommendations and outcomes reflect a particular study, and adaptations between cases, surgeons, and institutions will exist. As such, vascularized pedicle flaps can be utilized in grade 1 and 2 CSF leaks based on surgeon preference. It is also worth mentioning that some authors report the addition of a fascial inlay graft for larger transcribiform and transclival dural defects. This graft is placed inside the dural defect between the brain parenchyma and dura in these scenarios. However, they do not recommend this modification for transplanum transtuberculum defects, especially tuberculum sella meningiomas, as the optic nerve sheath is often exposed, and there is a risk of nerve compression with inlay grafting [23].

## Intranasal Vascularized Pedicled Flaps

### Nasoseptal Flap (Hadad-Bassagasteguy Flap)

The nasoseptal flap is by far the most commonly used and well-documented in the literature for endoscopic skull base repair. The posteriorly pedicled nasoseptal flap was first described in 2006 by Hadad et al. and named the Hadad-Bassagaisteguy flap (HBF) after its co-creators [24]. It entails incising the nasal septal mucosa and raising a mucoperichondrial flap that is pedicled posteriorly around the posterolateral nasal arteries of the sphenopalatine artery (Fig. 27.1). In their original article published in the Laryngoscope, they outline the steps to flap harvest and inset, which are detailed below (Fig. 27.2).

### Flap Design and Harvest

- The inferior and middle turbinates are out fractured to allow for visualization of the nasal septum from cribriform to nasal floor (to allow for bimanual technique during endoscopic endonasal approaches one of the middle turbinates can be removed; this also allows for visualization of the flap pedicle).
- The flap is designed based on the size and shape of the defect and is recommended to overestimate the size needed as trimming can be performed later.
- Two parallel incisions are then made in the sagittal plane, one along the maxillary crest and one superiorly below the olfactory epithelium (i.e., 1–2 cm below the most superior aspect of the septum).
- A vertical incision is then made connecting the two incisions at the mucocutaneous junction of the columella.

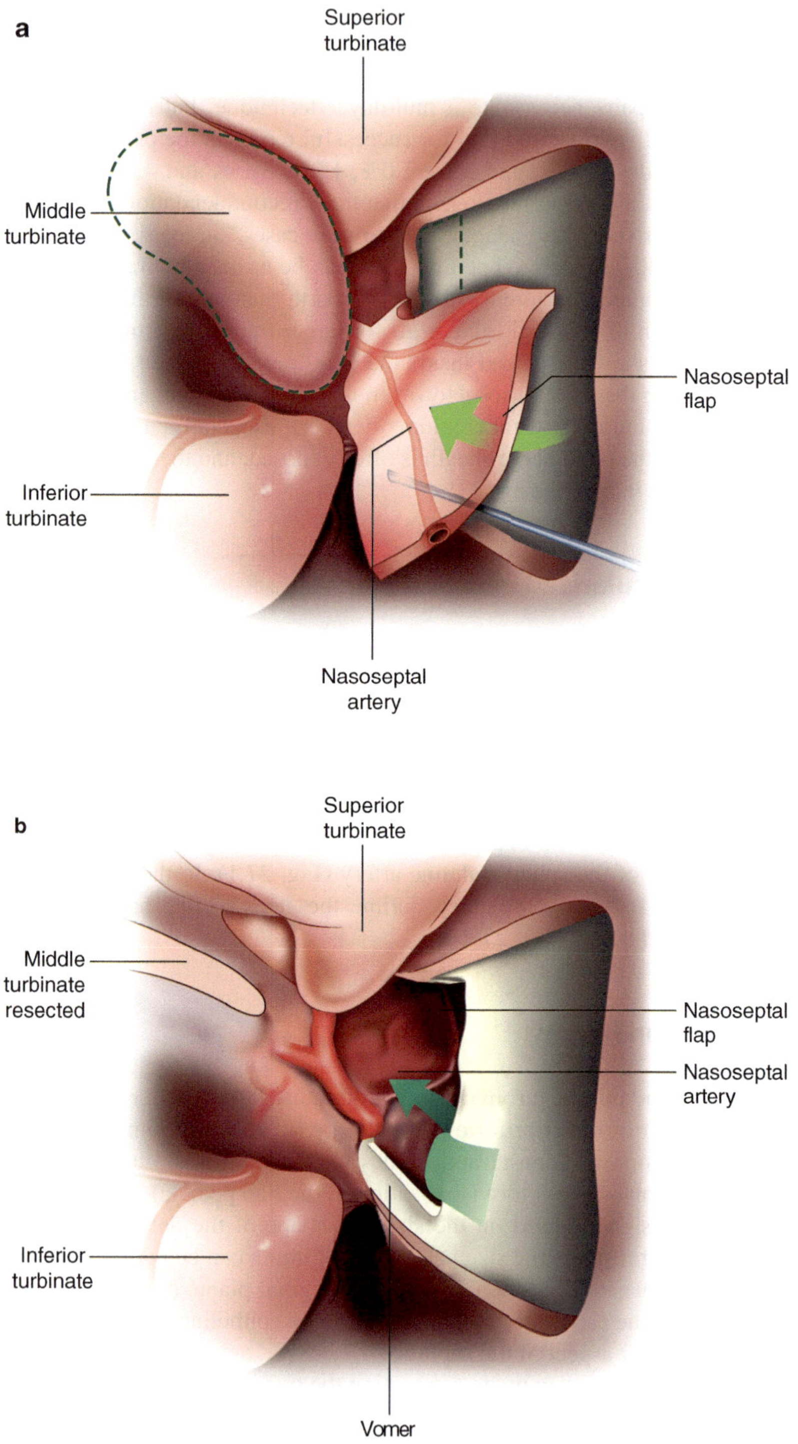


**Fig. 27.1** Vascular supply of the nasal septal mucosa. (This figure modified from Gutierrez et al. by Springer Nature. Gutierrez WR, Bennion DM, Walsh JE, Owen SR. Vascular pedicled flaps for skull base defect reconstruction. Laryngoscope Investig Otolaryngol. 2020;5(6):1029-1038)

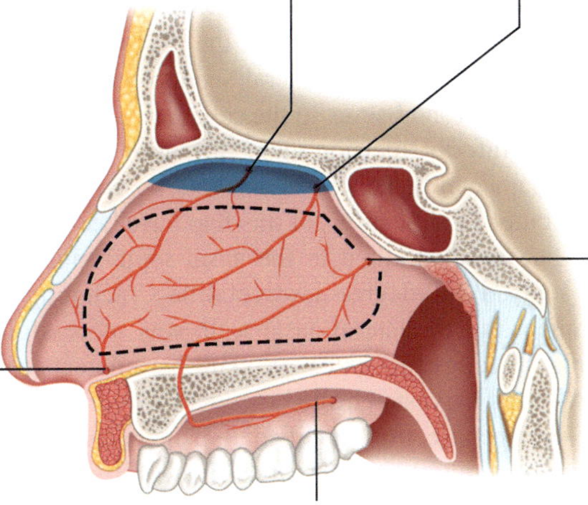


**Fig. 27.2** Illustration showing harvest and inset of the nasoseptal flap. (This figure modified from Laibangyang et al. by Springer Nature. Laibangyang A, Rodgers SD, Baron SL, et al. Pedicled nasoseptal flap reconstruction for craniopharyngiomas in pediatric patients. Childs Nerv Syst. 2020;36(3):491-496)

- At the posterior septum, the superior incision is extended laterally and with an inferior slant over the rostrum of the sphenoid sinus and crossing it horizontally at the level of the natural ostium.
- The inferior incision is then extended superiorly along the free posterior edge of the nasal septum and then laterally to cross the posterior choana below the floor of the sphenoid sinus.
- The flap is then elevated using a cottle dissector from anterior to posterior and completed once the flap is raised off of the face of the sphenoid sinus with preservation of the posterolateral pedicle. (It is recommended to complete all incisions prior to raising the flap because it is difficult to maintain orientation and tension once the flap is elevated).
- The flap can then be rotated down into the nasopharynx or placed against the lateral nasal wall until the ablative phase of the procedure is complete.
- The final defect is then reconstructed in a multilayer fashion as described in the previous section.

## Flap Advantages and Limitations

This flap is highly modifiable and can be sized to a varying degree of widths and lengths depending on the defect to be reconstructed. These capabilities make the nasoseptal flap the most versatile and superior vascularized pedicled flap for skull base reconstruction. If needed, the entirety of the mucoperichondrium and mucoperiosteum can be elevated off the ipsilateral septum to cover anterior skull base defects from the posterior frontal sinus to the sella turcica and span the orbits. It is possible to extend the inferior incision along the floor of the nose to gain extra width, and bilateral flaps can be harvested and interposed [25]. Since the original Hadad et al. article, other modifications of this flap have been reported.

The nasoseptal flap is not limited to the nasal septal mucosa and nasal floor either. In a recent study, a 360-degree nasoseptal flap, including the septum, nasal floor, and entire mucosa of the lateral nasal wall, was successfully harvested and used in five patients to reconstruct extensive skull base defects caused by invasive pituitary tumors. All flaps harvested healed successfully with no persistence of CSF rhinorrhea. However, because this modified flap includes the lateral nasal wall mucosa, one patient experienced nasolacrimal duct obstruction requiring dacryocystorhinostomy [25].

## Posterior Pedicle Inferior Turbinate Flap

The posterior pedicle inferior turbinate flap (PPITF), or inferior turbinate flap (ITF), is a local intranasal flap that is pedicled on the inferior turbinate artery. It can be used to repair the posterior aspect of the anterior cranial fossa for small-moderate-sized sellar or clival defects or as a secondary reconstructive method when the vascular supply of the nasoseptal flap has been compromised. This can occur secondary to tumor invasion and erosion of the vascular pedicle, previous septectomy, previous widened sphenoidotomy, or radiation therapy. ITF consideration is dependent on the anatomic location of the defect and the coverage required [18, 26]. Although it provides a reliable alternative to the HBF, it is important to consider other free grafts and local or regional reconstructive flaps.

To review, the vascular origin and route of the pertinent arteries will be described. The sphenopalatine artery is a terminal branch of the maxillary artery that leaves the pterygopalatine fossa via the sphenopalatine foramen to access the nasal cavity. Sphenopalatine artery branching is highly variable. The most clinically relevant pattern occurs as it bifurcates into the posterior lateral nasal artery and posterior septal nasal artery; the former is relevant to this technique [27].

The posterior lateral nasal artery supplies the majority of the lateral nasal wall, including the middle and inferior turbinates, by taking an anterior inferior route over the palatine perpendicular plate, during which it provides a medial branch to the middle turbinate. It descends on average 1.2 cm before piercing the inferior turbinate at the superior aspect of its lateral attachment 1.0–1.5 cm from the posterior margin. The posterior lateral nasal artery typically terminates by providing two inferior turbinate arteries that ultimately form a robust anastomotic connection with the anterior supply of the inferior turbinate [28].

## Flap Design and Harvest

- 1% lidocaine with 1:100,000 epinephrine is injected into the lateral nasal wall just anterior to the inferior turbinate to decongest the nasal cavity.
- After EEA has been completed, the inferior turbinate can be carefully medialized to provide optimal exposure of its entire medial surface.
- The uncinate process and ethmoid bulla are then removed to visualize the maxillary ostium. The sphenopalatine artery is visualized as it exits the sphenopalatine foramen and is followed until the posterior lateral nasal artery is identified, as this serves as the pedicle it is vital that it remains viable.
- The maxillary ostium can then be extended posteriorly; it is important to consider variations in the course of the posterior lateral nasal artery, as it may lie anterior to the posterior wall of the maxillary sinus.
- The submucoperiosteal mucosa is lifted from the anterior aspect of the palatine's ascending process posteriorly toward the crista ethmoidalis, sphenopalatine artery, and foramen.
- Two parallel incisions are made in the sagittal plane. A superior incision is made just above the inferior turbinate that extends from its posterior aspect, at the level of the middle meatal antrostomy, over its attachment to the lateral nasal wall. An inferior incision is made just below the inferior turbinate, along its caudal margin, in the posterior to anterior direction. A vertical incision is made connecting these two along the anterior head of the inferior turbinate.
- The mucoperiosteum is elevated from the floor of the inferior turbinate in an anteroposterior fashion. A variable amount of bone can be elevated depending on the ease of dissection.
- The flap is carefully unrolled so that the mucosal side faces externally and that the pedicle is free of kinks. After nonvascularized tissue, bone, and foreign body have been cleared in between the flap and defect margins, it can then be placed either directly to the dura, denuded bone or over a fat graft.
- After sealant or biological glue is applied over the flap, absorbable gelatin sponges are placed. To press the flap gently against the defect, a sponge nasal packing may be used. While a Foley catheter balloon can be used, some caution against its use to prevent untoward damage to the flap pedicle. Finally, silicone nasal splints are placed, and remain for 10–21 days postoperatively to protect the denuded lateral nasal wall [18, 26, 28, 29].

## Surgical Challenges of the ITF

A common technical challenge is the often difficult elevation of the ITF, especially after the inferior turbinate has been fractured. Additionally, because of the presence of the midline ridge overlying the mucosa of the inferior turbinate, the flap will often retain its shape. It may be necessary to make a small Y-shaped incision in the distal flap and flatten it for it to fit securely over the defect [26].

## Flap Advantages and Limitations

The ITF is a reliable option when the HBF is contraindicated. It eliminates risks associated with vascularized regional flaps such as parietal and pericranial flaps and minimizes healing time because of rapid mucosalization [29]. However, inherent limitations include shorter length, limited arc of coverage, and difficulty rotating the flap.

The estimated surface area provided by the ITF is not well described currently; several sources, even in recent literature, cite the 1999 Murakami et al. analysis of five cadavers, in which an average ITF was reported to be 4.97 $cm^2$ [18, 29, 30]. Regardless, surgeons in the field are aware of the limitations of the ITF and have since elaborated upon its design and capabilities. The extended ITF (EITF), described by Choby et al. 2014, incorporated nasal floor mucosa to supplement the ITF; this was further expanded upon with the addition of septal mucosa. They reported an EITF surface area of $27.26 \pm 3.65$ $cm^2$ and $40.53 \pm 6.45$ $cm^2$ with the addition of septal mucosa. For reference, the reported HBF surface area was 25 $cm^2$. The EITF also reduces the arc of rotation by providing a longer, further-reaching flap [28]. Fortunately, like the HBF, the ITF is modifiable, and its historical limitations are no longer absolute. The defects of the anterior skull base beyond the standard ITF's capabilities can be repaired effectively.

## Posterior Pedicle Middle Turbinate Flap

The posterior pedicle middle turbinate flap (PPMTF), or middle turbinate flap (MTF), is a local intranasal flap based on the middle turbinate artery, a medial branch of the posterior lateral nasal artery. The relevant vascular anatomy was described previously; however, the middle turbinate artery lies inferior to the middle turbinate and splits into anterior and posterior segments that vascularized the lateral and medial mucosa, respectively. As the MTF surface area is comparable to that of the ITF, similar limitations are found in both designs. However, the superior location of the vascular pedicle provides a means of reaching further into the anterior skull base. As such the MTF is a reliable option for reconstruction of the small-to-moderate-size defects of the planum sphenoidale, cribriform plate, or sella. If necessary, the flap can be used to repair clival defects, but the ITF is still considered the primary design if HBF is not an option [26, 30].

### Flap Design and Harvest

- To begin, a vertical incision is made along the anterior surface of the head of the middle turbinate. A second incision is made in the sagittal plane from anterior to posterior along the vertical attachment of the middle turbinate just inferior to the skull base.
- The mucoperiosteum is then elevated from the medial and lateral surfaces in a superior to inferior direction. To elevate the lateral aspect, a horizontal incision is made along the axilla that extends posteriorly to the level of the sphenopalatine foramen. A similar incision is made on the medial surface of the middle turbinate.
- By dissecting and elevating at the level of the sphenopalatine foramen, the reach and arch of rotation are increased.
- Finally, the flap is rotated and placed over the defect, and closure continues as previously described.
- When elevating the MTF, the posterior and superior attachments (ethmoid crest and vertical lamella, respectively) should be carefully considered. This is to prevent destabilization or fracturing of the middle turbinate. Such injuries can lead to CSF fistulae and associated complications [18, 26].

### Flap Advantages and Limitations

The MTF provides an additional option when the ITF or HBF are compromised. Like the ITF, the primary procedural challenge is faced when elevating the flap. In the presence of an unstable middle turbinate, anatomical variations such as concha bullosa, paradoxical turbinate, middle turbinate hypoplasia, or previous surgery, elevation becomes increasingly difficult. As such, MTF is generally contraindicated in these cases. In the case of previous sphenopalatine artery ligation, MTF is not an option [26, 30].

## Regional Vascularized Extranasal Flaps

### Endoscopic-Assisted Pericranial Flap

The pericranial flap is a versatile flap that has been proven reliable for the reconstruction of large skull base defects. The flap is an axial flap based on the supraorbital and supratrochlear arteries and can be harvested using an open approach as well as an endoscopically assisted approach utilizing two port scalp incisions. The endoscopic approach allows the surgeon to use durable vascularized tissue to repair large defects by transposing the pericranial tissue through a bony window tunnel into the nasal cavity without the need for an open, external flap harvest. Utilization of this flap is ideal for anterior cranial base defects because of the location of the pedicle and has been documented as a reliable flap for the reconstruction of cribriform and planar defects. With the extension of the flap, defects of the clivus have also been reported [31, 32].

## Flap Design and Harvest for Endoscopic Harvest

- A 2-cm midline incision and a 1-cm lateral port incision are marked along the coronal plane of the scalp.
- Identification of the supraorbital and supratrochlear arteries via a Doppler. Once identified, the artery locations are marked.
- A 3-cm wide pedicle is marked at the level of the supraorbital rim.
- The subgaleal plane is identified, and a subgaleal dissection is carried out until the anterior vascular pedicle is identified.
- Using an extended insulated needle tip cautery, the pericranium is incised, and the pericranial flap is elevated off the cranium.
- Next, the bony window tunnel is made by making a 1-cm transverse glabellar incision.
- This incision is carried down to the underlying nasion.
- A subperiosteal plane is made from the nasion up to the pedicle of the flap superiorly.
- The bone over the nasion is then drilled away until an opening into the nasal cavity is developed.
- The flap is then rotated into the nasal cavity using care to carefully place the pedicle without unneeded tension or strain.
- The flap should be applied with the superficial surface of the flap placed in contact with the dural defect.

## Flap Advantages and Limitations

The use of the endoscopic-assisted pericranial flap provides an option for minimally invasive reconstruction of skull base defects using durable, vascularized tissue. Outcomes of utilizing this flap have shown minimal donor site morbidity, high success rates without postoperative CSF leaks, and low complication rates [2, 17, 31]. It is a reliable option for skull base reconstruction in the event of intranasal tissue destruction by tumor or when prior intranasal surgery has eliminated intranasal vascular supply and is a good option when the need for postoperative radiotherapy is warranted. Some limitations of the flap include the need for bony osteotomy as well as limitations in posterior skull base defects because of the inability of the pedicle length.

## Temporoparietal Fascial Flap

The temporoparietal fascial flap is a regional flap based on the superficial temporal artery. It is a hardy flap that can provide extensive soft tissue coverage and can be used if no other reliable intranasal flap options are available. It is a good option when reconstruction of large clival and parasellar defects is needed [31].

## Flap Design and Harvest

- A total ethmoidectomy (anterior and posterior) is performed along with a large maxillary antrostomy.
- The sphenopalatine artery and posterior nasal artery are identified and clipped at the sphenopalatine foramen.
- The sphenopalatine artery is dissected posteriorly, and the posterior bony wall of the maxillary sinus is removed to expose the pterygopalatine fossa.
- Next, the infratemporal fossa is opened, and communication is formed with the nasal cavity by removing the lateral wall of the maxillary sinus.
- Within the infratemporal fossa, the descending palatine artery is identified, thus allowing the contents of the pterygopalatine fossa to be displaced inferiorly and laterally to expose the pterygoid plates.
- Reduction of the anterior pterygoid plates is performed with the drill to allow a wide opening for tunneling of the flap.
- Key anatomical structures within the pterygopalatine fossa include the internal maxillary artery, vidian nerve, and pterygopalatine ganglion. The internal maxillary artery and pterygopalatine artery should be preserved, but the division of the vidian nerve is required to separate the ganglion and allow it to be inferiorly displaced.
- Next, the temporoparietal fascial flap is harvested by utilizing a hemicoronal incision. It is key to preserve the superficial temporal artery and vein during the harvest. Extreme care should be taken as these lie superficial in the subcutaneous tissue and are at risk.
- After the hemicoronal incision is made, the fascia is incised laterally and is separated from the underlying muscle and deep fascia.
- The deep fascia is then removed from the underlying calvarium and dissected down to the pedicle creating a doorway for the flap to be tunneled.
- A lateral canthotomy can be performed to allow separation of the temporalis muscle from the lateral orbit and pterygomaxillary fissure.
- After the above is completed, there should be a tunnel that allows connection between the temporal fossa, the infratemporal fossa, and through the transpterygoid exposure to the skull base defect.
- The tunnel is sequentially dilated, and the flap is tunneled through to cover your skull base defect. After coverage, the flap can be stabilized with a sealant and/or gelfoam sponges.

## Flap Advantages and Limitations

The temporoparietal flap offers the ability for reconstruction of large skull base defects. It is a regional flap that can be used when intranasal flap options are limited or nonviable. It is ideal for clival and parasellar defects. Limitations of the flap include the need for an external incision, the risk of injury to the frontotemporal branch of the facial nerve, and a limit of axis of rotation limiting ability for reconstruction of the anterior skull base [17].

## Pearls for Reconstruction

Endoscopic skull base reconstruction can be technically challenging; however, adequate planning and adherence to the basic principles of skull base reconstruction, as outlined in this chapter, are key to producing a favorable outcome. A thorough understanding of the endoscopic anatomy, as well as the size and severity of the skull base defect, is of the utmost importance as it will dictate the technique and materials needed to perform a successful reconstruction. Regardless of the defect size, a multilayer closure technique should always be employed. The surgeon should always be ready to utilize multiple reconstructive options should certain options become unavailable. In the event a vascularized pedicle flap is indicated, it is prudent to harvest a larger flap than what may be needed to account for flap contraction and evolution of the skull base defect. This is of particular importance as many vascularized pedicled flaps are harvested prior to extirpation and creation of the defect. Meticulous attention to the flap inset is also crucial in mitigating postoperative complications such as mucocele formation. This applies specifically to the preparation of the defect as some authors recommend denuding ~1 cm of mucosa around the bony defect to prevent trapping of mucosa under the flap, which can result in the formation of a mucocele postoperatively [23].

Additionally, proper utilization of reconstructive options is crucial in the event of an unfavorable outcome with the need for revision surgery. In such a situation, the reconstructive surgeon must have backup options available, and if the feasible reconstructive options were overutilized during the initial surgery, it will greatly limit the reconstructive options available for revision surgery. Furthermore, the principles outlined in this chapter are intended to provide a general layout to the planning and execution of a successful skull base reconstruction with the understanding that these considerations must be applied on a case-by-case basis and variation in protocols based on institution and surgeons exist. The understanding of these principles and subsequent surgical planning must be openly communicated amongst the surgical specialties involved to ensure the best possible outcome.

## Postoperative Care

The postoperative care for endoscopic skull base repair is similar with or without a vascularized pedicle flap. Management includes avoiding activities that can raise the intracranial pressure, such as maintaining the head of the bed elevation, avoidance of nose blowing, heavy lifting, straining, and leaning forward. When a CSF leak is encountered intraoperatively, avoidance of these activities is recommended up to 4 weeks following surgery [33]. Adequate bowel regimen and stool softeners are also important to prevent straining during bowel movements [23, 24]. Nasal packing is typically maintained for 5 days on average but can be left in longer depending on risk factors, including high flow CSF leak, degree of arachnoid dissection, opening of a cistern, and patient body habitus [21, 24]. This can also be subject to surgeon preference as some authors recommend leaving packing in place for 10–12 days [23]. Once packing is removed, meticulous nasal hygiene with saline rinses and debridement is essential to mitigate nasal crusting. Debridement must be performed carefully so as not to disturb the flap positioning, inciting a CSF leak [24]. The use of postoperative antibiotics for the prevention of meningitis is controversial and highly variable among providers [34]. Though many surgeons will place patients on a course of postoperative antibiotics, including first to second and third to fifth generation cephalosporins [24, 25, 34]. Lumbar drain care is outside the scope of this chapter. However, meticulous maintenance and care of a lumbar drain, if used, is vital to prevent major complications, including tension pneumocephalus and meningitis. Some authors report the use of routine postoperative imaging within the first 24 h of surgery to screen for the presence of intracranial bleeding or developing tension pneumocephalus [24].

## References


1. Dehdashti AR, Ganna A, Witterick I, Gentili F. Expanded endoscopic endonasal approach for anterior cranial base and suprasellar lesions: indications and limitations. Neurosurgery. 2009;64(4):677–87.
2. Zimmer L, Theodosopoulos P. Anterior skull base surgery: open versus endoscopic; 2021.
3. Cappabianca P, Alfieri A, de Divitiis E, Tschabitscher M. Atlas of endoscopic anatomy for endonasal intracranial surgery. New York: Springer; 2001.
4. Moon HJ, Kim HU, Lee JG, Chung IH, Yoon JH. Surgical anatomy of the anterior ethmoidal canal in ethmoid roof. Laryngoscope. 2001;111(5):900–4. https://doi.org/10.1097/00005537-200105000-00027.
5. Castelnuovo P, Pistochini A, Locatelli D. Different surgical approaches to the sellar region: focusing on the "two nostrils four hands technique". Rhinology. 2006;44(1):2–7.
6. Cavallo LM, Somma T, Solari D, et al. Endoscopic endonasal transsphenoidal surgery: history and evolution. World Neurosurg. 2019;127:686–94. https://doi.org/10.1016/j.wneu.2019.03.048.
7. Kassam AB, Vescan AD, Carrau RL, et al. Expanded endonasal approach: vidian canal as a landmark to the petrous internal carotid artery. J Neurosurg. 2008;108(1):177–83. https://doi.org/10.3171/JNS/2008/108/01/0177.
8. Patel CR, Fernandez-Miranda JC, Wang WH, Wang EW. Skull base anatomy. Otolaryngol Clin North Am. 2016;49(1):9–20. https://doi.org/10.1016/j.otc.2015.09.001.

9. Kennedy D. Rhinology: diseases of the nose, sinuses, and skull base. New York: Thieme Medical Publishers; 2012. p. 631.
10. Razek AA, Huang BY. Lesions of the petrous apex: classification and findings at CT and MR imaging. Radiographics. 2012;32(1):151–73. https://doi.org/10.1148/rg.321105758.
11. Vescan AD, Carrau RL, Snyderman CH, Kassam AB, Mintz A, Gardner P. Minimally invasive techniques: endonasal endoscopic skull base surgery. In: Hanna EY, DeMonte F, editors. Comprehensive management of skull base tumors. 1st ed. Informa Health; 2009. p. 131.
12. Alokby G, Casiano RR. Endoscopic resection of sinonasal and ventral skull base malignancies. Otolaryngol Clin North Am. 2017;50(2):273–85. https://doi.org/10.1016/j.otc.2016.12.005.
13. Hanna EY, Kupferman M, DeMonte F. Surgical management of tumors of the nasal cavity, paranasal sinuses, orbit, and anterior skull base. In: Hanna EY, DeMonte F, editors. Comprehensive management of skull base tumors. 1st ed. Informa Health; 2009. p. 242.
14. Gan HW. Management of craniopharyngiomas in the era of molecular oncological therapies: not a panacea. J Endocr Soc. 2021;5(7):bvab094. https://doi.org/10.1210/jendso/bvab09.
15. Kasemsiri P, Carrau RL, Ditzel Filho LF, Prevedello DM, Otto BA, Old M, de Lara D, Kassam AB. Advantages and limitations of endoscopic endonasal approaches to the skull base. World Neurosurg. 2014;82(6 Suppl):S12–21. https://doi.org/10.1016/j.wneu.2014.07.022.
16. Snyderman CH, Wang EW, Zenonos GA, Gardner PA. Reconstruction after endoscopic surgery for skull base malignancies. J Neurooncol. 2020;150(3):463–8. https://doi.org/10.1007/s11060-020-03465-0.
17. Sigler AC, D'Anza B, Lobo BC, Woodard TD, Recinos PF, Sindwani R. Endoscopic skull base reconstruction: an evolution of materials and methods. Otolaryngol Clin North Am. 2017;50(3):643–53. https://doi.org/10.1016/j.otc.2017.01.015.
18. Zanation AM, Thorp BD, Parmar P, Harvey RJ. Reconstructive options for endoscopic skull base surgery. Otolaryngol Clin North Am. 2011;44(5):1201–22. https://doi.org/10.1016/j.otc.2011.06.016.
19. Green ST, Walkevar RR, Culicchia F, Nuss DW. Surgery of the anterior and middle cranial base. In: Flint PW, Haughey BH, Lund VJ, Thomas JR, Robbins KT, Francis HW, editors. Cummings otolaryngology: head and neck surgery, 7th ed. Elsevier; 2020. p. 2634–2661.
20. Fraser S, Gardner PA, Koutourousiou M, et al. Risk factors associated with postoperative cerebrospinal fluid leak after endoscopic endonasal skull base surgery. J Neurosurg. 2018;128(4):1066–71. https://doi.org/10.3171/2016.12.JNS1694.
21. Conger A, Zhao F, Wang X, et al. Evolution of the graded repair of CSF leaks and skull base defects in endonasal endoscopic tumor surgery: trends in repair failure and meningitis rates in 509 patients. J Neurosurg. 2018;130(3):861–75. https://doi.org/10.3171/2017.11.JNS172141.
22. Zwagerman NT, Wang EW, Shin SS, et al. Does lumbar drainage reduce postoperative cerebrospinal fluid leak after endoscopic endonasal skull base surgery? A prospective, randomized controlled trial [published online ahead of print, 2018 Oct 1]. J Neurosurg. 2018;131:1172–8. https://doi.org/10.3171/2018.4.JNS172447.
23. Liu JK, Schmidt RF, Choudhry OJ, Shukla PA, Eloy JA. Surgical nuances for nasoseptal flap reconstruction of cranial base defects with high-flow cerebrospinal fluid leaks after endoscopic skull base surgery. Neurosurg Focus. 2012;32(6):E7. https://doi.org/10.3171/2012.5.FOCUS1255.
24. Hadad G, Bassagasteguy L, Carrau RL, et al. A novel reconstructive technique after endoscopic expanded endonasal approaches: vascular pedicle nasoseptal flap. Laryngoscope. 2006;116(10):1882–6. https://doi.org/10.1097/01.mlg.0000234933.37779.e4.
25. Moon JH, Kim EH, Kim SH. Various modifications of a vascularized nasoseptal flap for repair of extensive skull base dural defects. J Neurosurg. 2019;132(2):371–9. https://doi.org/10.3171/2018.10.JNS181556.
26. Chakravarthi S, Gonen L, Monroy-Sosa A, Khalili S, Kassam A. Endoscopic endonasal reconstructive methods to the anterior skull base. Semin Plast Surg. 2017;31(4):203–13. https://doi.org/10.1055/s-0037-1607274.

27. Kuan EC, Palmer KN. Epistaxis. In: Flint PW, Haughey BH, Lund VJ, Thomas JR, Robbins KT, Francis HW, editors. Cummings otolaryngology: head and neck surgery, 7th ed. Elsevier; 2020. p. 733–744.
28. Choby GW, Pinheiro-Neto CD, de Almeida JR, et al. Extended inferior turbinate flap for endoscopic reconstruction of skull base defects. J Neurol Surg B Skull Base. 2014;75(4):225–30. https://doi.org/10.1055/s-0033-1358791.
29. Yip J, Macdonald KI, Lee J, Witterick IJ, Zadeh G, Gentili F, Vescan AD. The inferior turbinate flap in skull base reconstruction. J Otolaryngol Head Neck Surg. 2013;42(1):6. https://doi.org/10.1186/1916-0216-42-6.
30. Hachem RA, Beer-Furlan A, Jamshidi A, ElKhatib A, Carrau RL, Prevedello DM. Skull base reconstruction following resection of skull base chordomas and chondrosarcoma. In: Harsh IV GR, Vaz-Guimaraes F, editors. Chordomas and chondrosarcomas of the skull base and spine, 2nd ed. Academic; 2017. p. 259–270.
31. Kennedy D. Rhinology: diseases of the nose, sinuses, and skull base. New York: Thieme Medical Publishers; 2012. p. 699.
32. Kim GG, Hang AX, Mitchell CA, Zanation AM. Pedicled extranasal flaps in skull base reconstruction. Adv Otorhinolaryngol. 2013;74:71–80. https://doi.org/10.1159/000342282.
33. Tien DA, Stokken JK, Recinos PF, Woodard TD, Sindwani R. Comprehensive postoperative management after endoscopic skull base surgery. Otolaryngol Clin North Am. 2016;49(1):253–63. https://doi.org/10.1016/j.otc.2015.09.015.
34. Fang CH, Hawn VS, Agarwal V, et al. Antibiotic prophylaxis in anterior skull-base surgery: a survey of the North American Skull Base Society. Int Forum Allergy Rhinol. 2019;9(10):1196–204. https://doi.org/10.1002/alr.22396.

# Open (Anterior) Skull Base Repair

# 28

Yusuf M. Agamawi, Fiyin Sokoya, and Yadranko Ducic

## Introduction

The development of interdisciplinary skull base surgery started with the collaboration between otolaryngology and neurosurgery, and it has continued to change with the advancement in technology and techniques from ablative and reconstructive skull base surgeries [1]. These advancements have caused a paradigm shift from open techniques to endoscopic techniques, becoming the standard for skull base surgery. However, it is crucial not to let open skull base surgery become a "lost art" because open skull base reconstruction techniques for certain malignant tumors, larger composite defects, major craniofacial trauma, osteoradionecrosis, and failed previous endoscopic reconstructions are still often indicated [1].

The main goals of skull base reconstruction are to recreate a water-tight seal and separation between the intracranial and extracranial contents while also eliminating dead space and restoring reasonable form and function [1]. Anterior skull base reconstruction can be done with grafting of local tissues (e.g., free mucosal graft) and/or manufactured products (e.g., acellular matrices) in conjunction with or without local vascularized flap (e.g., pedicle-based nasoseptal flap) for minor defects that generally coincide with endoscopic skull base surgery. For larger skull base defects, the reconstructions can range from the minor ones mentioned above in

Y. M. Agamawi (✉)
Department of Otolaryngology—Head and Neck Surgery, Saint Louis University School of Medicine, Saint Louis, MO, USA

Otolaryngology and Facial Plastic Surgery Associates, Fort Worth, TX, USA

F. Sokoya
Wellstar Health Systems, Atlanta, GA, USA

Y. Ducic
Otolaryngology and Facial Plastic Surgery Associates, Atlanta, GA, USA



F. Sokoya, A. G. Vincent (eds.), *Manual of Head and Neck Reconstruction*,
https://doi.org/10.1007/978-3-031-65999-7_28

combination with larger pedicled muscle and/or fascia flaps (e.g., pericranium or temporalis muscle) and/or free tissue transfer or free flap.

## Anatomy

Skull base surgery offers a unique "bi-approach" capability with the option to approach endoscopically through the sinonasal cavities from below and/or approach externally or open through the skin via the scalp and/or forehead from above the skull base. To operate at full capacity, it is necessary to understand the anatomy and its relations when approaching from above and below the skull base.

The anterior skull base is composed of the frontal, ethmoid, and sphenoid bones, and this thin osseous structure separates the intracranial contents from the sinonasal and orbital contents. The frontal bone contributes to the posterior wall of the frontal sinus and the roof of the orbits, the ethmoid bone forms the ethmoid sinus roof and cribriform plate, and lastly, the posterior portion of the skull base is made up of the planum sphenoidale and anterior clinoid processes of the sphenoid bone (Fig. 28.1) [1]. Briefly in regards to sinonasal anatomy from below or inferior to the skull base, the anterior border is frontal sinus and/or agger nasi cell, the lateral border is the lateral sinonasal wall and medial orbital wall/orbit, the posterior border is the posterior sphenoid wall and/or sella turcica, and when unilateral the medial border is nasal septum and cribriform plate of the ethmoid bone. From the transnasal endoscopic approach, the oversimplified anatomical skull base layering is mucosa,

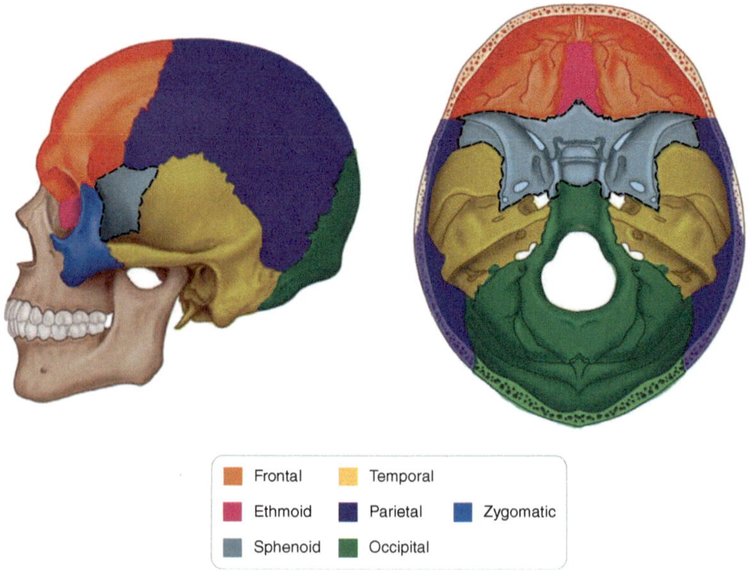


**Fig. 28.1** Skull base bony anatomy

periosteum, bone, meninges (dura mater, arachnoid, cerebrospinal fluid (CSF), pia mater), and then brain tissue.

For open skull base surgery, it is critical to understand scalp and forehead anatomy. The anatomic layers of the scalp, from superficial to deep, are the (S)kin, sub(C)cutaneous tissue, galea (A)poneurosis, (L)oose areolar tissue, and (P)ericranium, which form the mnemonic "SCALP" (Fig. 28.2) [2]. In regards to scalp reconstruction, there are "loose areas" of the scalp, which allow great mobility of the scalp for local tissue rearrangement, and there are "tight areas" with little to give. The area with the greatest mobility is at the temporoparietal fascia overlying the temporalis fascia, and the area with the least mobility is at the temporal line where the galea is adherent to the pericranium. However, this may be released to increase mobility [2]. Blood vessels and nerves that supply the skin of the scalp run superficially to the galea aponeurosis and frontalis muscle within the subcutaneous tissue layer [2].

The vasculature of the scalp and forehead originates from both the internal and external carotid arteries with an extensive network of terminal branches and the formation of collaterals to aid in redundant blood supply to the areas (Fig. 28.3). The forehead and anterior scalp blood supply comes from the supraorbital (laterally) and supratrochlear (medially) artery branches from the ophthalmic artery via the internal carotid artery. The lateral temporal and parietal scalp areas are supplied by the branches from the superficial temporal artery (STA) via the external carotid artery.

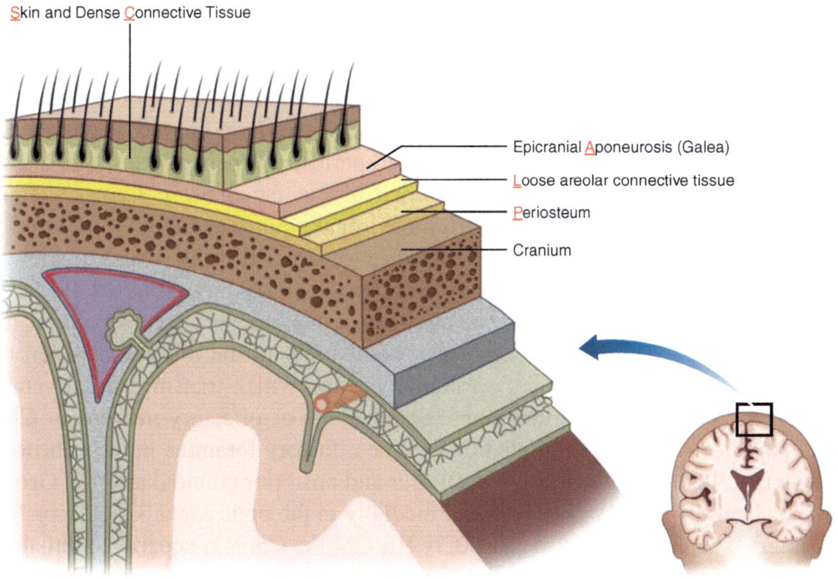


**Fig. 28.2** Scalp tissue anatomy

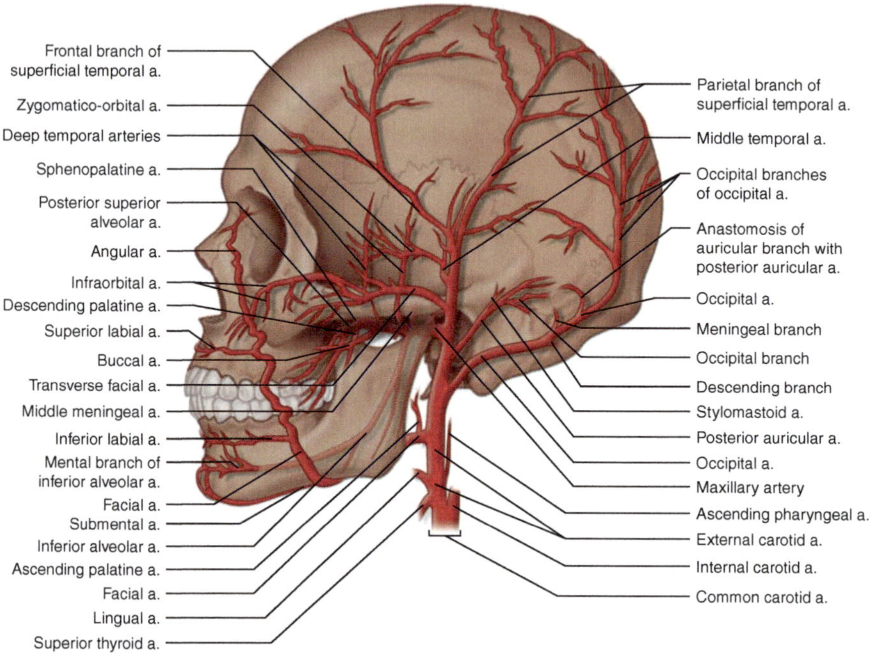


**Fig. 28.3** Vasculature anatomy of scalp and forehead

The temporal region is more anatomically complex given the more soft tissue covering layers of the temporal calvarium and clinical importance in regards to cranial nerve (CN) VII (facial nerve). The soft tissue layers from superficial to deep are the skin, subcutaneous tissue, superficial temporal fascia (temporoparietal fascia), superficial layer of the deep temporal fascia, temporal fat pad, deep layer of deep temporal fascia, temporalis muscle, and periosteum/pericranium. The classic path of the frontotemporal (frontal) branch of the facial nerve traverses along Pitanguy's Line, which is generally from the tragal pointer (1 cm anterior, inferior, and deep to tragus; approximates the location of CV VII trunk where it exits the stylomastoid foramen) to about 1.5–2 cm above the lateral brow (Fig. 28.4) [2, 3].

There are several other intracranial and extracranial neurovascular structures traversing the bony skeleton of the anterior skull base. In the midline between the crista galli and frontal bone is the foramen cecum, which transmits nasal venous drainage to the superior sagittal sinus. Smell fibers or olfactory neurons of CN I travel superiorly through multiple holes of the olfactory foramina in the cribriform plate to the olfactory bulb above the anterior and posterior ethmoid arteries. Orbital contents laterally travel posteriorly and medially in the optic canal (CN II, ophthalmic artery), superior orbital fissure (CN III, CN IV, CN V1, superior ophthalmic vein), and inferior orbital fissure (inferior ophthalmic vein) to converge toward the internal carotid arteries, cavernous sinus, and optic chiasm at the anterior clinoid process, which is the border between the anterior and middle cranial fossae.

Fig. 28.4 Pitanguy's line

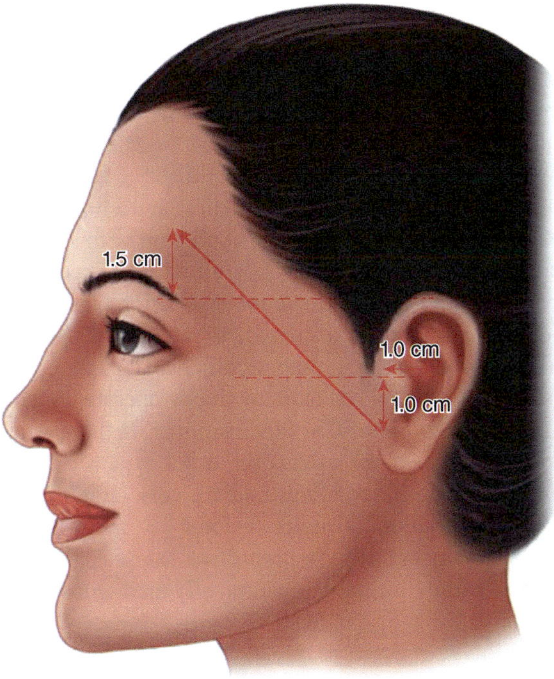


## Planning

The primary objective of skull base reconstruction is to recreate a durable watertight seal separating the intradural contents from external exposure [1]. This facilitates the prevention/reduction of possible high-risk complications from persistent CSF leak/fistula, such as meningitis, pneumocephalus, and the associated morbidity and mortality that increase over time [1]. The secondary objective is to eliminate dead space, return function, and restore cosmesis [1, 4]. The reconstruction strategy to attain these objectives requires careful consideration of various anatomic and patient-related factors. Furthermore, the strategy must incorporate multiple reconstruction options, including free tissue transfer or free flaps, to account for the unpredictability of ablative skull base surgery.

The utilization of three-dimensional (3D) reconstructions from fine-cut computed tomography (CT) and magnetic resonance imaging (MRI) for virtual surgical planning (VSP) is becoming more pronounced, especially with extensive defects, and the application of multiplanar imaging for surgical navigation is considered the standard of care [1, 5, 6]. VSP may help better define the extent of the tumor and/or defect to aid in reconstruction planning and prefabrication of customized hardware, implants, and prostheses [1, 7–11].

## Anatomic Factors

Anatomic factors to consider mainly pertain to the defect's location, size/volume, and the associated extent of the communication between the intradural and extradural spaces. Persistent CSF leaks have been associated with intraoperative CSF leaks, clival defects, and large dural openings [1, 12–15]. To minimize complications, the integrity of the dural reconstruction and eliminating dead space are critical. For anterior defects of the anterior skull base with small dural defect and/or intact bony ledge, underlay grafts or flaps with multilayered acellular alloplastic materials and free grafts may be adequate reconstruction, and potentially, the weight of the anterior intracranial contents may help seal the reconstruction [1, 16]. For large posteriorly portioned defects with significant dura defect and/or bony loss, vascularized tissue is often required along with postoperative medical management of CSF pressure with or without CSF diversion [1]. If there is persistent dead space along the skull base tissue reconstruction, dural expansion via duraplasty should be considered [1]. Skull base defects that are very large involve significant bone loss (especially orbitocranial and/or extend to middle cranial fossa), include orbital exenteration, and/or have high-flow CSF leaks likely to require free flap(s) for volume and allow for more anatomically analogous tissue reconstructions [1].

## Patient Factors

Patient factors to evaluate are history of radiation therapy, prior surgeries and reconstruction attempts, and availability of local tissues for reconstruction [1]. Radiation therapy prior to surgery has been associated with poor wound healing and central nervous complications (e.g., CSF leak and meningitis) in skull base reconstruction [1, 12, 17–19]. Prior head and neck surgeries and/or reconstruction attempts may have disrupted the local vasculature and subsequently lessened the reliability and/or availability of local or pedicled flaps. This, coupled with the unpredictability of ablative skull base surgery, further highlights the need to strategize multiple reconstruction options.

# Instruments and Equipment Setup

Facial trauma and plastic and/or head and neck basic tray(s) with varying-sized toothed pickups, dissecting scissors, scalpels, osteotomes, periosteal elevators, bipolar cautery, saw, and attachments.

Fixation system with appropriate drills, drill bits and attachments, various plate sizes/shapes, and associated screws. Consider having a Mitek mini bone anchor system, external nasal splints/casts (e.g., Aquaplast) and K-wire available for naso-orbitoethmoid (naso-orbital-ethmoid; NOE) complex reconstruction.

## Surgical Technique

Open skull base reconstruction is performed under general anesthesia with the patient/operative table turned 180° to allow the surgeon(s) full and uninhibited access to the patient's head, as well as to be sure that other potential tissue donor sites remain accessible if needed. Suppose the reconstruction is in coordination with ablation, and it is a two-team approach. In that case, the reconstruction team/surgeon(s) should routinely check in with the ablative team/surgeon(s) to assess the progress of the defect so that the reconstructive plan can be adjusted if needed. Reconstructive options range from nonvascular grafts and manufactured materials, local and regional flaps, and free tissue transfer or free flaps. It is critical to reestablish that water-tight seal between the intradural and extradural compartments and eliminate dead space, as well as a tension-free repair for locoregional and free flap reconstructions.

The main approach utilized for open skull base surgery is the coronal approach. For the coronal incisional approach, the patient's head is generally shaved, or a 1–2 cm width strip is shaved along the proposed incision(s). Local anesthetic (1% lidocaine with 1:100,000 epinephrine) is infiltrated along the proposed incision(s). Surgical sites, including all potential reconstructive donor sites, are then prepped (betadine paint) and draped sterilely. It is critical to be continuously cautious and cognizant of the eyes and to place eye corneal shields at the beginning of the case to protect the eyes and vision of the patients.

## Nonvascular and Manufactured Grafts

There are a wide variety of nonvascular autologous tissue grafts (e.g., nasal mucoperichondrium and mucoperiosteum, tensor fascia lata, temporoparietal fascia, calvarial bone, and abdominal adipose tissue) and acellular manufactured materials (e.g., DuraGen (Integra LifeSciences), AlloDerm (Allergan), DuraSeal (Integra LifeSciences), and hydroxyapatite cement) [1, 20–25]. They have been successfully used for skull base repair in combination with multiple layers, gasket-seal configuration, button, and/or underlay grafting. However, the defects are relatively small, with bony ledge present as described in endoscopic skull base surgery and commonly used in combination with vascularized flaps [1, 13, 26, 27].

## Local and Regional Flaps

The main pillar of anterior skull base reconstruction is vascularized locoregional flaps [1]. The nasal septal or Hadad-Bassagasteguy flap base off of the posterior septal artery is the main go-to flap in endoscopic reconstruction with decreased CSF leak rates [1, 12, 28]. However, the nasal septal flap has limited use for the reconstruction of large skull base defects and may not be an option with advanced tumors requiring resection of the nasal septum.

The pericranial flap is the workhorse for open craniofacial and skull base reconstruction surgery because of its wide surface area, significant length, and reliable vascularity [1, 29]. This flap receives its blood supply from the supratrochlear and supraorbital blood vessels and is ideal for patients with a history of and/or anticipating radiation therapy [1, 29]. Depending on the defect, the pericranial flap can be harvested unilaterally or bilaterally, and because of its thinness and pliability, it is a very functional option to restore a dural lining that will be used with other soft tissue or bony reconstructions [1, 30]. An osteo-pericranial composite flap using split calvarial bone grafts has been described to reconstruct defects needing a more rigid structure [1, 31].

The temporoparietal fascia flap (TPFF) has similar characteristics to the pericranial flap, which makes it an excellent choice in skull base reconstruction, especially for more lateral defects. The TPFF is superficial to the superficial layer of the deep temporalis fascia, and it is continuity with the adjacent and medial galea aponeurosis [32]. The superficial temporal artery (STA) from the external carotid system is the blood supply for the TPFF. The main trunk of the STA divides into multiple branches about 3 cm above the level of the zygomatic arch [32]. The STA also gives rise to the middle temporal artery and, if dissected with the STA, allows concomitant harvesting of deep temporal fascia, temporalis muscle, and/or adjacent calvarial bone [32–34]. Similar to pericranium with its versatility and pliability, TPFF may be tunneled through "keyholes" into the skull base [1].

The fan-shaped temporalis muscle transposition flap is another commonly used option for skull base reconstruction. It has a robust blood supply, mainly from the anterior and posterior deep temporal artery branches off of the internal maxillary artery from the external carotid artery, as well as an accessory supply from the middle temporal artery [35]. The temporal muscle spans the temporal fossa from the inferior temporal line superiorly to under the zygomatic arch to the coronoid process and ascending ramus of the mandible inferiorly [35, 36]. This muscle flap inherently provides more bulk than the pericranium and TPFF, which is useful for filling dead space, and muscle tissue has been shown to have improved healing properties [1, 37]. A composite flap with attached calvarial bone may be harvested to aid in bony reconstruction [1, 38, 39]. Skull base defects with orbital exenteration are excellent candidates for reconstruction with temporalis muscle flap because this flap can be tunneled through the lateral orbital wall or via the sphenoid keyhole technique [1, 35]. Because of its attachment at the coronoid process and ascending ramus of the mandible and its proximal blood supply, the reach/coverage of the temporalis muscle flap is somewhat limited and not ideal for medial or contralateral defects [1]. Other notable fasciocutaneous or myocutaneous regional flaps, but less commonly used due to reach/coverage limitations, are median or paramedian forehead flaps (supratrochlear artery) as local flap options, and trapezius, pectoralis, and latissimus as regional flap options [1].

## Free Tissue Transfer

Free tissue transfer or free flaps are a mainstay in anterior skull base reconstruction given the versatility with size (surface area, volume), composition (soft tissue and/or bony), and ability to shape. Free flaps provide a superior capacity to obliterate significant dead space and have been shown to reduce the risk of serious postoperative complications such as CSF leak, meningitis, and pneumocephalus [1, 40–42]. For substantial skull base dural defects and salvage cases, particularly with a history of extensive surgery and/or radiation therapy, free flaps are being considered the standard for reconstruction [1]. Soft tissue-free flap options include rectus abdominis, latissimus dorsi, anterolateral thigh (ALT), vastus lateralis, vascularized tensor fascia lata, and radial forearm. Bony-free flap options include fibula and scapula.

## Coronal Approach and Pericranial Flap

Prior to incision, the planned/marked incision is infiltrated subcutaneously with local anesthetic containing epinephrine (e.g., 0.5–2% lidocaine with 1:100,000 or 1:200,000 epinephrine).

For the coronal approach, incision placement and design will vary depending on the patient's hairline and/or balding pattern. Generally, most incisions will be from one superior helical root region to the other to allow adequate exposure, and the incisions will be a wave or zigzag/sawtooth geometric pattern rather than the traditional bow-like incision to better camouflage the incision scar [43]. Incisions can be extended inferiorly into the preauricular region bilaterally to allow for further exposure to the superior half of the maxilla if needed [44].

The initial incision should be between the upper origins of the temporal muscles, extending from one temporal line to the other and down to, but not through, the pericranium at the subgaleal plane [43, 44]. From the superior temporal line, the subgaleal plane continues deep to the temporoparietal fascia (superficial temporal fascia) but above the deep temporal fascia. The skin incision is continued laterally and inferiorly to the superior helical root or insertion area of the zygomatic arch. If considering TPFF, be cognizant of the STA and stay superficial to temporoparietal fascia in the subcutaneous layer. As a way to avoid incising the deep temporal fascia and temporalis muscle, which may cause brisk bleeding, undermining the skin soft tissue with scissors in the subgaleal plane on the deep temporal fascia can be done prior to incising the skin soft tissue [43]. The incision can then be further extended inferiorly into the preauricular region within a preauricular skin crease at the same subgaleal plane on the deep temporalis fascia. The coronal flap is then raised anteriorly in the subgaleal plane (within loose areolar tissue) above the pericranium and deep temporal fascia, with the dissection starting midline and then going out laterally on both sides to create a broad flap. The broad anterior dissection and raising of the coronal flap should be continued to the level of the supraorbital rims. The pericranium must be incised to develop and elevate the pericranial flap to expose the bony supraorbital rims and foramina with associated neurovascular bundles.

The pericranium is raised separately as an anteriorly pedicled vascularized flap for reconstructive purposes as needed. Prior to incising the pericranial flap posteriorly, the supra-pericranial dissection can be carried out posteriorly as far as the occiput. This would allow the posterior pericranial incision to be placed even further posteriorly and create an extended pericranial flap that could possibly double the length of the pericranial flap [44, 45]. The lateral incisions of the pericranial flap are at the superior temporal line from the posterior incision to the supraorbital rim. The pericranial flap is then elevated anteriorly from the posterior incision to expose the supraorbital rims. If the supraorbital foramen are true foramen, then a small osteotome can be used to chisel out the inferior portion of the foramen and convert the foramen to a notch, which then will release the supraorbital neurovascular bundle [43]. The coronal and pericranial flaps are then further elevated anteriorly and inferiorly to expose the bony mid-face as needed.

## Temporoparietal Fascia Flap (TPFF)

As mentioned earlier, the TPF and its blood supply are just deep into the subcutaneous fat layer. Once the appropriate plane just superior to the TPF and the desired area of TPF is exposed, the distal periphery of the flap from its pedicle can be sharply incised. The TPFF can then be elevated in a distal to proximal fashion. The middle temporal artery branch of the STA may be identified, dissected, and preserved if TPFF is to include deep temporal fascia, temporalis muscle, and/or adjacent calvarial bone [32–34]. Once the flap is fully elevated, it can be rotated and/or tunneled toward the defect for reconstruction. The tunneling may occur through the defect or a carefully made “keyhole” defect through the superolateral orbit or greater wing of the sphenoid bone at the zygomaticosphenoid suture line via a drill with a fluted burr [35].

## Temporalis Muscle Flap

Similar approach to TPFF, the temporalis muscle is identified, and its overlying fascia is incised superiorly. Dissection directly on top of the temporalis muscle is carried inferiorly and anteriorly toward the zygomatic arch and coronoid process. Being directly on top of the temporalis muscle allows you to preserve the frontal branch of CN VII and the temporal fat pads. After the temporalis muscle is fully exposed, the portion needed for reconstruction is elevated from the temporal fossa in a superior-posterior to inferior-anterior direction. The temporalis muscle flap can then be rotated and/or tunneled in a similar fashion as the TPFF toward the skull base defect for reconstruction.

## Postoperative Management

Postoperative management after repair of skull base defects should be carefully streamlined to avoid complications, such as pneumocephalus, graft migration, reactivation of CSF leak, and meningitis. A lumbar drain is often needed to decrease CSF pressure and allow time for the repair graft to heal. Head of bed elevation may be required to alleviate nasal congestion. Nasal precautions like no nose blowing, straining, and sneezing with mouth open are often important. Diet advancement, pain control, and seizure prophylaxis may be catered to individual patient indications.

## References


1. Kwon D, Iloreta A, Miles B, Inman J. Open anterior skull base reconstruction: a contemporary review. Semin Plast Surg. 2017;31(4):189–96.
2. Sokoya M, Inman J, Ducic Y. Scalp and forehead reconstruction. Semin Plast Surg. 2018;32(2):90–4.
3. Tolhurst DE, Carstens MH, Greco RJ, Hurwitz DJ. The surgical anatomy of the scalp. Plast Reconstr Surg. 1991;87(4):603–12; discussion 613–604.
4. Weber SM, Kim JH, Wax MK. Role of free tissue transfer in skull base reconstruction. Otolaryngol Head Neck Surg. 2007;136(6):914–9.
5. Zinreich SJ, Mattox DE, Kennedy DW, et al. 3-D CT for cranial facial and laryngeal surgery. Laryngoscope. 1988;98(11):1212–9.
6. Liu GTHHK. Three-dimensional display of human organs from computed tomograms. Comp Graphics Image Process. 1979;9(1):1–21.
7. Rosahl SK, Gharabaghi A, Hubbe U, Shahidi R, Samii M. Virtual reality augmentation in skull base surgery. Skull Base. 2006;16(2):59–66.
8. Markiewicz MR, Bell RB. The use of 3D imaging tools in facial plastic surgery. Facial Plast Surg Clin North Am. 2011;19(4):655–82, ix.
9. Levine JP, Patel A, Saadeh PB, Hirsch DL. Computer-aided design and manufacturing in craniomaxillofacial surgery: the new state of the art. J Craniofac Surg. 2012;23(1):288–93.
10. Schipper J, Ridder GJ, Spetzger U, Teszler CB, Fradis M, Maier W. Individual prefabricated titanium implants and titanium mesh in skull base reconstructive surgery. A report of cases. Eur Arch Otorrinolaringol. 2004;261(5):282–90.
11. Saigal K, Winokur RS, Finden S, Taub D, Pribitkin E. Use of three-dimensional computerized tomography reconstruction in complex facial trauma. Facial Plast Surg. 2005;21(3):214–20.
12. Zanation AM, Carrau RL, Snyderman CH, et al. Nasoseptal flap reconstruction of high flow intraoperative cerebral spinal fluid leaks during endoscopic skull base surgery. Am J Rhinol Allergy. 2009;23(5):518–21.
13. Patel MR, Stadler ME, Snyderman CH, et al. How to choose? Endoscopic skull base reconstructive options and limitations. Skull Base. 2010;20(6):397–404.
14. Harvey RJ, Nogueira JF, Schlosser RJ, Patel SJ, Vellutini E, Stamm AC. Closure of large skull base defects after endoscopic transnasal craniotomy. Clinical article. J Neurosurg. 2009;111(2):371–9.
15. Thorp BD, Sreenath SB, Ebert CS, Zanation AM. Endoscopic skull base reconstruction: a review and clinical case series of 152 vascularized flaps used for surgical skull base defects in the setting of intraoperative cerebrospinal fluid leak. Neurosurg Focus. 2014;37(4):E4.
16. Germani RM, Vivero R, Herzallah IR, Casiano RR. Endoscopic reconstruction of large anterior skull base defects using acellular dermal allograft. Am J Rhinol. 2007;21(5):615–8.
17. Ganly I, Patel SG, Singh B, et al. Complications of craniofacial resection for malignant tumors of the skull base: report of an international collaborative study. Head Neck. 2005;27(6):445–51.

18. Harvey RJ, Smith JE, Wise SK, Patel SJ, Frankel BM, Schlosser RJ. Intracranial complications before and after endoscopic skull base reconstruction. Am J Rhinol. 2008;22(5):516–21.
19. Paderno A, Piazza C, Bresciani L, Vella R, Nicolai P. Microvascular head and neck reconstruction after (chemo)radiation: facts and prejudices. Curr Opin Otolaryngol Head Neck Surg. 2016;24(2):83–90.
20. Wormald PJ, McDonogh M. The bath-plug closure of anterior skull base cerebrospinal fluid leaks. Am J Rhinol. 2003;17(5):299–305.
21. Leng LZ, Brown S, Anand VK, Schwartz TH. "Gasket-seal" watertight closure in minimal-access endoscopic cranial base surgery. Neurosurgery. 2008;62(5 Suppl 2):ONSE342–3; discussion ONSE343.
22. Wigand ME. Transnasal ethmoidectomy under endoscopical control. Rhinology. 1981;19(1):7–15.
23. Narotam PK, van Dellen JR, Bhoola KD. A clinicopathological study of collagen sponge as a dural graft in neurosurgery. J Neurosurg. 1995;82(3):406–12.
24. Cappabianca P, Esposito F, Cavallo LM, et al. Use of equine collagen foil as dura mater substitute in endoscopic endonasal transsphenoidal surgery. Surg Neurol. 2006;65(2):144–8; discussion 149.
25. Verret DJ, Ducic Y, Oxford L, Smith J. Hydroxyapatite cement in craniofacial reconstruction. Otolaryngol Head Neck Surg. 2005;133(6):897–9.
26. Soudry E, Turner JH, Nayak JV, Hwang PH. Endoscopic reconstruction of surgically created skull base defects: a systematic review. Otolaryngol Head Neck Surg. 2014;150(5):730–8.
27. Garcia-Navarro V, Anand VK, Schwartz TH. Gasket seal closure for extended endonasal endoscopic skull base surgery: efficacy in a large case series. World Neurosurg. 2013;80(5):563–8.
28. Hadad G, Bassagasteguy L, Carrau RL, et al. A novel reconstructive technique after endoscopic expanded endonasal approaches: vascular pedicle nasoseptal flap. Laryngoscope. 2006;116(10):1882–6.
29. Miles B, Davis S, Crandall C, Ellis E 3rd. Laser-Doppler examination of the blood supply in pericranial flaps. J Oral Maxillofac Surg. 2010;68(8):1740–5.
30. Snyderman CH, Janecka IP, Sekhar LN, Sen CN, Eibling DE. Anterior cranial base reconstruction: role of galeal and pericranial flaps. Laryngoscope. 1990;100(6):607–14.
31. Kantrowitz AB, Hall C, Moser F, Spallone A, Feghali JG. Split-calvaria osteoplastic rotational flap for anterior fossa floor repair after tumor excision. Technical note. J Neurosurg. 1993;79(5):782–6.
32. Jawad BA, Raggio BS. Temporoparietal fascia flaps. In: StatPearls. Treasure Island; 2022.
33. Jose A, Nagori SA, Arya S, Roy ID. Chimeric temporopareital osteofascial and temporalis muscle flap; a novel method for the reconstruction of composite orbito-maxillary defects. J Stomatol Oral Maxillofac Surg. 2019;120(3):250–4.
34. Denadai R, Raposo-Amaral CE, Marques FF, Raposo-Amaral CA. Posttraumatic eyebrow reconstruction with hair-bearing temporoparietal fascia flap. Einstein (Sao Paulo). 2015;13(1):106–9.
35. Sokoya M, Bahrami A, Cohn J, Kadakia S, Mourad M, Ducic Y. Orbital skull base reconstruction with temporalis muscle: the sphenoid keyhole technique. Craniomaxillofac Trauma Reconstr Open. 2018;2(1):s-0038-1669421.
36. Smith JE, Ducic Y, Adelson R. The utility of the temporalis muscle flap for oropharyngeal, base of tongue, and nasopharyngeal reconstruction. Otolaryngol Head Neck Surg. 2005;132(3):373–80.
37. Chan JK, Harry L, Williams G, Nanchahal J. Soft-tissue reconstruction of open fractures of the lower limb: muscle versus fasciocutaneous flaps. Plast Reconstr Surg. 2012;130(2):284e–95e.
38. Bakamjian VY, Souther SG. Use of temporal muscle flap for reconstruction after orbito-maxillary resections for cancer. Plast Reconstr Surg. 1975;56(2):171–7.
39. Smith JE, Ducic Y, Adelson RT. Temporalis muscle flap for reconstruction of skull base defects. Head Neck. 2010;32(2):199–203.
40. Moyer JS, Chepeha DB, Teknos TN. Contemporary skull base reconstruction. Curr Opin Otolaryngol Head Neck Surg. 2004;12(4):294–9.

41. Chang DW, Langstein HN, Gupta A, et al. Reconstructive management of cranial base defects after tumor ablation. Plast Reconstr Surg. 2001;107(6):1346–55; discussion 1356–1347.
42. Clayman GL, DeMonte F, Jaffe DM, et al. Outcome and complications of extended cranial-base resection requiring microvascular free-tissue transfer. Arch Otolaryngol Head Neck Surg. 1995;121(11):1253–7.
43. Cornelius C-P, Gellrich N, Hillerup S, Kusumoto K, Schubert W. Midface. https://surgeryreference.aofoundation.org/cmf/trauma/midface. Accessed 12 Jan 2022.
44. Ducic Y, Coimbra C. The subfrontal approach to the anterior skull base. Oper Techn Otolaryngol Head Neck Surg. 2010;21(1):9–18.
45. Smith JE, Ducic Y. The versatile extended pericranial flap for closure of skull base defects. Otolaryngol Head Neck Surg. 2004;130(6):704–11.

# Index




F. Sokoya, A. G. Vincent (eds.), *Manual of Head and Neck Reconstruction*,
https://doi.org/10.1007/978-3-031-65999-7

GPSR Compliance

*The European Union's (EU) General Product Safety Regulation (GPSR) is a set of rules that requires consumer products to be safe and our obligations to ensure this.*

*If you have any concerns about our products, you can contact us on ProductSafety@springernature.com*

In case Publisher is established outside the EU, the EU authorized representative is:

Springer Nature Customer Service Center GmbH
Europaplatz 3
69115 Heidelberg, Germany

**Batch number: 10732076**

Printed by Printforce, the Netherlands